Addressing Unhealthy Alcohol Use in Primary Care

Richard Saitz
Editor

Addressing Unhealthy Alcohol Use in Primary Care

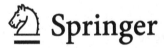 Springer

Editor
Richard Saitz
Section of General Internal Medicine
Boston Medical Center
Boston, Massachusetts
USA

ISBN 978-1-4614-4778-8   ISBN 978-1-4614-4779-5 (eBook)
DOI 10.1007/978-1-4614-4779-5
Springer New York Heidelberg Dordrecht London

Library of Congress Control Number: 2012952149

Preface

As a primary care physician I have seen the health and social consequences of excessive alcohol use and I have been frustrated by my inability to prevent them. After a few years in practice it became clear to me that my assumption that someone else was taking care of the problem was very wrong. It turns out that although there is a specialty care system that helps people who seek help, most people don't enter it (and it can't deliver all of the proven effective treatments anyway). The situation so impressed me that I decided to devote my career to figuring out how to address the problem as a generalist. Recently I saw that there was no resource for people like me trying to do the same, so I decided to deliver this book.

The vast majority of people with health risks and consequences related to alcohol use receive no attention at all from healthcare, despite the fact that alcohol is a leading cause of early preventable death. Early in the last century excessive alcohol use was addressed largely as a social and moral problem, and then people at the most severe end of the spectrum of unhealthy use—alcohol dependence or alcoholism—reaped the benefits of a social network, Alcoholics Anonymous (the small proportion who made it there and stuck with it). But attention to this health problem—both its prevention and treatment—has been notably absent from health care. The end of the last century brought recognition that health consequences from alcohol were not limited to alcoholism—that there was a spectrum of unhealthy use from amounts that risk consequences in people who have yet to have one, to drinking with consequences but no diagnosable disorder, to the alcohol use disorders including dependence (known also as alcoholism). Recognition of the spectrum came with the obvious understanding that it should be addressed, in part because most of the health consequences of drinking in a population accrue to those without dependence. Public health measures play a big role in addressing unhealthy alcohol use but the last four decades have brought results of clinical trials that demonstrate the efficacy of healthcare interventions.

Because there are known efficacious medical interventions—from screening and brief counseling, to pharmacotherapy, to referral for specialty care and coordination of care—generalist physicians have a very big role to play, just as they do for any other medical problem. Yet medical training and medical textbooks are generally weak in how they address unhealthy alcohol use. This book aims to provide clinically actionable information so that primary care clinicians can address unhealthy alcohol use in patients. This first edition does not address pregnant women or children—that remains for another time. But in these chapters, the generalist clinician will find information on how to identify, diagnose, and intervene in ways that help people with unhealthy use.

What is unhealthy alcohol use? Use that risks consequences (defined by amounts of consumption), use with consequences of that use, and the alcohol use disorders—currently called abuse and dependence (likely to be combined by the American Psychiatric Association in the fifth Diagnostic and Statistical Manual for Mental Disorders (DSM 5) under one alcohol use disorder). I think this definition is critical—*unhealthy use* is the only term that covers what doctors and other clinicians care and should care about—it is what we screen for, we can do something about it, and it is something our patients need us to care about.

In summary, this book is written for generalists and primary care clinicians in the hopes that it will provide clinically useful information for clinical practice—to identify and address unhealthy alcohol use as a medical condition that can be screened for and managed. I hope that this will lead to many patients being helped. I also hope to improve on this edition in the future. I welcome reader feedback.

Richard Saitz MD, MPH

Contents

Contributors

Daniel P. Alford, MD, MPH, FACP, FASAM, Associate Professor of Medicine, Section of General Internal Medicine, Clinical Addiction Research and Education Unit, Boston University School of Medicine and Boston Medical Center, Boston, MA

Maryann Amodeo, PhD, MSW, Professor of Clinical Practice; Co-Director, Center for Addictions Research and Services, Boston University School of Social Work, Boston, MA

Mohammadreza Azadfard, MD, Department of Family Medicine, University at Buffalo, Buffalo, NY

Douglas Berger, MD, General Medicine Service, VA Puget Sound Health Care System; Department of Medicine, University of Washington, Seattle, WA

Richard Blondell, MD, Department of Family Medicine, University at Buffalo, Buffalo, NY

Katharine Bradley, MD, MPH, Group Health Research Institute, Health Services Research and Development Northwest Center of Excellence in Substance Abuse Treatment and Education; Departments of Medicine and Health Services, University of Washington, Seattle, WA

Lauren Matukaitis Broyles, PhD, RN, Research Health Scientist, Center for Health Equity Research and Promotion (CHERP), VA Pittsburgh Healthcare System; Assistant Professor of Medicine, Division of General Medicine, University at Pittsburg Medical Center Montefiore Hospital, Pittsburgh, PA

Dylan Brock, University of Louisville School of Medicine, Louisville, KY

Chinazo Cunningham, MD, MS, Associate Professor of Medicine (Division of General Internal Medicine) and Family and Social Medicine, Albert Einstein College of Medicine and Montefiore Medical Center, Bronx, NY 10467, USA

Thomas J. Doyle, MD, Staff Physician, Primary Care and Hospitalist Services, Providence VA Medical Center; Clinical Assistant Professor of Medicine, Warren Alpert Medical School of Brown University, Providence, RI

Judd Fastenberg, MD, Albany Medical College, Albany, NY

Peter D. Friedmann, MD, MPH, FASAM, FACP, Reap Director, Research Service, Providence, VA Medical Center; Director, Research Section, Division of General Internal Medicine, Rhode Island Hospital; Professor of Medicine, Health Services, Policy and Practice, Warren Alpert Medical School of Brown University, Providence, RI

Adam J. Gordon, MD, MPH, FACP, FASAM, Associate Professor of Medicine, and Advisory Dean, University of Pittsburgh School of Medicine and VA Pittsburgh Healthcare System, Pittsburgh, PA, USA

Joanne M. Gordon, PhD, RN, Emeritus Professor of Biomedical Sciences, Missouri State University, Springfield, MO, USA

Ellie Grossman, MD, MPH, Assistant Professor, Deparment of Medicine, Division of General Internal Medicine, NYU School of Medicine, New York, NY

Erik W. Gunderson, MD, FASAM, Assistant Professor, Departments of Psychiatry and Neurobehavioral Sciences and Medicine, University of Virginia, Charlottesville, VA; Adjunct Associate Research Scientist, Department of Psychiatry, Division of Substance Abuse, Columbia University College of Physicians and Surgeons, New York, NY

Amy Harrington, MD, Assistant Professor, Department of Psychiatry, Division of Addiction Psychiatry, University of Massachusetts Medical School, Worcester, MA

Hilary Kunins, MD, MPH, MS, Program Director, Departments of Medicine (Division of General Internal Medicine) and Psychiatry and Behavioral Sciences, Albert Einstein College of Medicine and Montefiore Medical Center, Bronx, NY 10467, USA

Joshua D. Lee, MD, MSc, Assistant Professor, Departments of Population Health and Medicine, Division of General Internal Medicine, NYU School of Medicine, New York, NY

Luz Marilis López, PhD, MSW, MPH, Clinical Associate Professor, Boston University School of Social Work, Boston, MA

Jennifer McNeely, MD, MS, Assistant Professor, Departments of Population Health and Medicine, Division of General Internal Medicine, NYU School of Medicine, New York, NY

John Muench, MD, MPH, Associate Professor, Department of Family Medicine, Oregon Heath & Science University, Portland, OR

Timothy S. Naimi, MD, MPH, Clinical Addiction Research and Education Unit, Section of General Internal Medicine, Boston Medical Center; Associate Professor, Boston University Schools of Medicine and Public Health, Boston, MA

Steven J. Ondersma, PhD, Associate Professor, Departments of Psychiatry and Behavioral Neurosciences, Merill-Palmer Skillman Institute, Wayne State University, Detroit, MI

Darius A. Rastegar, MD, Associate Professor of Medicine, Department of Medicine, Johns Hopkins Bayview Medical Center, Baltimore, MD

Richard Saitz, MD, MPH, FACP, FASAM, Professor of Medicine and Epidemiology; Director, Clinical Addiction Research and Education Unit, Section of General Internal Medicine and Department of Medicine and Epidemiology, Boston University Schools of Medicine and Public Health, Boston Medical Center, Boston, MA

Department of Epidemiology, Boston University School of Public Health, Boston, MA, USA

Office of Clinical Research and Clinical Translational Science Institute, Boston University Medical Campus, Boston, MA, USA

Luis Sanchez, MD, Director, Physician Health Services, Inc., a subsidiary of the Massachusetts Medical Society, Waltham, MA

Babak Tofighi, MD, Lenox Hill Hospital, New York, NY

Golfo K. Tzilos, PhD, Postdoctoral Fellow, Center for Alcohol and Addiction Studies, Brown University, Providence, RI

Michael Weaver, MD, FASM, Associate Professor of Internal Medicine & Psychiatry, Virginia Commonwealth University School of Medicine, Richmond, VA

William H. Zywiak, PhD, Assistant Director and Research Scientist, Decision Sciences Institute, Pawtucket, RI; Adjunct Assistant Professor (Research) of Psychiatry and Human Behavior, Warren Alpert Medical School of Brown University, Providence, RI

Chapter 1
Unhealthy Alcohol Use: What is it? What Can and Should We be Doing About it in Primary Care Settings?

Richard Saitz

Identification of unhealthy alcohol use followed by brief counseling are among the most effective and cost-effective preventive services that can be delivered in primary medical care settings [1]. Despite the 85,000 preventable deaths each year in the United States attributable to alcohol use [2], the annual $ 235 billion cost attributable to alcohol in the United States [3], the well-known direct effects of heavy drinking as a cause of illnesses (e.g., liver disease, hypertension) and the effects of such drinking on the care of other medical and psychiatric conditions (e.g., medication adherence), only about 10 % of patients with alcohol dependence receive any care at all for the condition [4]. Furthermore, most patients with unhealthy use are not even identified by clinicians, and more than 90 % with an alcohol use disorder receive no specialty treatment for it [5]. In part this dismal state of affairs can be attributed to patients who do not seek help—they may not recognize the problem or they may recognize and either not be motivated to address it or not think of it as a health problem. Some seek help but find that the system of care for people with dependence is challenging to navigate and focused on acute care when the condition for some is chronic. They may also find a general lack of understanding of unhealthy alcohol use in medical settings, accompanied by stigmatization that is all too common in society.

However, there is hope that this situation can change, and I hope this book can be a part of the solution. Already, the U.S. Preventive Services Task Force recommends universal screening of adults and brief counseling for unhealthy alcohol use in primary care settings, based on numerous positive randomized controlled trials [6]. Pharmacotherapies for alcohol dependence that have also been proven efficacious in randomized trials are approved by regulatory agencies like the U.S. Food

R. Saitz (✉)
Clinical Addiction Research and Education (CARE) Unit,
Section of General Internal Medicine, Department of Medicine,
Boston Medical Center and Boston University School of Medicine, Boston, MA, USA
e-mail: rsaitz@bu.edu

Department of Epidemiology, Boston University School of Public Health, Boston, MA, USA

Office of Clinical Research and Clinical Translational Science Institute,
Boston University Medical Campus, Boston, MA, USA

and Drug Administration. Studies showing treatment efficacy have been done in primary care settings, and have shown efficacy for treatments that are feasible in primary care settings. Counseling that has the best efficacy can be delivered by a range of health professionals, including physicians, nurses, and health educators, in 10–15 min aliquots over several visits; traditional weekly one-hour psychotherapy sessions and 28-day residential programs featuring group therapy have not met the need and their superiority is questionable at best. Although these research-based advances have not yet led to major improvements in receipt of care by those who need it, some changes in health care delivery have the potential to deliver great improvements.

Two key conceptual advances place addressing unhealthy alcohol use squarely in the camp of primary care. The first was the Institute of Medicine's 1990 report that encouraged broadening the base of alcohol treatment [7]. The report points out that there is a range of excessive alcohol use that affects health and that our attention should not be focused solely on alcoholism. For more than a decade, for example, alcoholic beverages have been listed as known human carcinogens [8]. The second conceptual advance was a long time coming through the twentieth century, during which unhealthy alcohol use was often seen as a moral failing or simply bad behavior, and certainly not a medical problem. We now know that alcohol dependence has all the features of many other medical problems, and in some severe cases is a chronic disease [9]. Alcohol dependence is heritable (approximately 45 % genetic, 55 % environmental) [10], with a greater proportion attributable to genetics than other common medical disorders like hypertension and diabetes. Understanding alcohol dependence as a sometime chronic condition contributes to our understanding by allowing us to recognize that treatments may need to be long term; we should not be surprised, nor should we conclude that a treatment doesn't 'work' if the condition recurs when treatment is discontinued (e.g., just as we would not be surprised to see the blood sugar or blood pressure increase upon stopping medications for patients with diabetes or hypertension, respectively). Research also indicates that brain neurochemistry differs. For example, women with alcohol dependence who are abstinent have lower gamma-aminobutyric acid (GABA) receptor function than women without dependence, an observation that fits with our understanding of alcohol as a major actor at those receptors [11]. These scientific observations and conceptual advances suggest that taking a drink may be a behavior that can be prevented, but there is also a disorder of the brain, a treatable disease [12].

These advances also make obvious system changes needed to best help patients with these conditions. It stands to reason that care for medical, alcohol use, and mental health conditions should be integrated. People with unhealthy alcohol use often have medical and mental health conditions and other health issues. Unhealthy alcohol use causes medical and psychiatric illnesses, and complicates their effective treatment. Thus, it is no longer defensible to relegate care for alcohol use disorders to settings outside the healthcare system. It is also inefficient to send patients who commonly have conditions in all three areas to different practitioners for each. Even when specialists in each domain are needed, integrated care suggests such care at least be coordinated. Primary care settings and the patient-centered medical home are the logical places for this integrated coordinated care.

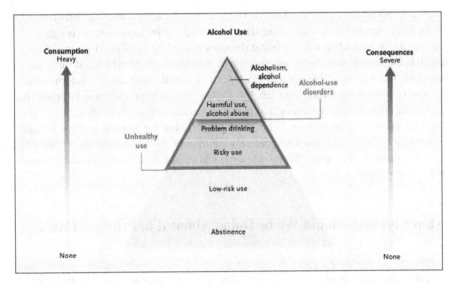

Fig. 1.1 The spectrum of unhealthy alcohol use. (Reproduced with permission from Saitz R. Unhealthy alcohol use. New Engl J Med. 2005;352:596–607, copyright ownership Massachusetts Medical Society)

What Exactly is 'Unhealthy Alcohol Use?'

Unhealthy alcohol use is what we are interested in as clinicians (see Fig. 1.1). It is any alcohol use that risks or has caused health consequences. We might also be interested in alcohol use associated with health benefits though this is a much more nuanced and complex issue than most think (see Chap. 13). Unhealthy alcohol use encompasses the spectrum of alcohol use that clinicians should identify and address. It is what is identified by good screening tests. It includes risky consumption amounts, problem use (use with consequences that does not meet criteria for an alcohol use disorder) and the alcohol use disorders, alcohol abuse (similar to harmful use as it is known internationally), and alcohol dependence (see Chap. 3). Risky consumption amounts have also been called 'hazardous alcohol use.' Of note, the World Health Organization has defined hazardous use as a repeated pattern of drinking that confers a risk of harm [13]. All of these latter terms—problem or hazardous use, alcohol abuse or harmful use, and dependence—are mutually exclusive. In other words, although harmful use is . . . harmful, once a patient has dependence, they are categorized as such. Risky or hazardous consumption amounts can be used by those anywhere on the spectrum of unhealthy use. Unhealthy alcohol use is the only term that encompasses risky consumption amounts, use below such limits that still may cause problems, and the alcohol use disorders.

Unhealthy alcohol use includes drinking that is associated with a risk of health consequences. Such drinking can be defined by amounts that are known to increase the risk of consequences (e.g., 3–6 drinks per week increase the risk for breast cancer) [14] or by other circumstances (e.g., any use during pregnancy, drinking when a medical condition or medication interaction contraindicates it, drinking and driving). There is no single study that could determine risky drinking amounts because of the varying thresholds across different diseases caused by alcohol. However, public health bodies worldwide agree that specifying thresholds above which risks increase, based on the best epidemiological evidence, is useful. And despite international variability in how such limits are set, thresholds tend to be in the same ballpark. In the United States, risky consumption is defined as more than 7 standard drinks per week on average or more than 3 drinks on an occasion for women and for anyone over 65 years of age (14 and 4 respectively for men of 21–65 years of age). Close to 30 % of adults in the United States drink risky amounts, 5 % meet criteria for abuse and 4 % for dependence.

What Can and Should We be Doing About it in Primary Care?

In primary care settings, there is much we can do. First, using questionnaires we should systematically screen all patients for unhealthy alcohol use. For those who screen positive, we should briefly assess their readiness to change and the severity of unhealthy use. That information is then used in brief counseling interventions. The goal of such interventions may be cutting down or abstinence, and may include recommendations for more specialized treatments (e.g., pharmacotherapy, evidence-based counseling) either in primary care or specialty settings by referral. For those with very heavy and daily drinking, we should manage withdrawal from alcohol with medications as needed, and in appropriate clinical settings. Practical and detailed information on all of these topics appears in chapters in this book, including electronic resources for patients and clinicians, and descriptions of practice systems and other ways to implement these services. In addition, we cover the role of the social network Alcoholics Anonymous, management of patients in recovery, and a number of issues that come up frequently in the management of patients with unhealthy alcohol use, such as other drug use, medical and psychiatric comorbidities, pain management, patient confidentiality, ethical and legal issues, hospital and perioperative management, and physicians themselves with unhealthy use.

The authors and I hope that this book becomes a practical tool for clinicians in primary care settings to improve the quality of care for people with unhealthy alcohol use. We hope it translates the best science that can be used in clinical practice, and that it supports clinicians wanting to use those scientific advances and improvements in health care delivery systems that are long overdue. Our patients deserve no less.

References

1. Solberg LI, Maciosek MV, Edwards NM. Primary care intervention to reduce alcohol misuse: ranking its health impact and cost effectiveness.Am J Prev Med. 2008;34(2):143–152.
2. Mokdad AH, Marks JS, Stroup DF, Gerberding JL. Actual causes of death in the United States, 2000. JAMA. 2004;291(10):1238–1245.

3. Rehm J, Mathers C, Popova S, Thavorncharoensap M, Teerawattananon Y, Patra J. Global burden of disease and injury and economic cost attributable to alcohol use and alcohol-use disorders. Lancet. 2009;373(9682):2223–2233.
4. McGlynn EA, Asch SM, Adams J, et al. The quality of health care delivered to adults in the United States. N Engl J Med. 2003;348:2635–2645
5. Substance Abuse and Mental Health Services Administration. Results from the 2010 National Survey on Drug Use and Health: Summary of National Findings, NSDUH Series H-41, HHS Publication No. (SMA) 11-4658. Rockville: Substance Abuse and Mental Health Services Administration; 2011.
6. U.S. Preventive Services Task Force. Screening and behavioral counseling interventions in primary care to reduce alcohol misuse, Topic Page. April 2004. http://www.uspreventiveservicestaskforce.org/uspstf/uspsdrin.htm. Accessed 5 Feb 2012.
7. Institute of Medicine. Broadening the base of treatment for alcohol problems. Report of a study by a Committee of the Institute of Medicine, Division of Mental Health and Behavioral Medicine. Washington, DC: National Academy Press, 1990.
8. NTP. Report on Carcinogens, 12th ed. Research Triangle Park: U.S. Department of Health and Human Services, Public Health Service, National Toxicology Program; 2011. p. 499.
9. McLellan AT, Lewis DC, O'Brien CP, Kleber HD. Drug dependence, a chronic medical illness: implications for treatment, insurance, and outcomes evaluation. JAMA. 2000;284(13):1689–1695.
10. Knopik VS, Heath AC, Madden PA, Bucholz KK, Slutske WS, Nelson EC, Statham D, Whitfield JB, Martin NG. Genetic effects on alcohol dependence risk: re-evaluating the importance of psychiatric and other heritable risk factors. Psychol Med. 2004;34:1519–1530.
11. Lingford-Hughes AR, Acton PD, Gacinovic S, Boddington SJA, Costa DC, Pilowsky LS, Ell PJ, Marshall EJ, Kerwin RW. Levels of GABA-benzodiazepine receptors in female abstinent alcohol dependent subjects: preliminary findings from an [123I]-iomazenil single photon emission tomography study. Alcohol Clin Exp Res. 2000;24:1449–55.
12. Infofacts: Understanding Drug Abuse and Addiction. http://www.drugabuse.gov/publications/infofacts/understanding-drug-abuse-addiction. Accessed 5 Feb 2012.
13. Saunders JB, Lee NK. Hazardous alcohol use: its delineation as a subthreshold disorder, and approaches to its diagnosis and management. Comprehensive Psychiatry. 2000;41(2) Suppl 1: 95–103.
14. Chen WY, Rosner B, Hankinson SE, et al. Moderate alcohol consumption during adult life, drinking patterns, and breast cancer risk. JAMA. 2011;306(17):1884–1890.

Chapter 2
Screening for Unhealthy Alcohol Use

Katharine Bradley and Douglas Berger

Principles of Alcohol Screening

Rationale for Screening

The purpose of alcohol screening is to identify patients with unhealthy alcohol use so that interventions can be provided to reduce drinking and prevent harm. From the 1960s to the 1990s, alcohol screening was aimed at identifying "alcoholism," now referred to as alcohol dependence. Alcohol use disorders are defined in the Diagnostic and Statistical Manual of Mental Disorders, Fourth Edition (DSM-IV) [1] and consist of alcohol abuse and dependence. Identification of alcohol use disorders remains central to alcohol screening as patients with these disorders can benefit from interventions including medical monitoring [2], medications for alcohol dependence [3], and referral to Alcoholics Anonymous and/or specialty addictions treatment.

However, many patients consume unhealthy amounts of alcohol without meeting criteria for abuse or dependence. Extensive epidemiologic research has defined unhealthy levels of alcohol consumption and has resulted in gender- and age-specific recommended drinking limits (Table 2.1) [4]. Drinking above these limits is referred to as "risky drinking." Risky drinking also includes drinking despite medical contraindications, such as pregnancy or trying to conceive, liver disease (e.g., chronic hepatitis C), taking medications that interact with alcohol, or previous diagnosis or treatment for alcohol use disorders. Even when it does not involve the psycho-social or other consequences indicative of abuse or dependence, risky drinking can cause

K. Bradley (✉)
Group Health Research Institute, Group Health Cooperative; Northwest Center of Excellence in Substance Abuse Treatment and Education and Health Services Research & Development, VA Puget Sound Health Care System, Department of Veterans Affairs; Departments of Medicine and Health Services, University of Washington, Seattle, WA, USA
e-mail: Bradley.k@ghc.org

D. Berger
General Medicine Service, VA Puget Sound Health Care System, Department of Veterans Affairs; Department of Medicine, University of Washington, Seattle, WA, USA
e-mail: Douglas.berger@va.gov

R. Saitz (ed.), *Addressing Unhealthy Alcohol Use in Primary Care,*
DOI 10.1007/978-1-4614-4779-5_2, © Springer Science+Business Media New York 2013

Table 2.1 Recommended drinking limits*

Recommended drinking limits[∂]	
Men up to age 65	14 drinks[§] a week, and 4 drinks[§] in a day
Women, or men over age 65	7 drinks[§] a week 3 drinks[§] in a day

* Recommended limits for drinking have been established by the National Institutes of Health (NIH) based on a large number of epidemiologic studies. People who drink above these limits are at higher risk of harm due to drinking. Recommended limits for women reflect their susceptibility to adverse consequences at lower levels of consumption than men, including adverse consequences of episodic heavy drinking with 4 (instead of 5) drinks in a day [19, 20], increased risk of liver disease above 1 drink per day on average [21], and increased risk of breast cancer at even lower levels of consumption [22]. This increased risk at lower levels of consumption than men is likely due to women's lower total body water due to their smaller size and higher percent body fat, and potentially other physiologic and hormonal factors [22]
[∂] These limits serve as a guide, but specific advice to a particular patient should reflect the patient's age, gender, specific health condition(s) and medication regimen. Men over 65 years old are generally advised to follow the guidelines for women. All patients should be advised not drink if they have medical contraindications such as a prior diagnosis of alcohol dependence, pregnancy or plans to conceive, medications that interact with alcohol, or liver disease
[§] 1 drink = 1 standard US drink size = 12 ounces (oz) of beer or 5 oz of wine or 1.5 oz of hard liquor or 8 oz of malt liquor [4]

injuries and gastrointestinal complications (e.g., gastritis and hepatitis), complicate management of chronic medical conditions [5, 6], impact medication adherence [7], complicate surgical procedures [8–11], and result in potentially preventable hospitalizations [12, 13] and death [14]. Risky drinking also contributes to the development of abuse and dependence. Moreover, risky drinking responds to interventions, ranging from one-time advice about drinking to sustained conversations, monitoring, and feedback [15–18].

As risky drinking can cause significant harms and is amenable to intervention, it is critical that alcohol screening identify patients with the full spectrum of unhealthy alcohol use, not only those with abuse or dependence. Indeed, from a population perspective, patients with non-dependent unhealthy alcohol use account for a greater burden of adverse alcohol-related consequences (e.g., injuries) than patients with alcohol abuse or dependence. This 'preventive paradox' results from the fact that although patients with alcohol dependence are more likely to suffer from adverse alcohol-related consequences than patients with non-dependent unhealthy use, the latter far outnumber the former [23]. In addition, as risky drinking often precedes alcohol use disorders, harm may be prevented by detection and intervention at this stage. Finally, patients with non-dependent unhealthy alcohol use are likely more responsive to brief interventions (BI) than patients with alcohol dependence [24].

Thus, primary care alcohol screening should aim to identify the full range of unhealthy drinking. Further, alcohol screening should be implemented in a manner that facilitates appropriate interventions when unhealthy alcohol use is identified. Since laboratory tests are not effective for screening for the spectrum of unhealthy drinking (see below), validated questionnaires are recommended for evidence-based alcohol screening.

Who to Screen and Screening Guidelines

All adult primary care patients should be assessed in a standardized manner for any alcohol use and screened for unhealthy alcohol use with a validated alcohol screening questionnaire. Although young patients and men are more likely to drink at risky levels or to have alcohol use disorders than older patients and women, unhealthy drinking is relatively common even in lower-risk groups. When alcohol screening is restricted to selected high risk sub-groups of patients, many patients with unhealthy drinking are missed. If screening is restricted to patients with evidence of drinking excessively (e.g., liver disease) the majority of screen-positive patients will have severe unhealthy drinking.

Routine alcohol screening is recommended by a number of organizations. The US Preventive Services Task Force (USPSTF) recommends screening and brief intervention (BI) (B recommendation) [15], and screening followed by BI has been identified as the 3rd highest prevention priority for US adults [25]. Several physician professional organizations have also recommended alcohol screening and BI: for all adults and pregnant women (American Academy of Family Physicians) [26]; annually for women and during the first trimester of pregnancy (American College of Obstetricians and Gynecologists) [27]; and annually for adolescents as part of screening for substance use (American Academy of Pediatrics) [28]. The Veterans Health Administration and Department of Defense also have clinical guidelines supporting alcohol screening and BI [26, 29].

Barriers to Screening

Time is a critical barrier to alcohol screening, and screening methods must be efficient [30]. However, implementation of alcohol screening has been limited by more than time constraints. Many clinicians are uncomfortable discussing alcohol use for fear of alienating patients. Yet most patients not only find it acceptable to be asked about alcohol use, they expect it and associate it with higher quality care [31]. Some providers lack knowledge of recommended drinking limits and their scientific basis and may feel that recommended drinking limits [4] are unrealistically low or may drink at unhealthy levels themselves. Others have a dichotomous view of alcoholism in which patients who are not alcoholic need not worry about their drinking.

Because of stigma surrounding unhealthy alcohol use, patients may fear that frank discussion of unhealthy drinking will undermine the doctor-patient relationship. Some patients under-report drinking due to embarrassment or fear of repercussions (e.g., uninsurability, employment or other discrimination). Others under-report average alcohol consumption because of a tendency to ignore episodic heavy drinking when reporting average alcohol consumption.

Thus, asking patients if they have problems with alcohol use or asking them to quantify average alcohol consumption is inadequate for identification of unhealthy drinking. Because people under-report average alcohol consumption, asking patients about their average alcohol consumption can miss almost half of those who drink

Table 2.2 Interpreting data from alcohol screening questionnaire validation studies—the fine print

Comparison standard	Alcohol screening questionnaires are evaluated compared to "gold" standard in-depth interviews. These interviews ask about each type of alcoholic beverage, typical and episodic drinking patterns and diagnostic criteria for a DSM diagnosis of alcohol use disorders. It is important to note whether the comparison standard is risky drinking, DSM-IV abuse and/or dependence, or another standard such as a specified level of daily alcohol consumption
Sensitivity	= *true positive rate* = the proportion of patients with unhealthy drinking (risky drinking or alcohol use disorders) based on in-depth interviews, who screen positive
Specificity	= *true negative rate* = the proportion of patients without unhealthy drinking, (risky drinking or alcohol use disorders) based on in-depth interviews, who screen negative
Screening threshold ("cut-point" for a positive screen)	= *the score used to define a "positive" screen* is often the screening score (threshold) that balances sensitivity and specificity. However, in certain settings such as those with a low prevalence of unhealthy drinking or limited resources to address unhealthy drinking, the cost of false positive screens outweighs the benefit of true positive screens and cut-points with lower sensitivity than specificity are optimal [33]. Several validation studies of alcohol screening questionnaires have used these concepts to choose a screening threshold [34], or to present optimal screening thresholds for a range of situations [60, 61].

above recommended average drinking limits [32]. When a standardized screen is not used, providers tend to ask general or vague questions, and patients are apt to respond vaguely such as "I just drink occasionally," or "I am just a social drinker," a process that takes more time and yields less clinically actionable results than asking standardized questions just as clinicians would implement a laboratory-based screening test. Ad hoc questions about problem drinking are especially likely to miss milder risky drinking.

Interpreting and Using Screening Results

Screening is not the same as diagnosis. Just as a positive mammogram does not diagnose breast cancer nor a negative mammogram exclude it, screening for unhealthy drinking does not definitively identify unhealthy alcohol use and by no means should a positive test be mis-interpreted as alcohol abuse or dependence or "alcoholism" (without further assessment). Instead, primary care alcohol screening questionnaires are intended as brief screens to alert clinicians to patients who should have further assessment of their drinking. Different tests have different characteristics, and even for the same test it may be possible to increase sensitivity at the expense of specificity by adjusting the screening threshold (Table 2.2). In some contexts it might make sense to choose a very sensitive screening method and then assess patients who screen positive in greater detail to eliminate false positives. On the other hand, in settings with limited resources to address unhealthy drinking, or in settings with a very low prevalence of unhealthy drinking (which makes false positives more common, e.g., among older women), clinicians might want to use a screen with a very low false positive rate (high specificity) knowing that some unhealthy drinking will be missed. In some cases, time constraints may not allow for full assessment and clinicians may move directly from the screening result to action, be it BI or referral for further assessment and/or treatment.

Although alcohol screening questionnaires are typically used (at least initially) as dichotomous screening tests (positive or negative), unhealthy drinking falls along a spectrum from drinking slightly above recommended limits to severe alcohol dependence. Some screening questionnaires provide information on the severity of unhealthy drinking and alcohol-related risks [35]. In addition, unhealthy drinking can change over time, and some screening questionnaires for unhealthy drinking can be used to monitor risk over time [36, 37].

Validated Alcohol Screening Questionnaires

The CAGE Questionnaire and other Screening Tests for Alcohol Use Disorders

The 4-item CAGE questionnaire, previously the favorite validated screening test for alcohol use disorders in the US [38, 39], was developed in the 1960s to identify patients with alcohol use disorders who might benefit from referral to treatment. Validated in primary care patients in the 1990s [40], the CAGE asks patients whether they had ever Cut-down, been Annoyed by criticism, felt Guilty about drinking or had an Eye-opener in the morning. Two affirmative answers are often considered a positive test, although one point may be optimal in some populations [41].

The CAGE remains widely taught and recommended (though not widely used), but it has several limitations as a screening test for unhealthy drinking. First, the CAGE questions refer to a lifetime ('Have you ever. . .') and do not distinguish current from prior disorders. Therefore, a positive screen on the CAGE can remain positive for life, and as a result, up to 50 % of older patients who screen positive on the CAGE no longer drink alcohol [42]. While it may be useful for primary care clinicians to know about past disorders, the CAGE questionnaire identifies many for whom there is no current issue to address. Second, the CAGE asks about factors that may be culturally specific (e.g., guilt, annoyance due to criticism) [43]. Finally, when used alone, the CAGE identifies alcohol use disorders, but it is not an accurate test for identifying the whole spectrum of unhealthy drinking [41, 44, 45]. Other older screening tests, such as the Michigan Alcohol Screening Test (MAST), were also designed to identify only alcohol abuse and dependence [46–50].

Additions to the CAGE can address some of these limitations. Questions about current alcohol consumption can be added to the CAGE to identify risky drinking. These "augmented CAGE" questionnaires were validated [44, 45] and used in the first primary care trials of BI [51, 52], and have been further validated [32], and used in subsequent implementation efforts [53].

Alcohol Use Disorders Identification Test (AUDIT)

In the 1980s, the World Health Organization (WHO) developed a 10-item questionnaire, the Alcohol Use Disorders Identification Test (AUDIT). The AUDIT was developed specifically to identify the entire spectrum of unhealthy drinking, including risky drinking as well as alcohol dependence, so that patients could be offered BIs (Table 2.3) [54–56]. The AUDIT has 3 domains: alcohol consumption, including a question about the frequency of drinking 6 or more drinks on an occasion (3 items); alcohol dependence (3 items); and consequences of risky drinking (4 items). The AUDIT is scored from 0 to 40. WHO recommends a cut-point of 8 or more points based on the original dataset in which the AUDIT was developed, but all US primary care validation studies that have included a gold standard of risky drinking and/or DSM diagnoses of alcohol use disorders (i.e., the whole spectrum of unhealthy drinking) based on detailed interviews have found that thresholds of ≥4 points balance sensitivity and specificity for most settings (Table 2.4) [57–61]. There is also increasing interest in using "zones" of AUDIT scores to suggest different levels of intervention and follow-up [62]. Recently, empiric evidence from a large ethnically diverse primary care sample supported the use of AUDIT zones in estimating the probability of alcohol dependence (Table 2.5), although the defined zones [35] differed from those originally proposed [62]. In a large primary care study, at AUDIT scores of over 10 points for men and over 8 in women, 43 % and 45 % of men and women, respectively, met diagnostic criteria for active alcohol dependence (Table 2.5). Therefore, diagnostic assessment should be offered to all patients who score above these levels.

When the AUDIT is used in the United States, the WHO recommends that the 3rd question ask about the frequency of drinking '5 or more drinks' on an occasion–instead of '6 or more drinks'–because the original AUDIT was developed based on smaller drink sizes [62]. However, US primary care validation studies of the AUDIT have mostly used the original AUDIT question 3 (Table 2.3), and a study of women comparing 2 versions of question 3 that asked about "4 or more" and "6 or more" drinks on an occasion revealed little impact, although the former was slightly more sensitive [61]. We recommend that question 3 ask about the frequency of drinking ≥5 drinks on an occasion for US primary care practices, or that a gender-specific version be used (≥4 drinks for women and ≥5 drinks for men) which matches recommended drinking limits for a single day.

The AUDIT Consumption Questions (AUDIT-C)

Although the AUDIT takes only a few minutes to complete, that is long for many primary care settings screening for multiple conditions. In the 1990s, efforts to identify briefer approaches to screening for unhealthy drinking led to recognition that the first three AUDIT questions, which ask about alcohol consumption, had comparable performance to the entire 10-item AUDIT. These three questions, referred to as the AUDIT-C (for "Consumption" questions), are scored 0–12 points. Screening

Table 2.3 The Alcohol Use Disorders Identification Test (AUDIT) and AUDIT-C* interview versions: [62]

"Because alcohol use can affect your health and can interfere with certain medications and treatments, it is important that we ask some questions about your use of alcohol. ....."

Q#1.   *How often did you have a drink containing alcohol in the past year?*[§]
       Never (0 points);[§] Monthly or less (1 point); 2–4 times a month (2 points); 2–3 times per week (3 points); 4 or more times a week (4 points)

Q#2.   *How many drinks containing alcohol did you have on a typical day when you were drinking in the past year?*
       0 drinks (0 points);* 1 or 2 (0 points); 3 or 4 (1 point); 5 or 6 (2 points); 7–9 (3 points); 10 or more (4 points)

Q#3.   *How often did you have 5*[§] *or more drinks on one occasion in the past year?*
       Never (0 points); Less than monthly (1 point); Monthly (2 points); Weekly (3 points); Daily or almost daily (4 points)

Q#4.   *How often during the last year have you found that you were not able to stop drinking once you had started?*
       Same response options as Q#3.

Q#5.   *How often during the last year have you failed to do what was normally expected of you because of drinking?*
       Same response options as Q#3.

Q#6.   *How often during the last year have you needed a first drink in the morning to get yourself going after a heavy drinking session?*
       Same response options as Q#3.

Q#7.   *How often during the last year have you had a feeling of guilt or remorse after drinking?*
       Same response options as Q#3.

Q#8.   *How often during the last year have you been unable to remember what happened the night before because of your drinking?*
       Same response options as Q#3.

Q#9.   *Have you or someone else been injured because of your drinking?*
       No (0 points); Yes, but not in the last year (2 points); Yes, during the last year (4 points)

Q#10. *Has a relative, friend, doctor, other health care worker been concerned about your drinking?*
       Same response options as Q#9

* Questions 1–3, the AUDIT consumption questions, when used by themselves are called the AUDIT-C. For the AUDIT-C, if patients are screened by interview and Question 1 is answered "never", scores of 0 can be validly imputed for Questions 2–3 [60]. If the AUDIT-C is administered on paper or online without a skip pattern for non-drinkers to skip questions 2–3, a "0 drinks" option is typically added to Question 2 [59].
§ For the full AUDIT, experts recommend that patients skip to Questions 9–10 if they report no alcohol use on Questions 1–3 [62].
∂ The AUDIT has a past year timeframe, but it has been validated both with and without explicit reference to a past year time frame. The version shown here was validated in a large primary care population in Texas. See text for gender-specific versions of AUDIT Question 3 [57].

thresholds (cut-points) that balance sensitivity are ≥ 2 or 3 points for women and ≥ 4 points for men for most settings (Table 2.4). The Department of Veterans Affairs medical centers use a higher cut-off (≥ 5 for men and women) to decrease the burden of false positive screens on providers [64].

There are two reasons that the AUDIT-C can be a valid screening test for unhealthy drinking when–as noted above–simply asking patients about their typical drinking is not effective. First, the third question of the AUDIT about the frequency of episodic

Table 2.4 Sensitivity and specificity of the 10-item AUDIT and AUDIT-C for identifying risky drinking or DSM-IV alcohol use disorders in primary care

Questionnaire, Sample, and Screening Threshold (in points)	Sensitivity/Specificity (%)		
	Men	Women	Total
Full 10-item AUDIT			
Texas primary care patients [57, 60]			
≥2	98/53	92/74	–/–
≥3	96/71	79/87	–/–
≥4	91/80	65/93	85/84
≥5	81/90	53/95	–/–
≥6	69/92	42/97	69/93
US Department of Veterans Affairs (VA) outpatients [59, 61]			
≥2	–/–	87/71	–/–
≥3	–/–	70/86	–/–
≥4	90/69	47/92	–/–
≥5	81/84	35/98	–/–
≥6	69/91	–/–	–/–
Georgia primary care patients [58]			
≥4	–/–	–/–	84/77
≥5	–/–	–/–	71/87
≥6	–/–	–/–	60/93
*AUDIT-C**			
Texas primary care patients [60]			
≥2	98/63	89/78	–/–
≥3	92/79	73/91	–/–
≥4	86/89	57/96	–/–
≥5	72/96	36/98	–/–
VA outpatients [59, 61]			
≥2	–	81/86	–/–
≥3	95/60	60/96	–/–
≥4	86/72	38/98	–/–
≥5	68/90	–	–/–
Georgia primary care patients [58]			
≥2	–/–	–/–	96/32
≥3	–/–	–/–	88/64
≥4	–/–	–/–	76/80
Boston primary care patients [63]			
≥4 (men and women)	–/–	–/–	74/83

"–" = not available

heavy drinking is strongly associated with the risk of alcohol dependence and identifies patients drinking in excess of recommended drinking limits [35]. Second, the scoring of the AUDIT-C does not depend on whether patients report drinking above average drinking limits (7 drinks a week for women and 14 for men). Reported average alcohol consumption on AUDIT-C questions 1–2 underestimates average consumption, just like other questions about typical quantity and frequency of drinking. However, screening with the AUDIT-C relies on the screening score (points) instead of reported typical drinking. This is an essential point for clinicians to

Table 2.5 Recommended zones for the AUDIT and AUDIT-C. (Adapted from those identified in a US Primary Care Population [35])

Zone		Men		Women	
		Screening Scores (in points)	Estimated prevalence of past-year alcohol dependence % (95 % CI)	Screening Scores (in points)	Estimated prevalence of past-year alcohol dependence % (95 % CI)
AUDIT	1—No intervention	0–3	1 (0–2)	0–1	0 (0–1)
	2—Brief intervention & follow-up	4	1 (3–8)	2–4	4 (1–6)
	3—Brief intervention & follow-up	5–10	18 (9–26)	5–8	16 (8–25)
	4—Diagnostic assessment	11–14	43 (22–65)	9–12	45 (28–63)
	5—Diagnostic assessment	15–40	87 (72–100)	13–40	94 (82–100)
AUDIT-C	1—No intervention	0–2	1 (0–2)	0–1	1 (0–1)
	2—Brief intervention & follow-up	3–4	9 (2–15)	2–3	5 (2–8)
	3—Brief intervention & follow-up	5–6	22 (10–34)	4–6	24 (15–33)
	4—Diagnostic assessment	7–9	45 (28–61)	7–9	42 (22–63)
	5—Diagnostic assessment	10–12	75 (51–99)	10–12	88 (58–100)

understand because patients can screen positive on the AUDIT-C while reporting drinking within recommended limits.

Like the AUDIT, the AUDIT-C score also reflects the probability of alcohol dependence (Table 2.5). Men and women with AUDIT-C scores of 7 or more, have a probability of current alcohol dependence of over 45 % and 42 %, respectively, and should therefore be offered diagnostic assessment. In addition, the association between AUDIT-C scores and health outcomes has been studied extensively in male Veterans, with higher AUDIT-C scores associated with decreased medication adherence (scores ≥ 4) [7], and increased risk of new onset gastrointestinal conditions and hospitalizations (scores ≥ 5 and 6) [12, 65], fractures and hospitalizations for trauma (scores ≥ 8) [66, 67], hospitalizations with potentially preventable diagnoses (scores ≥ 8) [13], post-operative complications (scores ≥ 5) [10, 11], and death (scores ≥ 10) [68].

Single-item Alcohol Screening Questions (SASQs)

During the 1990s, there was also increased recognition of the risks associated with episodic heavy drinking and the strong association between the frequency of episodic heavy drinking and the probability of alcohol dependence [69]. Furthermore, the majority of people who report drinking risky amounts also report heavy-drinking episodes. Several single-item alcohol screening questions (SASQs) were validated for unhealthy drinking all of which assess episodic heavy drinking (Table 2.6) [58, 59, 61, 63, 70, 71]. For medical settings, the National Institute of Alcohol Abuse and Alcoholism (NIAAA) recommends asking 'Do you sometimes drink alcohol?' [4] followed by the SASQ, 'How many times in the past year have you had X or more drinks in a day?' where 'X' is 5 for men and 4 for women, and 1 or more days is considered a positive screen (Table 2.6) [4].

Screening Questionnaires for Special Populations

Screening for alcohol use is of particular concern during pregnancy [27]. The TWEAK and the T-ACE are the most widely recommended screens in this setting [72–74], although questions about any alcohol use [27] and unhealthy drinking should be added. The AUDIT-C is an alternative, although it has only been evaluated among women who said they were pregnant in the National Epidemiologic Survey of Alcohol and Related Conditions (NESARC), not in a clinical sample of pregnant women, with scores of 3 or more associated with a sensitivity of 95 % and a specificity of 85 % for risky drinking [75]. The AUDIT, POSIT, CRAFFT [76], AUDIT-C, and 2-item screen [77], have been validated to screen for alcohol abuse and dependence in adolescents. The National Institute on Alcohol Abuse and Alcoholism (NIAAA) recommends asking children and adolescents two questions: one about alcohol consumption by the patient and one about alcohol consumption by friends (http://pubs.niaaa.nih.gov/publications/Practitioner/YouthGuide/YouthGuide.pdf).

Table 2.6 Sensitivity and specificity of single-item alcohol screening questions (SASQs) for identifying risky drinking and/or DSM-IV alcohol use disorders in primary care

Single-item Alcohol Screening Questionnaires (SASQs)*	Sensitivity/Specificity (%)		
	Men	Women	Total
"On any single occasion during the past 3 months, have you had more than 5 drinks containing alcohol?" [70] Yes response is considered positive.	–/–	–/–	62/93
"When was the last time you had more than X drinks in 1 day?" (X = 4 for women and 5 for men) [58]. Within the last 3 months is considered positive	81/63	78/81	80/74
NIAAA recommended: *"How many times in the past year have you had X or more drinks in a day?"* (X = 5 men and 4 women) Response of > 1 is considered positive. [4, 63]	83/72	81/84	82/79
AUDIT question #3: *How often have you had 6 or more drinks on one occasion in the past year? Ever in the past year considered positive.* Ever in the past year considered positive			
VA outpatients [59, 61]	77/83	45/96	–/–
Texas primary care patients [60]	87/84	60/92	–/–
Gender modified AUDIT question #3: *"How often .... 4 or more drinks...?"* Ever in the past year considered positive	–	69/94	–/–

'–' = not available

* These questions are typically asked after a screen for any alcohol use. To assess whether patients drink, a validated question should be used, such as: 'Do you sometimes drink alcohol?' [4]

The exact wording and order of the suggested questions vary by age, but unlike the validated screens for adolescents, the NIAAA questions assess whether the patient consumes *any* alcohol (more than a few sips). For adults, in settings where alcohol screening is desired as part of a broader screen for drug abuse, the ASSIST is an option though its length will likely preclude its widespread use except if it is self-administered by computer [78]. A single-item for drug screening provides a more practical alternative [79].

Laboratory-based Screening Tests

Given the limitations of patient report of alcohol consumption, ideally there would be a laboratory test that could be used as an alcohol use "vital sign" to identify unhealthy drinking, assess its severity, and monitor changes in unhealthy drinking over time. Unfortunately, there is currently no laboratory marker with sufficient sensitivity and specificity to be useful for primary care screening for unhealthy drinking [80]. Serum alcohol degrades rapidly, and therefore serum alcohol concentration is of little clinical use, except to confirm recent alcohol use or when present at levels indicative of physiologic tolerance. Routine laboratory tests including aspartate aminotransferase (AST), alanine aminotransferase (ALT), and mean corpuscular volume (MCV) often increase with chronic unhealthy alcohol use and certain patterns of these tests (e.g., AST/ALT ratio >2) are associated with alcoholic liver disease, but they are not effective for alcohol screening due to inadequate sensitivity and specificity for risky drinking [81]. The liver enzyme gamma-glutamyl-transferase (GGT) is the most commonly used alcohol biomarker and is widely available in primary care [82]. A newer marker, available in most commercial labs, percent carbohydrate-deficient transferrin (%CDT), has comparable sensitivity and higher specificity than GGT [82, 83]. Although high sensitivities for GGT and CDT have been reported when screening for very heavy drinking or the presence of an alcohol use disorder (up to 60–70 %) [84, 85], both tests are relatively insensitive for lower level risky drinking [86]. Sensitivities are also lower in women than in men. Ethyl-glucuronide (EtG) is an emerging marker of recent alcohol use (within 1–2 days) though not of risky amounts, and it is not yet widely available [87].

Some have suggested combining laboratory markers with screening questions as a way to identify additional risky drinkers. One computer simulation study found that the addition of the %CDT to screening questionnaires could be cost-effective for populations less than 60 years old with a prevalence over 15 % of unhealthy alcohol use (e.g., men) [88]. However, in an emergency room setting, adding %CDT and other lab markers to the AUDIT questionnaire did not improve sensitivity or specificity [89]. Laboratory markers may also be used to supplement or replace questionnaires in pre-operative settings or cases of critical illness or when patients are obtunded [80]. The best lab markers in the population of patients who deny risky drinking on questionnaires are unknown, as is the utility of brief intervention in this setting. A lab marker such as EtG, while not suggestive of risky drinking, might be used to confirm a patient's report of no recent alcohol consumption and self-report might be expected to be more reliable if patients knew that laboratory testing would also be performed.

Even though laboratory tests are not very accurate screening tests for unhealthy use, if abnormal, they *can* motivate patients to change by providing objective evidence of the physiologic impact of drinking. Moreover, monitoring abnormal laboratory tests and providing repeated feedback to patients on results, along with repeated BIs, has been shown to decrease drinking (and even alcohol-related mortality) and increase abstinence for patients with unhealthy drinking [2, 90, 91]. Thus, if abnormal, laboratory markers of unhealthy drinking can play a role in interventions for unhealthy drinking once it is identified by screening.

Putting it all Together

Choosing Which Validated Screening Questionnaire to Use

The CAGE questionnaire augmented with 3–4 other questions including consumption questions [32, 51, 52], the 10-item AUDIT, the AUDIT-C and SASQs have been extensively validated as screening tests for the spectrum of unhealthy alcohol use. While there are subtle variations in sensitivity and specificity across studies, the confidence limits around estimates of sensitivity are broad and many of the observed

Table 2.7 Pros and cons of single-item alcohol screens (SASQs) and AUDIT-C

Pros	Cons
Single item alcohol screening questions (SASQs)	
Easy to memorize screening question and threshold	If asked or recorded as a dichotomous screen (yes/no), SASQs provide no information on severity. However, the frequency of heavy episodic drinking (e.g., AUDIT question #3 and NIAAAs question) is an excellent measure of severity
Easily integrated into interviews	
Can promote education regarding maximum recommended drinking in a day	
	Does not provide information about typical alcohol use and some risks (e.g., surgical complications) are associated with regular heavy drinking (not heavy episodic)
Positive screen always reflects patient-report of drinking above recommended limits	Should be prefaced with a validated question about alcohol use in general
	Does not assess unhealthy use prior to past year
AUDIT-C	
Assesses typical quantity and frequency of drinking as well as the frequency of episodic heavy drinking	Response options hard to remember, so not easy for interviews if no paper questionnaires or electronic medical record (EMR) decision support
Provides a scaled measure of the severity of unhealthy drinking; highest scores indicate >75 % probability of dependence	Clinicians must add up the score, unless EMR scores it
	Clinicians and others conducting screening need more training in administration and interpretation
Documented association with health outcomes: medication adherence, new GI diagnoses and hospitalizations, surgical complications, post-operative inpatient utilization, and mortality	Patients can screen positive while reporting drinking within limits (see text).
	Does not assess unhealthy use prior to past year
Has been used as an outcome measure for monitoring responses to BI [37]	

differences are not clinically meaningful. Moreover, different settings may call for different balances between sensitivity and specificity. In short, there is no one screening questionnaire and threshold that is best for all settings. Therefore, as long as a validated screening test for unhealthy drinking is used, the choice of which test to use should be made based on other criteria including convenience, acceptability to clinicians, or institutional preference. Generally, given the many competing agendas in primary care, brief screens will be preferred; we therefore recommend that all primary care providers commit a SASQ to memory, although for reasons outlined below (Table 2.7), the AUDIT-C is often the preferred screen for implementation throughout a health care system [92, 93].

The Importance of Training

All personnel involved in administering alcohol screening questionnaires should receive training in the purpose of alcohol screening and the basis for recommended limits for alcohol use. Users of screening questionnaires should understand the importance of verbatim screening and how to interpret the results. They should also learn to approach the process in a way that minimizes stigma and invites honest responses. Training should include role playing if at all possible. Scripting introductions to alcohol screening that explain its relevance to health and medical care (e.g., medication interactions), and screening for unhealthy alcohol use immediately after asking about smoking may make alcohol screening feel routine. Asking permission (e.g., "Do you mind if I ask you some questions about your alcohol use?") may also make alcohol screening more comfortable to patients and providers. Just as with sexual history questions, it is also useful to inform patients that alcohol screening questions are asked of all patients, to avoid having them feel as if they have been singled out for some reason for questioning.

Two Practical Approaches to Screening in Primary Care

As above, the choice of a screening instrument for unhealthy drinking will depend in large part on the type of medical practice and clinical preference. In some practices, screening is incorporated into individual providers' medical history taking. In other practices, there will be routine systems for carrying out preventive screening on paper, electronically, or by support staff. Although the ideal screening interval is unknown, alcohol screening can be conducted annually, along with other annual preventive care, both because alcohol use changes with time and due to the imperfect sensitivity of validated screens. In this section we outline two practical approaches to using two different screening questionnaires: integration of alcohol screening with a single question into the primary care providers' (or designee's, e.g., medical assistant) medical interviews or routine alcohol screening of all patients by members of the primary care team with the AUDIT-C on paper, online, or prompted by the electronic medical record.

Using SASQs as Part of Medical History Taking

Single-item alcohol screening questions (SASQs) can be easily integrated into the medical history. Although SASQs have been validated with and without a lead-in question about any alcohol use [63], many clinicians find it most comfortable to first ask patients if they drink at all, before asking questions about episodic heavy drinking. Asking about any alcohol consumption also provides useful information for patients with contraindications to any alcohol use or for patients taking medications that interact with alcohol. If this is done, it is essential to ask a validated question about alcohol use. When patients are asked 'Do you drink?' they can interpret the question as asking 'Do you drink *a significant amount?*' or '*Do* you drink *daily?*' Asking 'Are you a drinker?' can be interpreted as 'Are you a *problem* drinker?' Therefore, asking a validated question about any alcohol use, such as 'Do you sometimes drink alcohol?' [4, 63] or the first question of the AUDIT (Table 2.3) is recommended.

We believe that all primary care providers should memorize one validated question about alcohol use and one of the validated SASQ's. These questions can also be used in urgent care settings or at the bedside of hospitalized patients. When patients screen positive using a SASQ, further assessment can include questions about typical frequency and quantity of drinking or additional questions or brief screening tests for alcohol dependence [94].

AUDIT-C as Part of a Program of Routine Preventive Screening

When alcohol screening is conducted on paper, online, interactive voice recording [95, 96], or by trained clinicians prompted by decision support in an electronic medical record (EMR), we recommend using the 3-item AUDIT-C. Although SASQs can also be used in these settings, there are several benefits to screening with the AUDIT-C, especially when results of alcohol screening can be stored in an EMR for easy retrieval by all clinicians participating in a patient's care. First, as above, the frequency and quantity of even low-level alcohol use is important for many patients, including those with contraindications to any alcohol use (e.g., adolescents, women who are pregnant or trying to conceive or patients with hepatitis C infection), patients taking medications that interact with alcohol, and patients with prior alcohol dependence or treatment. Second, the scaled AUDIT-C score provides important information about the severity of unhealthy alcohol use and alcohol-related symptoms as well as the probability of alcohol dependence (Table 2.5) [35, 97]. The AUDIT-C score also provides information on risk of medication non-adherence [7], and medical [12, 66, 67] and surgical complications of drinking [11, 98]. Finally, the AUDIT-C score can be used to monitor changes in drinking over time [37].

However, use of the AUDIT-C requires clinician education on several essential points to avoid poor quality screening and resistance from providers. As with other alcohol screening questionnaires, anyone administering the AUDIT-C must understand that it is only a valid screen when questions are asked verbatim. Because AUDIT-C questions 1–2 ask about typical frequency and quantity, it is tempting to just ask patients 'How much do you drink?' Without rigorous adherence to verbatim screening the majority of patients with unhealthy drinking can be missed [99]. If the questions are asked by interview, the interviewer will want to use a lead-in such as that used for the AUDIT (Table 2.3), followed by asking each question verbatim. After patients respond, if responses are not consistent with a response option, the interviewer asks 'Would you say that is closer to __ or __?' providing the response options closest to the patient's response. Finally, the AUDIT-C has been validated using a skip pattern for non-drinkers. When patients indicate they have never had a drink containing alcohol in the past year on question 1, the other 2 questions can be skipped and an AUDIT-C score of 0 assigned [60], although another option is to ask AUDIT 9–10 to assess past problems due to drinking [62]. For patients who drink, AUDIT-C questions 2–3 should be asked and the score calculated. Women scoring

3 or more points and men scoring 4 or more points are considered to have positive screens for unhealthy alcohol use in most settings.

Summary

Primary medical care should include routine alcohol screening to identify patients with unhealthy alcohol use, whether an alcohol use disorder or risky drinking. Screening should include all adult primary care patients as well as adolescents. Although it is important that screening be done with a validated instrument, there are a number of similarly accurate alcohol screening questionnaires for identifying the entire spectrum of unhealthy drinking, and some of them are very brief. We believe that primary care clinicians should commit two validated questions to memory: one to assess any alcohol use and one single-item alcohol screening question (SASQ). However, in settings with EMRs and systems for universal screening, we favor use of the AUDIT-C because of the information it provides on reported typical drinking and on the severity of unhealthy drinking, as well as the utility of a scaled marker for measuring the severity of unhealthy alcohol use and changes over time. Finally, primary care clinicians and others conducting screening must all be carefully trained about recommended drinking limits and risks associated with drinking above them, the purpose of alcohol screening and the efficacy of brief alcohol interventions, including practicing asking validated screening questions in a comfortable manner.

References

1. American Psychiatric Association. Diagnostic and statistical manual of mental disorders. 4th ed. Washington, DC: American Psychiatric Association; 1994.
2. Willenbring ML, Olson DH. A randomized trial of integrated outpatient treatment for medically ill alcoholic men. Arch Intern Med. 1999;159(16):1946–1952.
3. Willenbring ML. Medications to treat alcohol dependence: adding to the continuum of care. JAMA. 2007;298(14):1691–1692.
4. National Institute on Alcohol Abuse and Alcoholism. Helping patients who drink too much: a clinician's guide (updated 2005 edition). Washington, DC: National Institutes of Health, U.S. Department of Health and Human Services; 2007. NIH Publication 07-3769.
5. Ahmed AT, Karter AJ, Liu J. Alcohol consumption is inversely associated with adherence to diabetes self-care behaviours. Diabet Med. Jul 2006;23(7):795–802.
6. Ahmed AT, Karter AJ, Warton EM, Doan JU, Weisner CM. The relationship between alcohol consumption and glycemic control among patients with diabetes: the Kaiser Permanente Northern California Diabetes Registry. J Gen Intern Med. 2008;23(3):275–282.
7. Bryson CL, Au DH, Sun H, Williams EC, Kivlahan DR, Bradley KA. Alcohol screening scores and medication nonadherence. Ann Intern Med 2008;149(11):795–804.
8. Tonnesen H, Rosenberg J, Nielsen H, et al. Effect of preoperative abstinence on poor postoperative outcome in alcohol misusers: randomised controlled trial. Br Med J. 1999;318(7194):1311–1316.
9. Tonnesen H, Petersen KR, Hojgaard L, et al. Postoperative morbidity among symptom-free alcohol misusers. Lancet. 1992;340(8815):334–337.

10. Harris AH, Reeder R, Ellerbe L, Bradley KA, Rubinsky AD, Giori NJ. Preoperative alcohol screening scores: association with complications in men undergoing total joint arthroplasty. J Bone Joint Surg Am. 2011;93(4):321–327.

11. Bradley KA, Rubinsky AD, Sun H, et al. Alcohol screening and risk of postoperative complications in male VA patients undergoing major non-cardiac surgery. J Gen Intern Med. 2011;26(2):162–169.

12. Au DH, Kivlahan DR, Bryson CL, Blough D, Bradley KA. Alcohol screening scores and risk of hospitalizations for GI conditions in men. Alcohol Clin Exp Res. 2007;31(3):443–451.

13. Chew RB, Bryson CL, Au DH, Maciejewski ML, Bradley KA. Are smoking and alcohol misuse associated with subsequent hospitalizations for ambulatory care sensitive conditions? J Behav Health Serv Res. 2011;38(1):3–15.

14. Mokdad AH, Marks JS, Stroup DF, Gerberding JL. Actual causes of death in the United States, 2000. JAMA. 2004;291(10):1238–1245.

15. Whitlock EP, Polen MR, Green CA, Orleans T, Klein J. Behavioral counseling interventions in primary care to reduce risky/harmful alcohol use by adults: a summary of the evidence for the U.S. Preventive Services Task Force. Ann Intern Med. 2004;140(7):557–568.

16. Kaner EF, Dickinson HO, Beyer F, et al. The effectiveness of brief alcohol interventions in primary care settings: A systematic review. Drug Alcohol Rev. 2009;28(3):301–323.

17. Kaner E, Beyer F, Dickinson H, et al. Effectiveness of brief alcohol interventions in primary care populations. Cochrane Database Syst Rev. 2007(2):CD004148.

18. Saitz R. Clinical practice. Unhealthy alcohol use. N Engl J Med. 2005;352(6):596–607.

19. Wechsler H, Dowdall GW, Davenport A, Rimm EB. A gender-specific measure of binge drinking among college students. Am J Public Health. 1995;85:982–985.

20. Bradley KA, Bush K, Davis TD, et al. Binge drinking among female Veterans Affairs patients: prevalence and associated risks. Psychol Addict Behav. 2001;15:297–305.

21. Becker U, Deis A, Sorenson TIA, Gronbaek M, Borch-Johnsen K, Muller CF. Prediction of risk of liver disease by alcohol intake, sex and age: a prospective population study. Hepatology. 1996;23:1025–1029.

22. Bradley KA, Badrinath S, Bush K, Boyd-Wickizer J, Anawalt B. Medical risks for women who drink alcohol. J Gen Intern Med. 1998;13(9):627–639.

23. Spurling MC, Vinson DC. Alcohol-related injuries: evidence for the prevention paradox. Ann Fam Med. 2005;3(1):47–52.

24. Saitz R. Alcohol screening and brief intervention in primary care: absence of evidence for efficacy in people with dependence or very heavy drinking. Drug Alcohol Rev. 2010;29(6):631–640.

25. Solberg LI, Maciosek MV, Edwards NM. Primary care intervention to reduce alcohol misuse ranking its health impact and cost effectiveness. Am J Prev Med. 2008;34(2):143–152.

26. American Academy of Family Physicians. Alcohol Misuse. 2011. http://www.aafp.org/online/en/home/clinical/exam/alcoholmisuse.html. Accessed 10 Aug 2011.

27. American College of Obstetricians and Gynecologists. At-risk drinking and alcohol dependence: obstetric and gynecologic implications. Committee Opinion No. 496. Obstet Gynecol. 2011;118:383–388.

28. Committee on Substance Abuse. Policy Statement—Alcohol use by youth and adolescents: a pediatric concern. 2010. www.pediatrics.org/cgi/doi/10.1542/peds.2010-0438.

29. VA Office of Quality and Performance. VA/DoD Clinical Practice Guideline for the Management of Substance Use Disorders, Version 2.0. http://www.healthquality.va.gov/sud/sud_full_601f.pdf 2009.

30. Yarnall KSH, Pollak KI, Ostbye T, Krause KM, Micchener JL. Primary care: is there enough time for prevention? Am J Public Health. 2003;93(4):635–641.

31. Saitz R, Horton NJ, Cheng DM, Samet JH. Alcohol counseling reflects higher quality of primary care. J Gen Intern Med. 2008;23(9):1482–1486.

32. Bradley KA, Kivlahan DR, Bush KR, McDonell MB, Fihn SD. Variations on the CAGE alcohol screening questionnaire: strengths and limitations in VA general medical patients. Alcohol Clin Exp Res. 2001;25(10):1472–1478.

33. Cantor SB, Sun CC, Tortolero-Luna G, Richards-Kortum R, Follen M. A comparison of C/B ratios from studies using receiver operating characteristic curve analysis. J Clin Epidemiol. 1999;52(9):885–892.

34. Steinbauer JR, Cantor SB, Holzer CE, Volk JR. Ethnic and sex bias in primary care screening tests for alcohol use disorders. Ann Intern Med. 1998;129:353–362.

35. Rubinsky AD, Kivlahan DR, Volk RJ, Maynard C, Bradley KA. Estimating risk of alcohol dependence using alcohol screening scores. Drug Alcohol Depend. 2010;108(1–2):29–36.

36. Institute of Medicine. Improving the quality of mental health care for mental and substance-use conditions. Washington, DC: The National Academies Press; 2006.

37. Williams EC, Lapham G, Achtmeyer CE, Volpp B, Kivlahan DR, Bradley KA. Use of an electronic clinical reminder for brief alcohol counseling is associated with resolution of alcohol misuse. J Gen Intern Med. 2010;25(1):11–18.

38. Ewing JA. Detecting alcoholism: the CAGE questionnaire. JAMA. 1984;252:1905–1907.

39. Ewing JA. Screening for alcoholism using CAGE. JAMA. 1998;280:1904–1905.

40. Buchsbaum DG, Buchanan RG, Centor RM, Schnoll SH, Lawton MJ. Screening for alcohol abuse using CAGE scores and likelihood ratios. Ann Intern Med. 1991;115:774–777.

41. Bradley KA, Bush KR, McDonell MB, Malone T, Fihn SD. Screening for problem drinking: comparison of CAGE and AUDIT. J Gen Intern Med. 1998;13(6):379–388.

42. Bradley KA, Maynard C, Kivlahan DR, McDonell MB, Fihn SD. The relationship between alcohol screening questionnaires and mortality among male veteran outpatients. J Stud Alcohol. 2001;62(6):826–833.

43. Volk RJ, Cantor SB, Steinbauer JR, Cass AR. Item bias in the CAGE screening test for alcohol use disorders. J Gen Intern Med. 1997;12:763–769.

44. Wallace P, Haines A. Use of a questionnaire in general practice to increase the recognition of patients with excessive alcohol consumption. Br Med J. 1985;290:1949–1952.

45. Fleming MF, Barry KL. A three-sample test of a masked alcohol screening questionnaire. Alcohol Alcohol. 1991;26(1):81–91.

46. Selzer ML, Vinokur A, von Rooijen L. A self administered Short Michigan Alcohol Screening Test (SMAST). J Stud Alcohol. 1975;36:117–126.

47. Zung BJ. Psychometric properties of the MAST and two briefer versions. J Stud Alcohol. 1979;40(9):845–859.

48. Hedlund JL, Vieweg B. The Michigan Alcoholism Screening Test (MAST): a comprehensive review. J Oper Psych. 1984;15:55–65.

49. Magruder-Habib K, Stevens HA, Alling WC. Relative performance of the MAST, VAST, and CAGE versus DSM-III-R criteria for alcohol dependence. J Clin Epidemiol. 1993;46(5):435–441.

50. Pokorny AD, Miller BA, Kaplan HB. The brief MAST: a shortened version of the Michigan Alcoholism Screening Test. Am J Psychiatry. 1972;129(342–345).

51. Wallace P, Cutler S, Haines A. Randomised controlled trial of general practitioner intervention in patients with excessive alcohol consumption. Br Med J. 1988;297:663–668.

52. Fleming MF, Barry KL, Manwell LB, Johnson K, London R. Brief physician advice for problem alcohol drinkers: a randomized controlled trial in community-based primary care practices. JAMA. 1997;277(13):1039–1045.

53. Fihn SD, McDonell MB, Diehr P, et al. Effects of sustained audit/feedback on self-reported health status of primary care patients. Am J Med. 2004;116(4):241–248.

54. Babor TF, Grant M. From clinical research to secondary prevention—international collaboration in the development of the alcohol use disorders identification test (AUDIT). Alcohol Health Res World. 1989;13(4):371–374.

55. Saunders JB, Aasland OG, Babor TF, De la Fuente JR, Grant M. Development of the alcohol use disorders identification test (AUDIT): WHO collaborative project on early detection of persons with harmful alcohol consumption—II. Addiction. 1993;88:791–804.

56. Babor TF, Higgins-Biddle JC. Brief intervention for hazardous and harmful drinking: a manual for use in primary care. Geneva: World Health Organization; 2001.

57. Volk RJ, Steinbauer JR, Cantor SB, Holzer CEI. The alcohol use disorders identification test (AUDIT) as a screen for at-risk patients of different racial/ethnic backgrounds. Addiction. 1997;92(2):197–206.
58. Seale JP, Boltri JM, Shellenberger S, et al. Primary care validation of a single screening question for drinkers. J Stud Alcohol. 2006;67(5):778–784.
59. Bush K, Kivlahan DR, McDonell MB, Fihn SD, Bradley KA. The AUDIT alcohol consumption questions (AUDIT-C): an effective brief screening test for problem drinking. Ambulatory Care Quality Improvement Project (ACQUIP). Alcohol Use Disorders Identification Test. Arch Intern Med. 1998;158(16):1789–1795.
60. Bradley KA, De Benedetti AF, Volk RJ, Williams EC, Frank D, Kivlahan DR. AUDIT-C as a brief screen for alcohol misuse in primary care. Alcohol Clin Exp Res. 2007;31(7):1208–1217.
61. Bradley KA, Bush KR, Epler AJ, et al. Two brief alcohol-screening tests from the alcohol use disorders identification test (AUDIT): validation in a female veterans affairs patient population. Arch Intern Med. 2003;163(7):821–829.
62. Babor TF, Higgins-Biddle JC, Saunders JB, Monteiro MG. AUDIT: the alcohol use disorders identification test: guidelines for use in primary care. 2001. 2nd: http://www.dass.stir.ac.uk/DRUGS/pdf/audit.pdf.
63. Smith PC, Schmidt SM, Allensworth-Davies D, Saitz R. Primary care validation of a single-question alcohol screening test. J Gen Intern Med. 2009;24(7):783–788.
64. Lapham GT, Achtmeyer CE, Williams EC, Hawkins EJ, Kivlahan DR, Bradley KA. Increased documented brief alcohol interventions with a performance measure and electronic decision support. Med Care. 2010 Sep 28 [E-pub ahead of print].
65. Lembke A, Bradley KA, Henderson P, Moos R, Harris AH. Alcohol screening scores and the risk of new-onset gastrointestinal illness or related hospitalization. J Gen Intern Med. 2011;26(7):777–782.
66. Harris AH, Bryson CL, Sun H, Blough D, Bradley KA. Alcohol screening scores predict risk of subsequent fractures. Subst Use Misuse. 2009;44:1055–1069.
67. Williams EC, Sun H, Chew RB, Chew LD, Blough DK, Au DH, Bradley KA. Association between alcohol screening results and hospitalizations for trauma in veterans affairs outpatients. Am J Drug Alcohol Abuse. Am J Drug Alcohol Abuse. 2012;38:73–80.
68. Harris AH, Bradley KA, Bowe T, Henderson P, Moos R. Associations between AUDIT-C and mortality vary by age and sex. Popul Health Manag. 2010;13(5):263–268.
69. Dawson DA, Archer LD. Relative frequency of heavy drinking and the risk of alcohol dependence. Addiction. 1993;88(11):1509–1518.
70. Taj N, Devera-Sales A, Vinson DC. Screening for problem drinking: does a single question work? J Fam Pract. 1998;46(4):328–335.
71. Williams R, Vinson DC. Validation of a single screening question for problem drinking. J Fam Pract. 2001;50(4):307–312.
72. Chang G. Alcohol-screening instruments for pregnant women. Alcohol Res Health. 2001;25(3):204–209.
73. Russell M, Martier SS, Sokol RJ, et al. Screening for pregnancy risk-drinking. Alcohol Clin Exp Res. 1994;18(5):1156–1161.
74. Russell M, Martier SS, Sokol RJ, Mudar P, Jacobson SJJ. Detecting risk drinking during pregnancy: a comparison of four screening questionnaires. Am J Public Health. 1996;86:1435–1439.
75. Dawson DA, Grant BF, Stinson FS, Zhou Y. Effectiveness of the derived alcohol use disorders identification test (AUDIT-C) in screening for alcohol use disorders and risk drinking in the US general population. Alcohol Clin Exp Res. 2005;29(5):844–854.
76. Knight JR, Sherritt L, Harris SK, Gates EC, Chang G. Validity of brief alcohol screening tests among adolescents: a comparison of the AUDIT, POSIT, CAGE, and CRAFFT. Alcohol Clin Exp Res. 2003;27(1):67–73.
77. Newton AS, Gokiert R, Mabood N, et al. Instruments to detect alcohol and other drug misuse in the emergency department: a systematic review. Pediatrics. 2011;128(1):e180–192.

78. Babor TF. The alcohol, smoking and substance involvement screening test (ASSIST): development, reliability and feasibility. Addiction. 2002;91:1183–1194.

79. Smith PC, Schmidt SM, Allensworth-Davies D, Saitz R. A single-question screening test for drug use in primary care. Arch Intern Med. 2010;170(13):1155–1160.

80. Neumann T, Spies C. Use of biomarkers for alcohol use disorders in clinical practice. Addiction. 2003;98(Suppl 2):81–91.

81. Center for Substance Abuse Treatment. The role of biomarkers in the treatment of alcohol use disorders. Substance abuse treatment advisory. In: US Department of Health and Human Services SAMHSA, Center for Substance Abuse Treatment. www.samhsa.gov, ed5. US Department of Health and Human Services; 2006.

82. Miller PM, Anton RF. Biochemical alcohol screening in primary health care. Addict Behav. 2004;29(7):1427–1437.

83. Fleming MF, Anton RF, Spies CD. A review of genetic, biological, pharmacological, and clinical factors that affect carbohydrate-deficient transferrin levels. Alcohol Clin Exp Res. 2004;28(9):1347–1355.

84. Yersin B, Nicolet JF, Decrey H, Burnier M, Van Melle G, Pecoud A. Screening for excessive alcohol drinking. Arch Intern Med. 1995;155:1907–1911.

85. Bell H, Tallaksen CM, Try K, Haug E. Carbohydrate-deficient transferrin and other markers of high alcohol consumption: a study of 502 patients admitted consecutively to a medical department. Alcohol Clin Exp Res. 1994;18(5):1103–1108.

86. Conigrave KM, Degenhardt LJ, Whitfield JB, Saunders JB, Helander A, Tabakoff B. CDT, GGT, and AST as markers of alcohol use: the WHO/ISBRA collaborative project. Alcohol Clin Exp Res. 2002;26(3):332–339.

87. Jatlow P, O'Malley SS. Clinical (nonforensic) application of ethyl glucuronide measurement: are we ready? Alcohol Clin Exp Res. 2010;34(6):968–975.

88. Kapoor A, Kraemer KL, Smith KJ, Roberts MS, Saitz R. Cost-effectiveness of screening for unhealthy alcohol use with % carbohydrate deficient transferrin: results from a literature-based decision analytic computer model. Alcohol Clin Exp Res. 2009;33(8):1440–1449.

89. Neumann T, Gentilello LM, Neuner B, et al. Screening trauma patients with the alcohol use disorders identification test and biomarkers of alcohol use. Alcohol Clin Exp Res. 2009;33(6):970–976.

90. Kristenson H, Ohlin H, Hulten-Nosslin M, Trell E, Hood B. Identification and intervention of heavy drinking in middle-aged men: results and follow-up of 24–60 months of long-term study with randomized controls. Alcohol Clin Exp Res. 1983;7(2):203–209.

91. Fleming M, Brown R, Brown D. The efficacy of a brief alcohol intervention combined with %CDT feedback in patients being treated for type 2 diabetes and/or hypertension. J Stud Alcohol. 2004;65(5):631–637.

92. Bradley KA, Williams EC, Achtmeyer CE, Volpp B, Collins BJ, Kivlahan DR. Implementation of evidence-based alcohol screening in the Veterans Health Administration. Am J Manag Care. 2006;12(10):597–606.

93. Rose HL, Miller PM, Nemeth LS, et al. Alcohol screening and brief counseling in a primary care hypertensive population: a quality improvement intervention. Addiction. 2008;103(8):1271–1280.

94. Vinson DC, Kruse RL, Seale JP. Simplifying alcohol assessment: two questions to identify alcohol use disorders. Alcohol Clin Exp Res. 2007;31(8):1392–1398.

95. Rose GL, Skelly JM, Badger GJ, Maclean CD, Malgeri MP, Helzer JE. Automated screening for at-risk drinking in a primary care office using interactive voice response. J Stud Alcohol Drugs. 2010;71(5):734–738.

96. Rose GL, MacLean CD, Skelly J, Badger GJ, Ferraro TA, Helzer JE. Interactive voice response technology can deliver alcohol screening and brief intervention in primary care. J Gen Intern Med. 2010;25(4):340–344.

97. Bradley KA, Kivlahan DR, Zhou XH, et al. Using alcohol screening results and treatment history to assess the severity of at-risk drinking in Veterans Affairs primary care patients. Alcohol Clin Exp Res. 2004;28(3):448–455.

98. Rubinsky AD, Sun H, Blough DK, et al. AUDIT-C alcohol misuse screening results and postoperative inpatient health care utilization J Am Coll Surg. 2012;214:296–305.e1.
99. Bradley KA, Lapham GT, Hawkins EJ, et al. Quality concerns with routine alcohol screening in VA clinical settings. J Gen Intern Med. 2011;26(3):299–306.

Chapter 3
Assessment of Unhealthy Alcohol Use in Primary Care

Hillary Kunins and Chinazo Cunningham

Patient A: A 64 year old man states that his wife thinks he has a drinking problem. He is not sure, and asks your opinion.

Patient B: A 42 year old woman has persistently uncontrolled hypertension and a poor relationship with her husband who you believe is drinking in an unhealthy manner.

Patient C: A 54 year old man completes the NIAAA (National Institute on Alcohol Abuse and Alcoholism)-recommended single item alcohol screening test in your office. In answer to the question, "How many times in the past year have you had 5 or more drinks in a day," he has answered "20." In the follow-up questions, "On average, on how many days each week do you have an alcoholic drink?" he reports "4," and, "On a typical drinking day, how many drinks do you have?" he reports, "6." Based on the patient's responses, he is considered to have a "positive" screening test and to be drinking amounts that increase the risk of health consequences.

What Should the Clinician do After Identifying Potentially Unhealthy Alcohol Use?

These common scenarios in clinical practice provide an opportunity for the primary care clinician to address a spectrum of unhealthy alcohol use, and to provide an appropriate intervention or treatment recommendation. In patient A, similar to other

H. Kunins (✉)
Departments of Medicine (Division of General Internal Medicine) and Psychiatry and Behavioral Sciences, Albert Einstein College of Medicine and Montefiore Medical Center, Bronx, NY 10467, USA
e-mail: hkunins@gmail.com

C. Cunningham
Medicine (Division of General Internal Medicine) and Family and Social Medicine, Albert Einstein College of Medicine and Montefiore Medical Center, Bronx, NY 10467, USA
e-mail: ccunning@montefiore.org

R. Saitz (ed.), *Addressing Unhealthy Alcohol Use in Primary Care*, DOI 10.1007/978-1-4614-4779-5_3, © Springer Science+Business Media New York 2013

conditions, patients or their family/friends may suspect an illness, and clinicians must determine whether one exists. In patient B, a collection of symptoms may suggest an illness, and again, the clinician must assess whether an illness is causing the symptoms. Finally, in patient C, similar to procedures after other screening tests, clinicians must determine whether or not the patient who tests positive on a screening test actually has an illness or risk factor. Unlike illnesses which are not directly behaviorally related, the clinician also needs to determine whether the patient regards his/her alcohol use as a problem or risk, and whether s/he is ready to make a change regarding alcohol use. This two-component procedure: determining whether unhealthy alcohol use is occurring (and its severity) and determining the patient's readiness to address the alcohol use is what we will call an "assessment." Such an assessment provides the information needed for the clinician to offer an appropriate and effective intervention. Symptoms or a positive screening test should prompt an assessment. In this chapter, we will discuss strategies and tools to undertake an assessment.

An assessment of alcohol use, consequences and readiness helps the clinician answer the central questions which inform next steps and intervention. Specifically, the assessment seeks to answer:

1. Does the patient have unhealthy alcohol consumption, specifically drinking amounts that increase the risk for health consequences; "problem" alcohol use (use with consequences that do not meet disorder criteria), or an alcohol use disorder (the diagnoses abuse or dependence)?
2. What is the patient's level of readiness with respect to changing his/her drinking behavior?

In this chapter, we will discuss the components of an assessment, including how to make a differential diagnosis for unhealthy alcohol use, the features of diagnoses particularly relevant for primary care clinicians, and available tools to help with diagnosis, including assessing the severity of the unhealthy alcohol use and its consequences. We will also discuss the importance of assessing the patient's "readiness." The final goal of the assessment is to help the clinician ascertain what advice to give or treatment recommendations to make, and to enable her to deliver an appropriate and tailored intervention.

Structured strategies and tools can be helpful to guide the clinician in conducting an assessment that is brief and feasible. Unfortunately, these have infrequently been tested in primary care practice in terms of validity but they are very likely to be informative and useful for immediate clinical decision-making. We include some of these tools as a guide, as recommendations for practice.

How Does the Clinician Assess if the Patient has an Alcohol Use Disorder?

As clinicians know, patients A, B, and/or C above could have no disease, a risk factor or mild disease, or severe disease. In the case of alcohol, this may range from risky or hazardous drinking (use that risks consequences but with no consequences yet), problem drinking (i.e, risky drinking with some consequences that does not meet criteria for the disorders abuse or dependence), or the disorders of alcohol abuse or alcohol dependence (see below box) [1].

Box: Spectrum of Alcohol Use

No Use – Low-Risk Use – Hazardous Use – Problem Use – Alcohol Abuse – Alcohol Dependence

Definitions:

Low-Risk Use: Alcohol use quantity and frequency less than hazardous use, and without alcohol-related consequences. Not drinking when on a medication that interacts with alcohol, when there is a medical condition that is caused or exacerbated by drinking, or during pregnancy.

Hazardous Use: For women and patients > 65, drinks > 7 standard drinks weekly or > 3 drinks on an occasion; for men ≤ 65 years old, > 14 standard drinks weekly or > 4 drinks per occasion; drinking while taking a medication that interacts significantly with alcohol or when there is a medical condition caused or worsened by alcohol; or drinking during pregnancy.

Problem Use: Alcohol use with consequences, but which does not meet DSM criteria for a disorder, alcohol abuse or dependence.

A central clinical task is to distinguish alcohol dependence from anything else. Alcohol dependence, unlike other possible conditions in the differential diagnosis, typically requires specialty treatment. Furthermore, patients with alcohol dependence can benefit from pharmacotherapy to safely stop drinking. In counseling patients with alcohol dependence, clinicians therefore ought to advise referral to specialty treatment settings, although the manner in which such advice is given should be consistent with motivational interviewing principles—that is, asking permission to share information, and giving feedback in a neutral manner, waiting until the patient expresses that s/he is ready for change. Patients with alcohol dependence may be candidates for longer term pharmacotherapy, such as naltrexone or acamprosate, which may help patients with dependence maintain abstinence or reduce drinking.

Also, determining the diagnosis of the patient's condition helps the clinician understand the severity. The differential diagnoses carry prognostic value—that is, how likely the patient will go on to have additional physical and/or psychosocial problems from alcohol—and therefore implications for intervention and treatment intensity. For example, the hazardous drinker is at lower risk for physical consequences than the drinker who meets criteria for alcohol abuse or dependence; the clinician may choose therefore to vary frequency and intensity of intervention for such patients.

How to make a differential diagnosis for the patient with a positive screening test for unhealthy alcohol use?

To determine whether a patient has hazardous drinking alone, problem drinking, or an alcohol use disorder (alcohol abuse or alcohol dependence), the clinician needs to determine whether the patient has suffered either physical or psychosocial consequences from alcohol use, is experiencing tolerance or withdrawal, and whether the patient has lost control over his/her own drinking. The reference standard for such a differential is from the Diagnostic and Statistical Manual of Mental Disorders, fourth Edition (DSM-IV) criteria, which define both alcohol abuse and alcohol dependence [2]. Patients who do not fulfill these criteria may be drinking hazardously, which is defined according to NIAAA determined amounts (amounts associated with health risks or drinking when alcohol interacts with a medication, affects a medical condition or any amounts during pregnancy). When the patient meets NIAAA hazardous drinking criteria (based on amounts) and has consequences, without meeting DSM-IV criteria for abuse or dependence, the clinician may categorize the condition as "problem" drinking (see Box on previous page) [1].

A clinician determines whether a patient has alcohol abuse or dependence by assessing whether the patient meets criteria set forth in the DSM-IV. While the diagnosis is made clinically, tools that facilitate a structured approach to making this diagnosis are available. An example of one such tool is the Alcohol Use Disorder and Associated Disabilities Interview Schedule (AUDADIS), which has been developed and validated for use by non-clinicians [3]. Another resource, "Helping Patients Who Drink Too Much: A Clinician's Guide," provides a helpful checklist and suggested questions adapted from DSM-IV criteria to assist clinicians in determining whether the patient meets criteria for alcohol abuse or dependence (see Tables 3.1 and 3.2) [4].

Increasingly, researchers are investigating whether shorter assessment strategies can effectively and efficiently identify patients with alcohol dependence (e.g., those who may benefit from referral to specialty care or from pharmacological management) and to characterize non-dependent but still unhealthy drinkers.

One approach to this portion of the assessment is to use the screening test itself to characterize a patient's severity of illness, and specifically, risk for alcohol abuse or dependence. Tools developed to screen for unhealthy alcohol use can sometimes be used to conduct assessments. For example, patients with higher scores on the AUDIT (15–40), or the shorter AUDIT-C (7–10 or greater), have greater likelihood of alcohol dependence than patients with lower scores [5]. In this case, a questionnaire originally designed as a screening test can help the clinician efficiently characterize the severity of the alcohol use.

Similarly, the Alcohol, Smoking and Substance Involvement Screening Test (AS-SIST), developed as a screening tool, can also provide information relevant to assessing a patient's severity of illness. Developed by the World Health Organization (WHO), the ASSIST has good test characteristics to categorize the severity of use, including dependence, in primary care settings [6]. The strength of the ASISST

Table 3.1 Assessing patients for alcohol abuse or dependence. (From: Helping Patients who Drink Too Much: A Clinician's Guide. Source: http://pubs.niaaa.nih.gov/publications/practitioner/clinic-ansguide2005/guide.pdf)

Determine whether, in the past 12 months, your patient's drinking has *repeatedly* caused or contributed to:
Risk of bodily harm (drinking and driving, operating machinery, swimming)
Relationship trouble (family or friends)
Role failure (interference with home, work, or school obligations)
Run-ins with the law (arrests or other legal problems)
If yes to *One or more* your patient has *Alcohol abuse*
In either case, proceed to assess for dependence symptoms
Determine whether, in the past 12 months, your patient has
Not been able to stick to drinking limits (repeatedly gone over them)
Not been able to cut down or stop (repeated failed attempts)
Shown tolerance (needed to drink a lot more to get the same effect)
Shown signs of withdrawal (tremors, sweating, nausea, or insomnia when trying to quit or cut down)
Kept drinking despite problems (recurrent physical or psychological problems)
Spent a lot of time drinking (or anticipating or recovering from drinking)
Spent less time on other matters (activities that had been important or pleasurable)
If yes to *Three or more* your patient has *Alcohol dependence*

is its ability to distinguish among substance use that is low risk, moderate risk (problem use/abuse) and high risk (dependence). The ASSIST is available on the WHO website, with a manual explaining its use and scoring [7]. The ASSIST may be particularly helpful in primary care settings that have infrastructure (such as non-physician personnel to administer it, or an electronic health record into which it can be embedded), as it has skip patterns and is lengthy to administer routinely.

A Two-Question Assessment Strategy

Shorter evidence-based strategies for assessment may promote more widespread implementation of strategies to identify dependent drinkers, and those who would benefit from specialty referral. In an intriguing study of a two-question assessment for alcohol use disorders, Vinson and colleagues developed and validated the use of a short assessment [10]. Their questions are:

1. In the past year, have you sometimes been under the influence of alcohol in situations where you could have caused an accident or gotten hurt?
2. Have there often been times when you had a lot more to drink than you intended to have?

This two-question assessment was between 72–96 % sensitive and 80–95 % specific for detecting alcohol abuse or dependence in people who had been screened positive for unhealthy use. As the authors note, if the patient screens positive in an initial

Table 3.2 Assessing patients with at-risk alcohol use: Sample questions from National Institutes on Alcohol Abuse and Alcoholism. (Source: http://www.niaaa.nih.gov/Publications/EducationTraining Materials/Documents/AssessmentSupport.pdf)

A diagnosis of alcohol *abuse* requires that the patient meet *one* or more of the following criteria, occurring at any time in the same 12-month period, and *not* meet the criteria for alcohol dependence. All questions are prefaced by "In the past 12 months..."

Recurrent drinking in hazardous situations:
Have you more than once driven a car or other vehicle while you were drinking? Or after having had too much to drink?
Have you gotten into situations while drinking or after drinking that increased your chances of getting hurt—like swimming, using machinery, or walking in a dangerous area or around heavy traffic?

Continued use despite recurrent interpersonal or social problems:
Have you continued to drink even though you knew it was causing you trouble with your family or friends?
Have you gotten into physical fights while drinking or right after drinking?

Failure to fulfill major role obligations at work, school, or home because of recurrent drinking:
Have you had a period when your drinking—or being sick from drinking—often interfered with taking care of your home or family? Caused job troubles? School problems?

Recurrent legal problems related to alcohol:
Have you gotten arrested, been held at a police station, or had any other legal problems because of your drinking?

A diagnosis of alcohol *dependence* requires that the patient meet *three* or more of the following criteria, occurring at any time in the same 12-month period. All questions are prefaced by "In the past 12 months..."

Drinking more or longer than intended:
Have you had times when you ended up drinking more than you meant to? Or kept on drinking for longer than you intended?

Impaired control:
Have you more than once wanted to stop or cut down on your drinking? Or tried more than once to stop or cut down but found you couldn't?

Tolerance:
Have you found that you have to drink much more than you once did to get the effect you want? Or that your usual number of drinks has much less effect on you than it once did?

Withdrawal syndrome or drinking to relieve withdrawal:
When the effects of alcohol are wearing off, have you had trouble sleeping? Found yourself shaking? Nervous? Nauseous? Restless? Sweating or with your heart beating fast? Have you sensed things that aren't really there? Had seizures?
Have you taken a drink or used any drug or medicine (other than over-the-counter pain relievers) to keep from having bad aftereffects of drinking? Or to get over them?

Continued use despite recurrent psychological or physical problems:
Have you continued to drink even though you knew it was making you feel depressed or anxious? Or causing a health problem or making one worse? Or after having had a blackout?

Time spent related to drinking or recovering:
Have you had a period when you spent a lot of time drinking? Or being sick or getting over the bad aftereffects of drinking?

Neglect of activities:
In order to drink, have you given up or cut down on activities that were important or interesting to you or gave you pleasure?

screening test, but negative in the two-question assessment, then brief advice is appropriate. If the assessment is positive, then additional assessment, exploration of consequences, and treatment or referral are indicated. As in Vinson et al.'s example of incidentally discovered hypertension in a patient presenting with knee pain, he suggests that further alcohol assessment could be scheduled for a subsequent visit, arranged specifically for that purpose.

Exploring Consequences—A Key Component of Assessment

A main task of assessment and narrowing the differential diagnosis for unhealthy alcohol use is to determine whether the patient has suffered adverse physical, mental, or social consequences from alcohol. Primary care clinicians, who develop longitudinal relationships with patients, and provide comprehensive care, may be uniquely positioned to conduct this portion of the assessment. Denial, a hallmark of the precontemplative patient with an alcohol use disorder, can sometimes be breached by the astute clinician, who is accustomed to taking a broad history and to making connections among seemingly unrelated problems.

The primary care clinician typically diagnoses and treats common physical problems that can also be complications of alcohol use, such a gastro-esophageal reflux, insomnia, depression, along with potentially life threatening complications such as cirrhosis. In the patient about whom the primary care clinician is concerned, whether because of a positive screening test, or concerns raised by the patient or family, the primary care clinician can assess the connection between the alcohol use and the patient's other health problems. For example, poorly controlled hypertension may be explained by a patient's unhealthy drinking. Primary care clinicians are also often aware of patients' interpersonal and social problems, such as family conflicts, arrests for drunken driving or fights, or job losses. These problems may be consequences of unhealthy alcohol use. The goal for the assessment for alcohol use is to identify these parts of the history as potentially connected to the alcohol use, and for the primary care clinician to incorporate knowledge about the patient's history into an assessment for consequences of alcohol use.

Tools to Assess Consequences of Alcohol Use in Primary Care Settings

The DSM-IV checklist, the AUDIT-C, and the ASSIST, among other tools, help the clinician assess the severity and consequences of patients' unhealthy alcohol use. Additional structured tools exist which ask patients to consider drinking consequences specifically. These can provide some structure for primary care clinicians to assess consequences of patients' alcohol use. For example, the 15-item Short Inventory of Problems, adapted from a longer assessment of drinking consequences, may be

Table 3.3 Short inventory of problems. (Source: Miller 2005)

During the *Past 3 Months*, about how often has this happened to you? Choose one answer (0 = never; 1= once or a few times; 2 = once or twice weekly; 3 = daily or almost daily)

1. I have been unhappy because of my drinking
2. Because of my drinking, I have not eaten properly
3. I have failed to do what is expected of me because of my drinking
4. I have felt guilty or ashamed because of my drinking
5. I have taken foolish risks when I have been drinking
6. When drinking, I have done impulsive things that I regretted later

Now answer these questions about things that may have happened to you. During the *Past 3 Months*, how much has this happened? Choose one answer: (0 = not at all; 1= a little; 2 = somewhat; 3 = very much)

7. My physical health has been harmed by my drinking
8. I have had money problems because of my drinking
9. My physical appearance has been harmed by my drinking
10. My family has been hurt by my drinking
11. A friendship or close relationship has been damaged by my drinking
12. My drinking has gotten in the way of my growth as a person
13. My drinking has damaged my social life, popularity, or reputation
14. I have spent too much or lost a lot of money because of my drinking

Has this happened to you during the *Past Months*? Choose one answer: 0 = No; 1 = Almost; 2 = 3 once; Yes; 3 = Yes, more than once

15. I have had an accident while drinking or intoxicated

helpful for use as a written questionnaire for patients who screen positive for problem alcohol use to identify any consequences of alcohol use and to initiate a discussion about them (see Table 3.3) [8, 9].

Exploring Readiness, Importance and Confidence

Why Explore Readiness Importance and Confidence?

In addition to the assessment of the patient's severity of alcohol use and consequences, the assessment of readiness, confidence, and importance can help the clinician provide a patient-centered and effective motivational or brief intervention [11].

As conceptualized by the transtheoretical model, individuals move among five states or stages of 'readiness' with respect to behavior change: precontemplation, contemplation, preparation, action, and maintenance [12]. Frequently depicted as a circular model, individuals move among these readiness states. The assessment task for the clinician preparing to address unhealthy alcohol use with a patient is to identify the patient's current stage of change in order to deliver a stage-of-change-specific intervention, which potentially assists the patient to move to another stage of change, or if ready, to enact behavior change.

Second, the clinician needs to assess how important the patient feels it is to make the prospective behavior change [11, 17, 18]. To provide an appropriately tailored intervention, the clinician ought to assess the patient's sense of importance about a recommended behavior change—if the patient feels the potential behavior change is unimportant, the clinician may need to start the intervention by using motivational strategies to promote the patient's sense of importance in making change.

To further understand the patient's relationship to the behavior change, and for the clinician to provide an appropriate intervention, the clinician can assess the patient's sense of confidence to carry out prospective behavior change. An individual's sense of confidence, or self-efficacy, has been associated with reductions in alcohol consumption and improvements in treatment outcomes in patients with alcohol use disorders [11, 13–15]. In a primary care-based study, Williams et al. found that patients' confidence in their ability to change was associated with decreased alcohol consumption [16]. In addition to its predictive ability for behavior change, assessing a patient's confidence, prior to delivering a brief intervention or referring to specialty treatment, can help the clinician to tailor a motivational intervention that will improve patient's confidence and therefore ability to implement the behavior change.

Tools to Assess Readiness, Importance, and Confidence

A simple way to get started can be to ask the patient what they think about the results of a screening test or assessment. The patient will state whether or not they perceive they are drinking too much or not. This statement can help the clinician know whether to work on problem recognition versus confidence and behavior change strategies.

Structured measures of readiness, importance, and confidence may help clinicians assess patients in a systematic fashion in order to provide patient-centered and readiness-informed counseling; results of some of these measures have been associated with change in drinking behavior prospectively. The 19-item SOCRATES scale and the 12-item Readiness to Change Questionnaire are examples of such structured measures [19, 20]. Although the length of each may limit utility for routine use in primary care, these scales highlight examples of questions about readiness, confidence, and importance. We have included these as tables in this chapter, as the questions may help the clinician with phrasing of questions or inquiry to determine patients' readiness (see Tables 3.4 and 3.5).

Another approach to assessing readiness is to simply ask the patient directly. As described in Rollnick and colleagues' practical book, *Health Behavior Change for Practitioners*, the clinician might use a visual analogue scale to ask the patient, "On a scale of 1–10, with 1 being not at all ready, to 10 being quite ready, how ready do you feel to make a change in your drinking?" [11] Using the answer to that question, with additional exchange of information, the clinician can tailor any subsequent advice to the patient's current readiness to change. Rollnick et al. also proposed the use of visual analogue scales to assess patient's confidence, and importance. In this efficient and easy-to-use strategy, the clinician asks the patient, on a scale of 1 to 10, how important do you feel it is (or how ready or confident are you) to change your behavior, with one being not at all ready (or confident, or important) and ten being

Table 3.4 SOCRATES: Tool for assessing readiness to change alcohol use. (Source: Miller WR, Tonigan JS. Assessing drinkers' motivation for change: The Stages of Change Readiness and Treatment Eagerness Scale (SOCRATES). Psychol Addict Behav. 1996;10:89–81.)

Answer Scale: 1 (*NO!* Strongly Disagree); 2 (*No* Disagree); 3 (*?* Undecided Or Unsure); 4 (*Yes* Agree); 5 (*YES!* Strongly Agree)

1. I really want to make changes in my drinking
2. Sometimes I wonder if I am an alcoholic
3. If I don't change my drinking soon, my problems are going to get worse
4. I have already started making some changes in my drinking
5. I was drinking too much at one time, but I've managed to change my drinking
6. Sometimes I wonder if my drinking is hurting other people
7. I am a problem drinker
8. I'm not just thinking about changing my drinking, I'm already doing something about it
9. I have already changed my drinking, and I am looking for ways to keep from slipping back to my old pattern
10. I have serious problems with drinking
11. Sometimes I wonder if I am in control of my drinking
12. My drinking is causing a lot of harm
13. I am actively doing things now to cut down or stop drinking
14. I want help to keep from going back to the drinking problems that I had before
15. I know that I have a drinking problem
16. There are times when I wonder if I drink too much
17. I am an alcoholic
18. I am working hard to change my drinking
19. I have made some changes in my drinking, and I want some help to keep from going back to the way I used to drink

Table 3.5 Readiness to change questionnaire. (Source: Rollnick S, Heather N, Gold R, Hall W. Development of a short 'Readiness to Change' questionnaire for use in brief opportunistic interventions. Br J Addict. 1992;87:754–743.)

Answers: Strongly Disagree (-2), Disagree (-1), Unsure (0), Agree (1), Strongly Agree (2)

1. I don't think I drink too much
2. I am trying to drink less than I used to
3. I enjoy my drinking, but sometimes I drink too much
4. Sometimes I think I should cut down on my drinking
5. It is a waste of time thinking about drinking
6. I have just recently changed my drinking habits
7. Anyone can talk about wanting to do something about drinking
8. I am at the stage where I should think about drinking less alcohol
9. My drinking is a problem sometimes but I am actually doing something about it
10. There is no need for me to think about changing my drinking
11. I am actually changing my drinking habits right now
12. Drinking less alcohol would be pointless for me

very ready (or confident or important) [11]. As a variation of these visual analogue-type rulers, Heather et al. developed the Readiness Ruler in which the behavioral stages of change were given as answer choices [21]. After being asked, "Which of the following best describes how you feel right now?" participants had the choice of answering, "never think about drinking less; sometimes I think about drinking less; I have decided to drink less; I am already trying to cut back on my drinking."

Using the Readiness Ruler could be another efficient strategy for clinicians to assess and then open a conversation with a patient about readiness. Another strategy to assess readiness is described in a study that evaluates whether three questions can assess a patient's stage of change (compared with the lengthier Readiness to Change Questionnaire in Table 3.5). Researchers examined the following three questions:

1. Has the amount you drink changed in the past 3 months?
2. Are you interested in drinking less?
3. Do you think you drink more than you should?

Positive answers to the first two questions indicated that the patient is in the "action" stage of change; positive answers to the second and third questions above indicate that the patient is in the "contemplative" stage of change; negative answers to all three questions indicate that the patient is in the "pre-contemplation" stage of change [22]. The brevity of these questions may be appealing to primary care clinicians seeking to efficiently assess patients' readiness to change drinking behavior.

Assessment Guides Next Steps

The assessment guides the clinician to next steps in intervention. She will be able to determine whether the patient has consequences of drinking and/or an alcohol use disorder. If the patient has alcohol dependence, specialty treatment is recommended. After assessing readiness, the clinician may recommend referral to such treatment if the patient is ready, or explain it is a medically appropriate course of action to be considered when ready. If the patient is physiologically dependent on alcohol, remember that safely tapering off alcohol ought to be attempted with medical supervision and pharmacotherapy, to prevent the untoward and potentially life-threatening exposure to alcohol withdrawal syndrome. The way in which the provider recommends referral should be tailored to the patient's readiness, confidence, and sense of importance for making the behavior change. In making this recommendation, the clinician should acknowledge the patient's choice in carrying it out, and after asking the patient's permission to share information. If the patient has hazardous drinking, or consequences (but does not meet criteria for abuse or dependence), s/he can benefit from a brief intervention with a goal to reduce harm (consumption that causes or risks consequences); otherwise the brief intervention goal may be better directed to recognition of the severity of the problem and towards seeking additional help.

References

1. Saitz R. Clinical practice. Unhealthy alcohol use. N. Engl. J Med. 2005;352(6):596–607.
2. American Psychiatric Association. Diagnostic and statistical manual of mental disorders. 4th ed. (text revision). Washington, DC: American Psychiatric Association; 2000.
3. Grant BF, Harford TC, Dawson DA, Chou PS, Pickering RP. The Alcohol Use Disorder and Associated Disabilities Interview schedule (AUDADIS): reliability of alcohol and drug modules in a general population sample. Drug Alcohol Depend. 1995;39(1):37–44.

4. National Institute on Alcohol Abuse and Alcoholism. Helping patients who drink too much, A clinician's guide, 2005 edition. U.S. Department of Health & Human Services, National Institutes of Health; 2007. http://pubs.niaaa.nih.gov/publications/Practitioner/CliniciansGuide2005/clinicians_guide.htm. Accessed 2 June 2011.

5. Rubinsky AD, Kivlahan DR, Volk RJ, Maynard C, Bradley KA. Estimating risk of alcohol dependence using alcohol screening scores. Drug Alcohol Depend. 2010;108(1–2):29–36.

6. Humeniuk R, Ali R, Babor TF, et al. Validation of the Alcohol, Smoking And Substance Involvement Screening Test (ASSIST). Addiction. 2008;103(6):1039–1047.

7. Humeniuk RE, Henry-Edwards S, Ali R, Poznyak V, Monteiro M. The Alcohol, Smoking and Substance Involvement Screening Test (ASSIST): manual for use in primary care. Geneva: World Health Organization; 2010. http://whqlibdoc.who.int/publications/2010/9789241599382_eng.pdf. Accessed 2 June 2011.

8. Vinson DC, Kruse RL, Seale JP. Simplifying alcohol assessment: two questions to identify alcohol use disorders. Alcohol. Clin. Exp. Res. 2007;31(8):1392–1398.

9. Alterman AI, Cacciola JS, Ivey MA, Habing B, Lynch KG. Reliability and validity of the alcohol short index of problems and a newly constructed drug short index of problems. J Stud Alcohol Drugs. 2009;70(2):304–307.

10. Miller W, Tonigan J, Longabaugh R. The Drinker Inventory of Consequences (DrInC): an instrument for assessing adverse consequences of alcohol abuse (test manual). Bethesda: National Institute on Alcohol Abuse and Alcoholism; 1995.

11. Rollnick S, Mason P, Butler C. Health behavior change: a guide for practitioners. Edinburgh: Churchill Livingstone; 1999.

12. DiClemente CC, Prochaska JO. Toward a comprehensive, transtheoretical model of change: stages of change and addictive behaviors. In: Miller WR, Heather N, editors. Treating addictive behaviors. 2nd ed. New York: Plenum; 1998. p. 3–24.

13. Butler C, Rollnick S, Stott N. The practitioner, the patient and resistance to change: recent ideas on compliance. CMAJ. 1996;154(9):1357–1362.

14. Miller WR, Rollnick SP. *Motivational interviewing, second edition: preparing people for change*. 2nd ed. New York: Guilford; 2002.

15. Demmel R, Beck B, Richter D, Reker T. Readiness to change in a clinical sample of problem drinkers: relation to alcohol use, self-efficacy, and treatment outcome. Eur Addict Res. 2004;10(3):133–138.

16. Moos RH, Moos BS. Rates and predictors of relapse after natural and treated remission from alcohol use disorders. Addiction. 2006;101(2):212–222.

17. Blume AW, Lostutter TW, Schmaling KB, Marlatt GA. Beliefs about drinking behavior predict drinking consequences. J Psychoactive Drugs. 2003;35(3):395–399.

18. Williams EC, Kivlahan DR, Saitz R, et al. Readiness to change in primary care patients who screened positive for alcohol misuse. Ann Fam Med. 2006;4(3):213–220.

19. Miller WR, Tonigan JS. Assessing drinkers' motivations for change: The Stages of Change Readiness and Treatment Eagerness Scale (SOCRATES). Psychology of Addictive Behaviors. 1996;10(2):81–89.

20. Rollnick S, Heather N, Gold R, Hall W. Development of a short readiness to change questionnaire for use in brief, opportunistic interventions among excessive drinkers. Br J Addict. 1992;87(5):743–754.

21. Heather N, Smailes D, Cassidy P. Development of a readiness ruler for use with alcohol brief interventions. Drug and Alcohol Dependence. 2008;98(3):235–240.

22. Heather N, Rollnick S, Bell A. Predictive validity of the readiness to change questionnaire. Addiction. 1993;88(12):1667–1677.

Chapter 4
Brief Intervention for Unhealthy Alcohol Use

Richard Saitz

Efficacy of Brief Intervention

Brief counseling interventions for patients identified by screening as having un-healthy alcohol use are among the most cost-effective preventive interventions in primary care settings. The US Preventive Services Task Force recommends alcohol screening and brief intervention for adults in primary care [1]. Brief intervention (BI) has efficacy for patients with non-dependent unhealthy alcohol use [2–6]. In one meta-analysis of randomized trials in primary care settings (2,784 patients) BI decreased the proportion of patients drinking risky amounts in one year (from 69 % in the usual care group to 57 % among those assigned to receive a BI) [6]. Another meta-analysis found that BI decreased drinking by about 3 drinks per week [5]. BI has also had efficacy among pregnant women [7].

In several randomized trials, BI has reduced healthcare utilization and costs [8–11]. For example, Fleming et al. studied BI in 17 primary care practices in Wisconsin and found that, compared to usual care, two 10–15-min physician discussions and a nurse follow-up phone call decreased drinking, days of hospitalization over 3 years and saved $ 546 in healthcare costs (and $ 7780 costs from a societal perspective mainly due to motor vehicle crashes) [9]. In a population-based study of middle-aged men who drank at least two drinks a day and had elevated serum gamma-glutamyl transferase (GGT) levels, repeated BIs by a physician and nurse including feedback on GGT levels was associated with fewer sick days taken from work, and lower alcohol-related mortality 16 years later (48 % of deaths were alcohol-related) [8, 11].

Although evidence for efficacy for patients with alcohol dependence is lacking [12], BI may be the trigger for a referral to specialty care, the first step in short-term motivational or other counseling, or even a prelude to pharmacotherapy.

R. Saitz (✉)
Clinical Addiction Research and Education (CARE) Unit,
Section of General Internal Medicine, Department of Medicine,
Boston Medical Center and Boston University School of Medicine, Boston, MA, USA
e-mail: rsaitz@bu.edu

Department of Epidemiology, Boston University School of Public Health, Boston, MA, USA

R. Saitz (ed.), *Addressing Unhealthy Alcohol Use in Primary Care,*
DOI 10.1007/978-1-4614-4779-5_4, © Springer Science+Business Media New York 2013

Although clinicians sometimes believe patients do not wish to be asked or advised about drinking, the opposite is generally true. Patients want to be asked, and on average, patients who receive BI for unhealthy alcohol use report having received higher quality of care from their physician [13]. In fact the best evidence for efficacy of BI in primary care comes from randomized trials in which the patient's primary care physician delivered the BI [2–6]. As BI becomes more widely disseminated, however, systems and other health professionals may be used to extend its reach. For example, waiting room or even home screening (telephone or web) might be used, or in-person screening by the medical assistant recording vital signs. The physician might briefly emphasize the importance of the issue and refer to a nurse or behavioral colleague for additional brief counseling. BI has not usually been implemented by substance abuse counselors. Although they could do successful BIs, they are often unfamiliar with patients who do not suffer from alcohol dependence, and are less familiar with brief motivational counseling techniques that clinicians are trained in specifically to do BIs.

What is Brief Intervention?

Brief intervention (BI) is counseling by a health professional, at least once for 5–15 min, but most efficacy studies have included more than one contact. BI counseling includes personalized feedback about the patient's drinking, specific advice, and discussion of the patient's goals and follow-up [14]. The goal of brief intervention is to open a conversation that could lead to a reduction in alcohol use, avoidance of use in hazardous situations (e.g., before driving) or abstinence.

Some readers will be familiar with motivational interviewing (MI) [15–17]. BI can draw on the principles of MI, though MI is a less-structured approach that requires more training than a straightforward BI. MI helps patients recognize discrepancy between their health behaviors and their goals and values. The key features, also key for successful BI, are listening to the patient, expression of empathy, and respect for the patient's autonomy. To state the obvious, the patient is the only one that can change his or her behavior. Sometimes it is useful to state this obvious fact as part of BI, to let the patient know it is their responsibility to change their alcohol use, and therefore they will be more likely to succeed if they decide how to proceed. Furthermore, it is important to tell the patient that you believe they can succeed (support their self-efficacy or confidence that they can make the changes they plan to make).

Personalized Feedback

BI often starts with feedback about the patient's alcohol use, including risks of such use and any consequences that have occurred or may occur. The source of information for this feedback is the result of any screening test or assessments, and any physical examination or laboratory test findings or of relevance.

Specific Advice

After giving feedback, the next step is to ask what the patient thinks of it or even what they might be thinking about doing to change, if anything. Prior to providing advice, which should be clear and specific, it is useful to ask permission ("Is it OK if I give you some advice?" "In my best medical judgment the safest course would be to... (cut down; avoid drinking in hazardous situations; abstain)."

Discussion of Goals

Although "best medical advice" should be clear, it is important to elicit the patient's goals, how they might go about achieving them, and also what they think of the advice given. The clinician should then discuss a menu of options, giving priority to those most consistent with the patient's ideas.

Follow-Up

In follow-up, the clinician checks on progress (by reassessing drinking and consequences, including laboratory tests such as GGT or carbohydrate deficient transferrin, if initially elevated), checks on the patient's goals and readiness to pursue them, helps the patient learn from successes and failures, provides additional advice, and revisits the menu of options. Clinicians should tell patients that they should follow-up regardless of whether they are still drinking too much or not.

How Should BI be Done?

BI should be done empathically. To demonstrate empathy, the clinician should listen, and show that they have heard what the patient has said and that they understand. Reflective listening is an important counseling skill that can demonstrate empathy; it helps the patient feel like they have been heard and understood.

Reflective listening involves either repeating what the patient has said, rephrasing it, paraphrasing it, or restating what the patient has said while adding inferred meaning or emotion. Part of the skill of reflective listening is choosing what to reflect. The clinician should reflect any talk of change or talk of ability to change. A reflection is a statement, not a question.

Talk of change, or "change talk," is when the patient says they want to change, they can change, they have reasons to change, they need to change or they are going to change.

An example is—if the patient says "I have been thinking about drinking less; my wife doesn't like it," the clinician might say "You've been thinking about cutting down. Your wife doesn't like it." Or the clinician might say "Drinking is causing some trouble at home so you want to change that." Or, "You are feeling guilty about your drinking." In any of these cases, the patient is likely to respond by explaining further. In addition, it is powerful for the patient to hear their own words coming from the clinician.

Reflective listening helps to reinforce the patient's plans to change and can also simply keep the conversation going when it seems stuck. Reflecting can lead the patient to talk further to explain.

A second component of how to do BI is to tailor the BI to the patient's readiness to change. Asking about readiness is an assessment that can help inform the BI, but the process of asking can also be part of the BI. For example, if a patient rates their readiness to change at a 2 on a scale from 1 to 10, the clinician might ask why they rated themselves at a 2 and not a 1. The patient will likely respond with a reason to change their drinking that is important to them. Reflecting that reason will reinforce the idea of change, and the clinician could also then ask what would need to happen to increase readiness.

Knowing the patient's readiness to change can also guide the BI. For example, if a patient does not recognize that they have a problem with alcohol ("precontemplation" stage), it would be pointless and likely counter-productive to spend time counseling them about specific ways to change (like recommending specialty treatment or Alcoholics Anonymous). Instead the physician should state that they are concerned about the patient's drinking in a non-judgmental way, agree to disagree about the existence of a problem, give some specific advice (e.g., about cutting down or quitting), and ask the patient to follow-up even if they haven't made a change.

For patients who think they may need to change but are unsure ("contemplation"), it is useful to discuss what they like and don't like about drinking, and what they might like and not like about not drinking (listing the pros and cons). The goal is to emphasize the pros of not drinking (or of cutting down) and the cons of drinking (too much) such that eventually the patient sees that the harms of drinking (too much) outweigh the benefits to them, and they choose to make a change. As above, advice and follow-up make sense.

For patients who have decided to make a change, it is still important to support their ability to do so as they may lack confidence. They may also remain ambivalent about changing so reminding them of their reasons for change can help. But at this stage ("determination" or "action"), patients need help deciding on the best course, with a menu of options from which to choose so that they can select the one they will most likely pursue successfully. Again, follow-up regardless of progress remains important. Once patients cut down or quit drinking, it is important to re-assess to see if drinking less is difficult (either symptoms of withdrawal, craving or loss of friends). They may need support to continue to drink less or abstain, and to recognize situations or triggers that might make them return to drinking too much. If they do return to drinking too much, they should be made to feel welcome to return to see the physician, and to use the relapse as a learning experience.

Ideal BI Drinking Goals

Abstinence is the preferred option (best medical advice) for those under age 21 years, those who have been unable to cut down, pregnant women or those trying to conceive, when there is another health condition caused by drinking, a medication that interacts with alcohol, and when the patient meets criteria for alcohol dependence. Others can aim for cutting down their alcohol use, though for those at risk for dependence or who have already experienced consequences, abstinence may be best.

For those with dependence, in addition to drinking less or abstaining and avoiding consequences, BI can also have the goal of engaging the patient in more intensive or specialized treatments or supports. These may include treatment with pharmacotherapy, group or individual counseling, admission to a treatment facility, and/or referral to a 12-step program. For patients with dependence who do not avail themselves of these options, repeated brief intervention may help increase their motivation to seek further help.

Resources to Support BI for Clinicians and Patients

Several websites have video and other teaching resources available free of charge to help clinicians learn BI. These are available at www.mdalcoholtraining.org and www.niaaa.nih.gov/Publications/EducationTrainingMaterials/Pages/CME_CE.aspx

For patients, they can be referred to www.alcoholscreening.org to be screened. Those who screen positive are given personalized feedback and advice. Similarly another website provides assessment of drinking (www.drinkerscheckup.com), and www.moderatedrinking.com provides help for changing drinking. Although not yet widely and freely available, some websites have shown efficacy as stand-alone online BIs [18] and may become more common in the future as adjuncts to or replacements for initial office-based in-person screening and BI.

Http://rethinkingdrinking.niaaa.nih.gov provides materials that can help patients as they contemplate and make changes including drinking diaries, worksheets to list pros and cons, and worksheets to help patients make a plan to change. Books have also been found effective for helping patients change their drinking. One book shown effective in a clinical trial can be recommended as a result: Miller WR, Muñoz RF. Controlling your drinking: tools to make moderation work for you, Guilford Press, New York 2005.

Outpatient Management of Alcohol Withdrawal

A detailed discussion of the management of alcohol withdrawal appears in Chap. 18. But the question of withdrawal arises sometimes when the goal of BI is abstinence for a patient with alcohol dependence. Although physicians are accustomed to seeing patients with symptomatic withdrawal in hospital settings, from a population perspective, most people with dependence withdraw from alcohol without medical attention and with few symptoms. On the other hand, symptomatic withdrawal can have significant morbid and mortal consequences. When recommending abstinence therefore, withdrawal risk should be assessed. Patients who report prior alcohol withdrawal seizures or delirium tremens should have withdrawal from alcohol done in a medically supervised inpatient setting and receive benzodiazepines there. The same is true for patients with acute medical, surgical or psychiatric conditions and those who present with substantially symptomatic withdrawal. Consideration of inpatient withdrawal should be given for those with a history of multiple prior detoxifications, use of illicit drugs, elderly patients, particularly if there is prior symptomatic withdrawal or medical conditions that could affect the risk from hyperautonomic symptoms (e.g., coronary artery disease) or the risk of benzodiazepine treatment (e.g., obstructive lung disease, cirrhosis). For patients who have only mild, or no past symptomatic withdrawal, outpatient management is often best.

Management of withdrawal as an outpatient is feasible in primary care as long as the patient has a stable home situation with a significant other willing to help, and if daily contact in person or by telephone is possible with the physician or other qualified clinician. Some patients will be able to abstain all at once with no symptoms of withdrawal. Others may prefer to cut down their drinking at their own pace over several days. Those who develop symptoms should be treated with medications.

For outpatient management it would seem to be ideal to use a medication that has low or no addictive potential, and that is associated with little sedation or central nervous system impairment, but the best choice is still a benzodiazepine. Although many medications have efficacy for reducing withdrawal symptoms (e.g., gabapentin, carbamazepine), none aside from benzodiazepines prevent seizures or delirium. For outpatients, the best course is to educate the patient and partner regarding symptoms of withdrawal (see Chap. 18) and then provide a daily prescription of benzodiazepine. If and when symptoms arise, the patient should take a dose, and repeat it every 1–2 h until symptoms are minimal, resuming dosing if they recur or worsen again. Particularly with use of long-acting medication there is no need of a scheduled taper. On average, symptoms will abate on the first day. Some will experience symptoms for 2–3 days and symptoms beyond that would be unusual for outpatient withdrawal. Preferred medications (provide 4–5 doses in a daily prescription) are chlordiazepoxide (25–50 mg doses), or lorazepam (0.5–2 mg doses) or oxazepam (15–30 mg doses) for patients with hepatic synthetic dysfunction, obstructive lung disease or the elderly. Diazepam is not preferred because although it is long-acting, it has rapid onset and greater abuse potential. Patients should be monitored daily by phone or in person to assess symptoms of withdrawal and if present, benzodiazepines can be continued, though one should not expect symptoms to continue beyond several days. Benzodiazepines should not be prescribed for more than several days in the outpatient setting. A failure of symptoms to resolve should prompt more thorough in person examination and possible admission to an inpatient facility. When symptoms of withdrawal have resolved, brief counseling should encourage engagement with treatment for alcohol dependence.

Summary

Brief intervention is the next step when patients are identified by screening as having unhealthy alcohol use. Brief intervention involves 10–15 min of personalized feedback, advice and goal setting done in a nonjudgmental empathic manner, supported by the skill of reflective listening. Reflective listening can keep the conversation going and reinforce the patient's reasons for change and course of action towards change. BI should be tailored to the patients level of readiness to change their drinking. Those with dependence or other reasons why drinking is contraindicated should abstain, and others can be advised to cut down or abstain. Those with dependence should have withdrawal risk considered and managed, and should have pharmacotherapy, referrals to Alcoholics Anonymous and/or specialty counseling among the menu of recommended options. Web and text resources can help support patients as they contemplate change and take action towards cutting down or abstaining from alcohol.

References

1. U.S. Preventive Services Task Force. Screening and behavioral counseling interventions in primary care to reduce alcohol misuse: recommendation statement. Ann Intern Med. 2004;140:554.
2. Kaner EF, Dickinson HO, Beyer F, et al. The effectiveness of brief alcohol interventions in primary care settings: a systematic review. Drug Alcohol Rev. 2009;28:301.
3. Jonas DE, Garbutt JC, Amick HR, et al. Behavioral counseling after screening for alcohol misuse in primary care: a systematic review and meta-analysis for the U.S. Preventive Services Task Force. Ann Intern Med 2012;157:645–654.
4. Ballesteros J, Duffy JC, Querejeta I, et al. Efficacy of brief interventions for hazardous drinkers in primary care: systematic review and meta-analyses. Alcohol Clin Exp Res. 2004;28:608.
5. Bertholet N, Daeppen JB, Wietlisbach V, et al. Reduction of alcohol consumption by brief alcohol intervention in primary care: systematic review and meta-analysis. Arch Intern Med. 2005;165:986.
6. Beich A, Thorsen T, Rollnick S. Screening in brief intervention trials targeting excessive drinkers in general practice: systematic review and meta-analysis. Br Med J. 2003;327:536.
7. O'Connor MJ, Whaley SE. Brief intervention for alcohol use by pregnant women. Am J Public Health. 2007;97:252.
8. Kristenson H, Ohlin H, Hultén-Nosslin MB, et al. Identification and intervention of heavy drinking in middle-aged men: results and follow-up of 24–60 months of long-term study with randomized controls. Alcohol Clin Exp Res. 1983;7:203.
9. Fleming MF, Mundt MP, French MT, et al. Brief physician advice for problem drinkers: long-term efficacy and benefit-cost analysis. Alcohol Clin Exp Res. 2002;26:36.
10. Solberg LI, Maciosek MV, Edwards NM. Primary care intervention to reduce alcohol misuse ranking its health impact and cost effectiveness. Am J Prev Med. 2008;34:143.
11. Kristenson H, Osterling A, Nilsson JA, Lindgärde F. Prevention of alcohol-related deaths in middle-aged heavy drinkers. Alcohol Clin Exp Res. 2002;26:478.
12. Saitz R. Alcohol screening and brief intervention in primary care: Absence of evidence for efficacy in people with dependence or very heavy drinking. Drug Alcohol Rev. 2010;29:631.
13. Saitz R, Horton NJ, Cheng DM, Samet JH. Alcohol counseling reflects higher quality of primary care. J Gen Intern Med. 2008;23:1482.

14. Bien TH, Miller WR, Tonigan JS. Brief interventions for alcohol problems: a review. Addiction. 1993;88:315.
15. Miller WR, Rollnick S. Motivational Interviewing: preparing people for change. New York: Guilford; 2002.
16. Rollnick S, Heather N, Bell A. Negotiating behavior change in medical settings: the development of brief motivational interviewing. J Mental Health. 1992;1:25.
17. Rollnick S, Mason P, Butler C. Health behavior change. Edinburgh: Churchill Livingstone; 1999.
18. Kypri K, Langley JD, Saunders JB, et al. Randomized controlled trial of web-based alcohol screening and brief intervention in primary care. Arch Intern Med. 2008;168:530.

Chapter 5
Alcohol Pharmacotherapies

Dylan Brock, Babak Tofighi, Joshua D. Lee and Judd Fastenberg

Increasingly, some cases of alcohol use disorders can be conceptualized as chronic diseases that can be controlled and managed with the help of effective medications. These can be used in concert with comprehensive psychosocial therapies and other specialized addiction treatments, but also within more simplified, medical management (MM) models in primary care settings. While few individuals with alcohol dependence and fewer still with alcohol abuse or hazardous drinking access alcohol pharmacotherapies [1], there is robust evidence that these medications should be in much wider use. National screening and brief intervention guidelines for primary care settings now emphasize these pharmacotherapy options [2].

This chapter will review the pharmacology and clinical evidence for the four Food and Drug Administration (FDA)-approved alcohol dependence medications and briefly consider other medications not FDA-approved or labeled for the treatment of alcohol dependence that likely have efficacy. These medications have been reviewed in much greater detail elsewhere, and here we briefly summarize the evidence base [3–5]. We then consider common practical issues related to all of the medications, including adherence enhancement strategies, ancillary and complementary psychosocial treatments, use in non-dependent "problem" drinkers, and cost and comparative effectiveness data. Primary care physicians and other practitioners, who may not consider themselves experts in addiction disorders, can and should prescribe these medications routinely.

J. D. Lee (✉)
Departments of Population Health and Medicine, Division of General Internal Medicine,
NYU School of Medicine, New York, NY, USA
e-mail: Joshua.lee@nyumc.org

D. Brock
University of Louisville School of Medicine, Louisville, KY, USA

B. Tofighi
Lenox Hill Hospital, New York, NY, USA

J. Fastenberg
Albany Medical College, Albany, NY, USA

R. Saitz (ed.), *Addressing Unhealthy Alcohol Use in Primary Care,*   49
DOI 10.1007/978-1-4614-4779-5_5, © Springer Science+Business Media New York 2013

Medications for the Treatment of Alcohol Dependence (Table 5.1)

Four medications (acamprosate, disulfiram, oral naltrexone, and extended-release naltrexone) are FDA-approved for the treatment of alcohol dependence. While topiramate is not FDA-approved for this indication, there is evidence for its efficacy, and topiramate is now routinely prescribed off-label for alcohol dependence. Conceptually, these medications counter several major biological mechanisms that are shown to be associated with relapse and alcohol-seeking behavior, including alcohol re-exposure (aversion/negative reinforcement, disulfiram; diminished positive reward, naltrexone), conditioned cue re-exposure (reduced cravings, naltrexone), and nonspecific stress (acamprosate, topiramate) [6].

Naltrexone

Naltrexone in both the oral (brand name Revia) and the more recently introduced injectable, extended-release formulation (abbreviated herein as XR-NTX, brand name Vivitrol) provides a complete antagonist blockade of the mu opioid receptors. Mu opioid receptors are highly concentrated in the brain's corticomesolimbic system, where agonism by endogenous endorphins or exogenous opioid medications produce dopamine release at the nucleus accumbens, resulting in perceived reward. Like prescribed and illicit opioids (i.e., morphine, heroin, oxycodone), alcohol has significant mu opioid receptor agonist effects, though the precise mechanism of action (e.g., direct receptor agonism or increased endogenous opioid release) is unknown. Alcohol's opioid agonist effects may be particularly important in persons, homo/heterozygous for a mu opioid receptor single nucleotide polymorphism "G allele" (OPRM1 Asp40 A118G) [7]. The limbic mu opioid system likely contributes strongly to the acute, pleasurable effects of alcohol ingestion, including euphoria and a favorable perception of taste. Further, the phenomenon of alcohol craving, which may simplistically be described as an individual's persistent memories or longings for prior alcohol-induced rewards, are also likely mu opioid receptor-mediated. Naltrexone's full mu receptor antagonism appears to: (1) reduce alcohol-related euphoria based on dopamine release at the nucleus accumbens, (2) blunt craving and reduce the risk of relapse to drinking and heavy drinking, and, (3) reduce heavy drinking episodes when slips or lapses occur [8–10]. Clinically, patients treated with naltrexone and achieving drinking reductions report less interest in alcohol when not drinking, less pleasure from alcohol when drinking does occur, and decreased occasions of heavy drinking (4 or more drinks, females; 5 or more drinks, males). These beneficial naltrexone effects appear to be more likely to occur in patients with the OPRM1 Asp40 A118G polymorphism [11, 12], which is more common in Caucasian and less common in African American ethnicities [13]. While routine testing for the polymorphism is not recommended or available, a therapeutic trial of naltrexone for alcohol dependence presents minimal risks and can be offered to any interested patient, regardless of ethnicity, provided there is no medical contraindication.

Table 5.1 Alcohol dependence, pharmacotherapies

Medication	Trade name	Dose	Dosing considerations	Contraindications*	Drug–drug interactions	Monthly retail cost*	Mechanism of action
Acamprosate	Campral	2 × 330 mg tablets, three times a day (1980 mg/day)	Avoid in renal failure. For creatinine clearance 30–50, reduce dose to 990 mg daily (1 tab, three times a day). Consider same half-dose during week 1 to avoid gastrointestinal side effects	Severe renal impairment (Creatinine CL < 30 ml)	None known	$ 163	NDMA agonist, taurine analog, glutamate inhibitor
Disulfiram	Antabuse	1 × 250 mg tablet, once daily (250 mg/day)	Initiate after at least 12 h of abstention from alcohol; monitor liver function in 14 days and every 12 months	Coronary artery disease, liver failure; avoid aftershave, mouthwash, and other products containing alcohol	Many, including warfarin, phenytoin, isoniazid	$ 120	Aldehyde dehydrogenase inhibitor
Naltrexone	Revia	1–2 × 50 mg tablet, once daily (50–100 mg/day)	100 mg daily dose may compensate for imperfect daily adherence; monitor liver function every 6 months	Opioid dependence or anticipated opioid treatment; liver failure	Opioid medications	$ 104	Mu opioid receptor full antagonist
Extended-release Naltrexone	Vivitrol	380 mg IM injection, every 4 weeks	Monitor liver function every 6 months	Opioid dependence or anticipated opioid treatment; liver failure	Opioid medications	$ 1102	Mu opioid receptor full agonist
Topiramate	Naltrexone	1 × 100 mg tablet, AM; 2 × 100 mg, PM (300 mg/day)	Titrate slowly (25 mg/week) to full dose over several weeks to avoid paresthesias; dose adjustment in renal failure	Increased risk of metabolic acidosis if in renal or liver disease	Major: carbonic anhydrase inhibitors, valproic acid	$ 83	Gamma-aminobutyric acid (GABA) agonist, reduced glutamate inhibitor

*All medications are pregnancy category C, meaning the agents have demonstrated potential fetal toxicity in animal studies and have not been extensively studied in human pregnancy

*Retail costs: www.drugstore.com, accessed Feb 13, 2012. Costs are for the lowest priced generic equivalent, when available

The bulk of the clinical trial literature to date concerns oral naltrexone, as opposed to XR-NTX. By far the most important recent single clinical trial favoring the use of oral naltrexone was the National Institute of Alcoholism and Alcohol Abuse supported Combined Pharmacotherapies and Behavioral Interventions (COMBINE) study, the largest alcohol pharmacotherapy randomized controlled trial (RCT) ever conducted [14]. In COMBINE, oral naltrexone was associated with a greater percent of days abstinent and fewer heavy drinking days compared to the placebo or acamprosate arms, and naltrexone within a MM counseling model was more effective than other combinations of pharmacotherapy and behavioral treatment. A Cochrane Database systematic review of 50 RCTs across 7793 patients yielded meta-analysis results for naltrexone (50–150 mg oral or 150–380 mg XR, majority of trials reviewed used 50 mg/day oral naltrexone) as reducing the risk of heavy drinking to 83 % of the risk in the placebo group (Relative Risk, 0.83; 95 % CI, 0.76–0.90), and decreased drinking days by about 4 % [15, 16].

In the COMBINE trial, a 100-mg daily oral dose was employed, as opposed to the standard 50-mg daily dose recommended by the package insert. This was done to maximize naltrexone's treatment effects in the face of less than 100 % daily adherence, an expected feature of all oral alcohol medications and naltrexone in particular. A 2001 Veterans Administration (VA) RCT showed daily adherence of 43 % and 44 %, respectively, in participants randomized to 3 and 12 months of oral naltrexone [17]. Regarding retention and persistence of oral naltrexone treatment, commercial HMO prescription data has shown < 15 % rates of persistent oral naltrexone refills through 6 months [18, 19], while one analysis of New England VA pharmacy data reported < 25 % of oral naltrexone prescriptions persisting through this same time frame [20]. Thus, achieving sustained, highly adherent, daily oral naltrexone therapy is a real-world challenge, and extended-release naltrexone was a direct result of decades of government-industry medication development intent on bringing sustained-release, effective addiction medications to market [21].

XR-NTX has been shown to be efficacious compared to placebo, in delaying time to heavy drinking in a pivotal RCT, which provided the basis for XR-NTX's FDA approval in 2006 [22]. Research at our center has supported its feasibility within a simplified, primary care, MM delivery model similar to the COMBINE MM intervention [23]. However, comparative effectiveness trials comparing oral to XR-NTX, or data for a stepped up care strategy such as using XR-NTX after an oral naltrexone treatment trial, are needed. XR-NTX is more expensive on a retail basis than oral naltrexone, and while a sustained-release adherence strategy may prove more effective, XR-NTX's cost-effectiveness is unknown.

Both oral and XR-naltrexone are contraindicated in patients with chronic pain requiring opioid pain control. Acute, unanticipated painful events are clearly more concerning following a monthly XR-NTX dose, which provides a 4–5 week mu opioid receptor blockade and therefore complicates the treatment of acute pain more so than oral naltrexone, which can be immediately discontinued. Treatment of acute, severe pain using escalating doses of opioid medications ("overcoming the XR-NTX blockade") should only be conducted by medical personnel in a monitored setting. Otherwise, non-opioid pain medications, such as NSAIDS or acetaminophen, are unaffected by naltrexone and should be used as first-line agents for pain control. Both oral and XR-naltrexone carry a "black box" warning of hepatotoxicity related to past trials of very high-dose oral naltrexone for weight loss among obese participants, in which transient elevations of liver enzymes were observed. Additionally, both are contraindicated in liver failure. In practice, liver function (AST, ALT) should be monitored every 6 months during naltrexone therapy, but hepatotoxicity at the doses used in alcohol treatment are rare, and XR-NTX's injectable formulation bypasses first-pass liver metabolism. XR-NTX should be used with caution in obese patients or in persons with excessive hip and buttock adiposity due to the risk of severe injection site reaction; mis-injection into subcutaneous tissue has been associated with painful swelling and subcutaneous necrosis [24].

Acamprosate

Acamprosate (brand name Campral) is a taurine amino acid analog with multiple central nervous system effects, and was FDA-approved in 2004 for the treatment of alcohol dependence based on multiple positive European trials showing its superiority over placebo in promoting abstinence and decreasing the frequency of heavy drinking. Acamprosate has effects on GABA neurotransmission (agonism) and, likely more crucial for alcohol dependence therapy, dampens glutamate/NMDA-receptor hyperactivity in chronic heavy drinkers. Heightened glutamate-mediated excitatory tone contributes to excessive alcohol withdrawal and alcohol abstinence symptoms, which, for many who drink heavily chronically, is an intolerable syndrome triggered by sudden alcohol abstinence. Most European trials leading up to acamprosate's FDA approval enrolled participants abstinent and recently detoxified at baseline, and in a meta-analysis of 20 studies, 36 % of acamprosate vs. 23 % of placebo patients had achieved continuous abstinence at 6 months [25]. Acamprosate was not superior to placebo, was inferior to naltrexone, and acamprosate plus naltrexone did not improve outcomes over naltrexone alone in the US COMBINE trial [14]. Similar negative results in other US trials have prompted analysis of the differences between United States and international studies, such as less lead-in abstinence and less baseline heavy drinking among US trial participants [26].

Acamprosate is unique in that it is not metabolized in the liver and excretion is entirely renal. Thus, it should be used with caution and in adjusted doses in patients with kidney disease. Its side-effect profile is relatively benign (diarrhea and pruritus are uncommon). Diarrhea, if it occurs, usually resolves with continued use. However, acamprosate is dispensed as 333 mg capsules, with a usual dose of two capsules three times a day. This relatively intensive daily medication schedule, as with any drug dosed multiple times per day, is a clear barrier to medication adherence.

Disulfiram

Disulfiram (brand name Antabuse) is a direct aldehyde dehydrogenase inhibitor approved for treatment of alcohol dependence in the United States since 1951. Disulfiram promotes the build-up of acetaldehyde, the first byproduct of alcohol's hepatic metabolism by alcohol dehydrogenase. Acetaldehyde is toxic at elevated levels, producing symptoms of nausea, vomiting, flushing, tachycardia, hypotension, dyspnea, throbbing headache, and anxiety, among a long list of unpleasant reactions triggered by alcohol re-exposure in disulfiram-loaded individuals. This is an aversion therapy, negative reinforcement approach to treatment, and disulfiram is used to promote extended abstinence and minimize drinking during a slip. Patients should be explicitly cautioned prior to disulfiram therapy about these potential reactions, they should abstain from any alcohol for at least 12 h before an initial dose, and be clearly motivated toward complete abstinence. Disulfiram is contraindicated in patients with ischemic heart disease and liver failure, interacts widely with common prescription medications (e.g., warfarin and phenytoin), and is associated with hepatotoxicity and optic and peripheral neuropathies.

Disulfiram was essentially "grandfathered" into regular use without rigorous evidence of efficacy or effectiveness. It is unique in psychiatry and medicine, as an agent of pharmacologic negative reinforcement; physical discomfort triggered by alcohol intake prevents future drinking. The largest US trial of disulfiram, a Veterans Administration Cooperative multi-site RCT of disulfiram vs. placebo, did not demonstrate effectiveness in increasing abstinence, and daily medication adherence to the blinded, 250 mg daily disulfiram dose was low [27]. But it is not clear that a blinded RCT is the correct study design when the efficacy of the medication depends on the patient knowing they are taking it and knowing they will become ill if they drink. Other trials have indicated moderate effects of disulfiram on abstinence and heavy drinking, including in combination with acamprosate [28, 29]. Studies showing greatest efficacy have been those in which disulfiram ingestion is monitored closely by a health professional or supportive other. Optimal outcomes are likely achieved among highly motivated patients able to commit to observed daily dosing [30]. Disulfiram, then, suffers, compared to naltrexone or acamprosate from a risk/benefit perspective and is simply harder to use successfully given its potential toxicity and medication interactions, yet it should be considered for otherwise healthy patients with alcohol dependence who are able to abstain from alcohol prior to treatment, are committed to complete alcohol abstinence and the avoidance of alcohol-containing products (e.g., mouthwash), and preferably have partnered with family or treatment professionals surrounding strict daily adherence.

Topiramate and Other Medications not FDA-Labeled for Treatment of Alcohol Dependence

Topiramate (brand name Topamax) is an anti-convulsant shown to be efficacious compared to placebo at reducing heavy drinking rates in a recent multi-site U.S. RCT, which also observed common topiramate adverse events including paresthesia, taste perversion, anorexia, and poor concentration [31]. Efficacy was in the range similar to the approved alcohol dependence medications. Topiramate and other anti-convulsants possibly efficacious for alcohol dependence treatment, including gabapentin, likely function similarly to acamprosate in increasing GABAergic activity and reducing glutamatergic tone [32]. Topiramate's dosing requires titration upward to a usual maintenance dose of 300 mg/day, which is taken in divided doses of 100/200 mg, twice daily. Thus, similar to acamprosate and in addition to a robust side effect profile, topiramate also presents the adherence challenge of multiple daily doses.

Many other neuroactive agents have been assessed for their potential alcohol dependence treatment efficacy, including baclofen, pregabalin, selective serotonin reuptake inhibitors (SSRI), and neurokinin 1 antagonists [33]. SSRIs can have benefit among those with depression, and baclofen may have promise for treating those with liver disease though results of trials are mixed. Clearly, as our understanding of alcohol's complex effects throughout the brain and on the corticomesolimbic system evolve, continues to the emergence of new alcohol pharmacotherapies should likewise, continue.

Are these Medications Under-Prescribed?

Much of the gap between a perceived need among millions of persons with alcohol dependence and the number of alcohol pharmacotherapy prescriptions dispensed annually relates to historically very low rates of alcohol dependence treatment initiation and retention. For the minority of all alcohol dependence patients who do access traditional specialty treatment, prescribing rates of these medications have also been low, and even lags behind the prescription of other medications like SSRIs for depression [34]. In primary care settings, alcohol use disorders are often overlooked and not routinely screened for; thus, opportunities for pharmacotherapy interventions are lost. National screening and brief intervention guidelines now recommend routine consideration of alcohol pharmacotherapies by primary care clinicians for patients with dependence, yet trials assessing the feasibility and effectiveness of linking patients with dependence who are identified by screening to alcohol pharmacotherapy are lacking [2]. In total, these effective medications for a common chronic condition appear to be greatly under-prescribed by specialty and primary care clinicians alike.

Historically, alcohol specialty treatment has emphasized behavioral, psychosocial, and 12-step approaches to recovery, and not medications. Individual addiction counselors themselves likely did not use medications as part of their own recovery process. Biases against addiction maintenance medications, including methadone for opioid disorders, or even more recent agendas such as pharmacologic smoking cessation interventions, are common [35–37]. Finally, while the estimated numbers needed to treat (NNT) to achieve a beneficial outcome for one person for alcohol medications, estimated at 7 for oral naltrexone [15], compare favorably to those of SSRIs or statins, the effects sizes for alcohol medications in most RCTs are modest. This is in part due to the quite high rates of favorable outcomes in placebo arms, and likely indicates a "healthy volunteer" effect across most large alcohol clinical trials. In clinical practice, many patients will in fact not experience substantial,

obvious benefit from a particular alcohol medication, and can be expected to often self-discontinue the medication, possibly after experiencing various side effects
known to occur at low but predictable rates. From a "glass half full," primary care
perspective, however, alcohol medications are again not unlike SSRIs, which are not
universally or always dramatically helpful, yet provide overall effectiveness across
a general patient population while being relatively simple to prescribe and monitor.

Medication Adherence Enhancement and Behavioral Therapies

On-going alcohol and drug use are well-known detractors from medication compliance in many chronic disease states (e.g., HIV, HTN, schizophrenia). It is not
surprising that adherence to alcohol medications themselves presents a common
challenge to patients and clinicians alike. Patient-level barriers to adherence include
cognitive deficits, mood complaints, limited social support, and medication side effects [38]. Directly observed dosing by a health professional or family member is a
clear response to low expected adherence, and this is the underlying rationale of XR-
NTX, injected monthly by a treatment provider, and network therapy approaches,
which recruit collateral support to encourage daily, "at-home" oral medication dosing
[30]. Minimizing pill burden is a general principle within all chronic disease management, and from this perspective monthly XR-NTX or once daily oral naltrexone
or disulfiram may be preferable to acamprosate or topiramate [39].

Medical management (MM), as defined in the COMBINE trial as a longitudinal medication adherence enhancement strategy delivered by physicians, nurses,
physician assistants, or pharmacists during 20-min continuity visits, was effective at
delaying relapse to heavy drinking when paired with oral naltrexone or additional
individual counseling [14]. MM is essentially primary care medicine itself; it consists of education surrounding the diagnosis of alcohol dependence and treatment
goals including reduced heavy drinking or alcohol abstinence, encouragement and
support surrounding medication adherence, assessment of medication side effects,
and support for 12-step (AA) participation. Model intake and follow-up progress
notes are provided within the National Institute on Alcohol Abuse and Alcoholism's
(NIAAA) Clinician's Guide [2]. MM is a model of care based on effective medications and sustained provider–patient rapport and partnership, and is an appropriate
psychosocial foundation when prescribing any of these medications.

It is our perspective that, in addition to MM, "the more, the better" in regards to
alcohol pharmacotherapies and psychosocial treatments. MM plus pharmacotherapy
provides a recurring and relatively low-intensity minimum level of care, on top of
which more comprehensive behavioral treatment can be pursued by interested patients. In COMBINE, individual counseling was an amalgam of cognitive behavioral
therapy, 12-step facilitation, and motivational interviewing, three standard alcohol
counseling approaches [40], which are feasibly paired with any of the alcohol pharmacotherapies, and are usually delivered by specialist counselors trained to deliver
these manualized therapies. In our center's observational study of XR-NTX with primary care MM, participants also involved in specialty alcohol behavioral treatment
completed 3 months of XR-NTX therapy at higher rates compared to participants
not receiving other ancillary psychosocial treatment [23].

Use of Medications Across the Spectrum of Unhealthy Alcohol Use: Beyond Alcohol Dependence

A small number of studies have examined alcohol pharmacotherapies among patients with unhealthy alcohol use but not meeting DSM-IV criteria for alcohol dependence. This describes the majority of persons with unhealthy use, who are hazardous drinkers (at risk for consequences, or with consequences that do not meet criteria for the disorders abuse or dependence, the latter known as "problem" drinkers), or have alcohol abuse but do not have alcohol dependence. In an 8-week trial among 150 early problem drinkers, most (83 %) of whom had a treatment goal focusing on reduced drinking (as opposed to total abstinence), oral naltrexone reduced the frequency of heavy drinking compared to placebo [41], a result which is similar to an earlier study in a similar population of early problem drinkers [42], a study of hazardous drinkers who were not advised to change their drinking [43], and hazardous drinkers treated with naltrexone within a smoking cessation trial who were not otherwise seeking alcohol treatment [44]. One application for these medications, particularly oral naltrexone, is "targeted therapy," in which naltrexone is dosed in anticipation of high-risk drinking situations, but not necessarily maintained on a daily basis [41, 45]. Similar results for topiramate and disulfiram offer evidence that alcohol pharmacotherapies can be considered as harm reduction interventions among broad populations of hazardous and problem drinkers and those with alcohol abuse.

Good Clinical Outcomes: What is the Optimal Outcome in Real-World Alcohol Pharmacotherapy?

A long-standing issue within the treatment and research community concerns what should be considered a good clinical outcome in alcohol dependence treatment, and how clinicians ought to integrate this into a realistic and worthwhile treatment plan. Total alcohol abstinence has historically been the primary treatment goal in many specialized alcohol treatment facilities in the United States, and is prized above all in 12-step, self-help traditions (e.g., AA). Total abstinence, however, is a high standard for evaluating the success in both community treatment and clinical trials, as a patient who is generally doing well but has occasional drinking slips would not meet a dichotomous endpoint of complete abstinence; yet such an outcome is clearly better than continued frequent heavy drinking [46].

Reducing the frequency of drinking days, heavy drinking days, and alcohol-related problems are also worthwhile clinical goals and have become the focus of recent clinical trials, including the COMBINE study. Composite 'good clinical outcomes' are primary end-points with high clinical relevance, and are typically defined as not exceeding recommended daily drinking limits (reduced heavy drinking) and not experiencing alcohol-related problems (e.g., trauma). Heavy drinking thresholds typically follow NIAAA guidelines (5 or more drinks in a day for men, 4 or more drinks in a day for women), and better translate to an overall improvement in a patient's global function and quality of life than do markers of complete abstinence [47]. Similarly, alcohol medications might be used to control heavy drinking in a patient with high blood pressure, with reduced heavy drinking and improved blood pressure control constituting a worthwhile good clinical outcome that involves decreased risk of cardiovascular disease but not necessarily alcohol abstinence.

The available evidence indicates that all the approved alcohol pharmacotherapies are more closely associated with these types of good clinical outcomes and reduced rates of heavy drinking than with complete abstinence. In addition to better informing the physician and patient's expectations, this fact more closely reflects our basic understanding of alcohol and addiction disorders as chronic conditions that wax and wane, and in which lapses and continued drinking are to be anticipated and minimized using the menu of effective medications.

Cost, Value, and Cost-Effectiveness

Several studies have demonstrated the cost-effectiveness of medication-based interventions. Naltrexone and acamprosate, specifically, have been shown to be cost-effective when compared to medical management alone approximately three years after treatment initiation [48]. Research has also demonstrated the potential for alcohol pharmacotherapies to generate significant social cost-savings by reducing the costs associated with health care utilization, crime, motor vehicle accidents, and labor-market outcomes. Patients receiving medication-based treatments may utilize less health care services than untreated patients—this includes detoxification admissions, alcoholism-related inpatient care, and emergency department visits [49]. The magnitude of health care cost-savings is most closely associated with patient adherence and the likelihood that patients will persist through a clinically relevant course of treatment. In this respect, XR-NTX has shown an observed advantage over oral, daily medications [50]. Overall, effective medication-based interventions appear to significantly reduce the burden that alcohol dependence imposes on patients, providers, and society.

Summary

Alcohol dependence is under-treated, and increased use by primary care physicians of alcohol pharmacotherapies would potentially greatly increase the proportion of patients accessing effective treatment. All alcohol pharmacotherapies can be used in the context of primary care MM counseling, which emphasizes medication adherence, regular follow-up, and partnership surrounding reduced alcohol intake and alcohol-related harm. A patient's failure to achieve complete alcohol abstinence should not be interpreted as a treatment failure, rather, substantial reductions in the quantity and frequency of alcohol over several months of treatment are good clinical outcomes linked to improved function, lower costs, and decreased mortality. Comparative effectiveness data from the COMBINE trial favor naltrexone as the initial first-line pharmacotherapy agent compared to acamprosate; either medication is safer and easier to monitor than disulfiram, which should be reserved for patients motivated toward complete abstinence and with no evidence of cardiovascular or severe liver disease. XR-NTX is the most recently approved medication option and should be considered in patients interested in naltrexone and in whom medication non-adherence is a concern. Topiramate is not approved by the FDA for the treatment of alcohol dependence, but is representative of a broad array of potentially effective psychotropic agents either in development or currently approved for other indications.

References

1. National Institute on Alcohol Abuse and Alcoholism. Alcohol use and alcohol use disorders in the United States: main findings from the 2001–2002 National Epidemiologic Survey on Alcohol and Related Conditions NESARC. US Alcohol Epidemiologic Data Reference Manual 8(1). Bethesda: National Institutes of Health; 2006. NIH Publication no. 05-5737.
2. National Institute on Alcohol Abuse and Alcoholism. Helping patients who drink too much: A clinician's guide, Updated 2005 Edition. 2007; NIH Publication No. 07–3769. http://pubs.niaaa.nih.gov/publications/Practitioner/CliniciansGuide2005/guide.pdf. Accessed 4 Aug 2011.
3. Rosenthal R. Alcohol abstinence management. In: Ruiz P, Strain E, Wolters, editors. Lowinson and Ruiz's Substance Abuse: A Comprehensive Textbook. 5th ed. Philadelphia; 2011.
4. Kranzler H, Ciraulo D, Jaffe J. Medications for use in alcohol rehabilitation. In: Ries R, Fiellin D, Miller S, Saitz R. Wolters, editors. Principles of Addiction Medicine. 4th ed., Philadelphia; 2009.
5. Garbutt JC. The state of pharmacotherapy for the treatment of alcohol dependence. J Subs Abuse Treatment. 2009;36(S1):S15–S23.
6. McBride WJ, Le AD, Noronha A. Central nervous system in alcohol relapse. Alcohol Clinical Exp Res. 2002;26:280–286.
7. Arias A, Feinn R, Kranzler HR. Association of an Asn40Asp (A118G) polymorphism in the mu-opioid receptor gene with substance dependence: a meta-analysis. Drug Alcohol Depend. 2006;83(3):262–268.
8. Myrick H, Anton RF, Li X, Henderson S, Randall PK, Voronin K. Effect of naltrexone and ondansetron on alcohol cue-induced activation of the ventral striatum in alcohol-dependent people. Arch Gen Psychiatry. 2008;65(4):466–475.
9. McCaul ME, Wand GS, Stauffer R, Lee SM, Rohde CA. Naltrexone dampens ethanol-induced cardiovascular and hypothalamic-pituitary-adrenal axis activation. Neuropsychopharmacol. 2001;25(4):537–547.
10. Davidson D, Palfai T, Bird C, Swift R. Effects of naltrexone on alcohol self-administration in heavy drinkers. Alcohol Clin Exp Res. 1999;23(2):195–203.
11. Oslin DW, Berrettini W, Kranzler HR, Pettinati H, Gelernter J, Volpicelli JR, O'Brien CP. A functional polymorphism of the mu-opioid receptor gene is associated with naltrexone response in alcohol-dependent patients. Neuropsychopharmacology. 2003;28(8):1546–1552.
12. Anton RF, Oroszi G, O'Malley SS, Couper D, Swift R, Pettinati H, Goldman D. An evaluation of mu-opioid receptor (OPRM1) as a predictor of naltrexone response in the treatment of alcohol

dependence: results from the Combined pharmacotherapies and behavioral interventions for alcohol dependence (COMBINE) study. Arch Gen Psychiatry. 2008;65(2):135–144.

13. Gelernter J, Kranzler H, Cubells J. Genetics of two mu opioid receptor gene (OPRM1) exon I polymorphisms: population studies, and allele frequencies in alcohol- and drug-dependent subjects. Mol Psychiatry. 1999;4(5):476–83.

14. Anton RF, O'Malley SS, Ciraulo DA, Cisler RA, Couper D, Donovan DM, et al. Combined pharmacotherapies and behavioral interventions for alcohol dependence: the COMBINE controlled study: a randomized trial. JAMA. 2006;295(17):2003–2017.

15. Rösner S, Hackl-Herrwerth A, Leucht S, Vecchi S, Srisurapanont M, Soyka M. Opioid antagonists for alcohol dependence. Cochrane Database Syst Rev. 2010;(12):CD001867.

16. Srisurapanont M, Jarusuraisin N. Naltrexone for the treatment of alcoholism: a meta-analysis of randomized controlled trials. Int J Neuropsychopharmacol. 2005;8(2):267–280.

17. Krystal JH, Cramer JA, Krol WF, Kirk GF, Rosenheck RA. Naltrexone in the treatment of alcohol dependence. NEJM. 2001;345(24):1734–1739.

18. Kranzler HR, Stephenson JJ, Montejano L, Wang S, Gastfriend DR. Persistence with oral naltrexone for alcohol treatment: implications for health-care utilization. Addiction. 2008;103(11):1801–1808.

19. Harris KM, DeVries A, Dimidjian K. Datapoints: trends in naltrexone use among members of a large private health plan. Psychiatr Serv. 2004;55(3):221.

20. Hermos JA, Young MM, Gagnon DR, Fiore LD. Patterns of dispensed disulfiram and naltrexone for alcoholism treatment in a veteran patient population. Alcohol Clin Exp Res. 2004;28:1229–1235.

21. National Institute on Drug Abuse. Narcotic antagonists: naltrexone pharmacochemistry and sustained-release preparations. In: Willette R, Barnett G, editors. DHS, NIDA research monograph, Vol. 28;1981.

22. Garbutt JC, Kranzler HR, O'Malley SS, Gastfriend DR, Pettinati HM, Silverman BL, et al. Efficacy and tolerability of long-acting injectable naltrexone for alcohol dependence: a randomized controlled trial. JAMA. 2005;293(13):1617–1625.

23. Lee JD, Grossman E, DiRocco D, Truncali A, Hanley K, Stevens D, Rotrosen J, Gourevitch MN. Extended-release Naltrexone for treatment of alcohol dependence in primary care. J Subst Abuse Treat. 2010;39(1):14–21.

24. Food and Drug Administration. Naltrexone Injection Site Reactions [naltrexone for extended-release injectable suspension (marketed as Vivitrol)]–Healthcare Professional Sheet. FDA Alert. http://ww.fda.gov/Drugs/DrugSafety/PostmarketDrugSafetyInformationforPatientsand-Providers/ucm126446.htm. Accessed 8 Dec 2008.

25. Mann K, Lehert P, Morgan MY. The efficacy of acamprosate in the maintenance of abstinence in alcohol-dependent individuals: results of a meta-analysis. Alcohol Clin Exp Res. 2004;28:51–63.

26. Mason BJ, Goodman AM, Chabac S, Lehert P. Effect of oral acamprosate on abstinence in patients with alcohol dependence in a double-blind, placebo-controlled trial: the role of patient motivation. J Psychiatric Res. 2006;40:383–393.

27. Fuller Rk, Branchey L, Brightwell DR, et al. Disulfiram treatment of alcoholism: a veterans administratinon cooperative study. J Am Med Assoc. 1986;256:1449–1455.

28. Chick J, Gough K, Falkowski W, Kershaw P, Hore B, Mehta B, Ritson B, Ropner R, Torley D. Disulfiram treatment of alcoholism. Br J Psychiatry. 1992;161:84–89.

29. Besson J, Aeby F, Kasas A, Lehert P, Potgieter A. Combined efficacy of acamprosate and disulfiram in the treatment of alcoholism: a controlled study. Alcohol Clin Exp Res. 1998;22(3):573–579.

30. Krampe H, Ehrenreich H. Supervised disulfiram as adjunct to psychotherapy in alcoholism treatment. Curr Pharm Des. 2010;16(19):2076–2090.

31. Johnson BA, Rosenthal N, Capece JA, Wiegand F, Mao L, Beyers K, McKay A, Ait-Daoud N, Anton RF, Ciraulo DA, Kranzler HR, Mann K, O'Malley SS, Swift RM. Topiramate for Alcoholism Advisory Board; Topiramate for Alcoholism Study Group. Topiramate for treating alcohol dependence: a randomized controlled trial. JAMA. 2007;298(14):1641–1651.

32. Anton RF, Myrick H, Wright TM, Latham PK, Baros AM, Waid LR, Randall PK. Gabapentin combined with naltrexone for the treatment of alcohol dependence. Am J Psychiatry. 2011;168(7):709–717.

33. Addolorato G, Leggio L, Ferrulli A, Cardone S, Bedogni G, Caputo F, Gasbarrini G, Landolfi R. Baclofen Study Group, dose-response effect of baclofen in reducing daily alcohol intake in alcohol dependence: secondary analysis of a randomized, double-blind, placebo-controlled trial Alcohol Alcohol. 2011;46(3):312–317.

34. Knudsen HK, Abraham AJ, Roman PM. Adoption and implementation of medications in addiction treatment programs. J Addict Med. 2011;5(1):21–27.

35. Fitzgerald JP, McCarty D. Understanding attitudes towards use of medication in substance abuse treatment: a multilevel approach. Psychol Serv. 2009;6(1):74–84.

36. Abraham AJ, Rieckmann T, McNulty T, Kovas AE, Roman PM. Counselor attitudes toward the use of naltrexone in substance abuse treatment: a multi-level modeling approach. Addict Behav. 2011;36(6):576–583.

37. Knudsen HK, Studts CR, Studts JL. The implementation of smoking cessation counseling in substance abuse treatment. J Behav Health Serv Res. 2011, *E pub ahead of print*.

38. Weiss RD. Adherence to pharmacotherapy in patients with alcohol and opiod dependence. Addiction. 2004;99:1382–1392.

39. Peterson AM. Improving adherence in patients with alcohol dependence: a new role for pharmacists. Am J Health Syst Pharm. 2007;64(5 Suppl 3):S23–29.

40. Project MATCH research group. Matching alcoholism treatments to client heterogeneity: Project MATCH three-year drinking outcomes. Alcohol Clinical Exp Res. 1998;22:1300–1311.

41. Kranzler HR, Armeli S, Tennen H, Blomqvist O, Oncken C, Petry N, Feinn R. Targeted naltrexone for early problem drinkers. J Clin Psychopharmacol. 2003;23(3):294–304.

42. Kranzler HR, Tennen H, Penta C, Bohn MJ. Targeted naltrexone treatment of early problem drinkers. Addict Behav. 1997;22(3):431–436.

43. Tidey JW, Monti PM, Rohsenow DJ, Gwaltney CJ, Miranda R Jr, McGeary JE, MacKillop J, Swift RM, Abrams DB, Shiffman S, Paty JA. Moderators of naltrexeone's effects on drinking, urge, and alcohol effects in non-treatment-seeking heavy drinkers in the natural environment. Alcohol Clin Exp Res. 2008;32(1):58–66.

44. O'Malley SS, Krinhnan-Sarin S, McKee SA, et al. Dose-dependent reduction of hazardous alcohol in a placebo-controlled trial of naltrexone for smoking cessation. Int J Neuropsychoparmacol. 2009;12(5):489–497.

45. Heinälä P, Alho H, Kiianmaa K, Lönnqvist J, Kuoppasalmi K, Sinclair JD. Targeted use of naltrexone without prior detoxification in the treatment of alcohol dependence: a factorial double-blind, placebo-controlled trial. J Clin Psychopharmacol. 2001;21(3):287–292.

46. Falk D, Wang XQ, Liu L, Fertig J, Mattson M, Ryan M, Johnson B, Stout R, Litten RZ. Percentage of subjects with no heavy drinking days: evaluation as an efficacy endpoint for alcohol clinical trials. Alcohol Clin Exp Res. 2010;34(12):2022–2034.

47. Donovan D, Mattson ME, Cisler RA, Longabaugh R, Zweben A. Quality of life as an outcome measure in alcoholism treatment research. J Stud Alcohol Suppl. 2005;15:119–139.

48. Zarkin GA, et al. The effect of alcohol treatment on social costs of alcohol dependence. Medical Care. 2010; 48(5):396–401.

49. Mark TL, et al. Comparison of healthcare utilization among patients treated with alcohol medications. Am J Managed Care. 2010; 16(12): 879–68.

50. Baser O, Chalk M, Rawson R, Gastfriend DR. Alcohol dependence treatments: comprehensive healthcare costs, utilization outcomes, and pharmacotherapy persistence. Am J Manag Care. 2011;17(8 Suppl):S222–S234.

Chapter 6
Making Effective Referrals to Specialty Care

Darius A. Rastegar

Primary care clinicians play a vital role in the identification and treatment of patients with alcohol use disorders; however, there are times—particularly for patients with alcohol dependence—when a referral to specialty care is appropriate; in these situations, the primary care clinician's role in helping a patient find the best treatment is no less essential. These types of referrals should be like any other referrals to specialists: Primary care practitioners should be as familiar with what happens to their patients as when they refer them to a cardiologist. Unfortunately, primary care clinicians often have little knowledge of or familiarity with the available resources. This is partly because they have little (if any) exposure to these types of services during their training. It is also because these services are generally provided in locations and by institutions that are separate from mainstream medical care. The development of formal linkages between primary care and addiction treatment, or integrated treatment programs can help overcome these barriers.

This chapter will review general strategies for making referrals to specialty care and briefly review some of these options. It should be noted that these resources are primarily for patients with alcohol dependence or those with recurrent or ongoing consequences and are generally not appropriate for patients with less severe unhealthy alcohol use. In addition, such resources are usually most appropriate for those who have some recognition that alcohol is harming their health.

Active vs. Passive Referrals

Ideally, referrals are done with a patient who is motivated to make changes; primary care clinicians can help patients get to this stage (see Chap. 4). However, even when patients are motivated, simply encouraging them to get treatment may not

D. A. Rastegar (✉)
Department of Medicine, Johns Hopkins Bayview Medical Center,
Baltimore, MD 21224, USA
e-mail: drasteg1@jhmi.edu

R. Saitz (ed.), *Addressing Unhealthy Alcohol Use in Primary Care,*
DOI 10.1007/978-1-4614-4779-5_6, © Springer Science+Business Media New York 2013

be sufficient and more active strategies appear to offer additional benefit. Having available and discussing a menu of appropriate treatment options is helpful so that the patient can have choice and autonomy, and be more likely to enter and persist with treatment. As with other types of referrals, a "warm hand-off," where the referring practitioner, the patient and the specialty clinician are all involved, is often the best approach. An example of this would be making a phone call to a specific program in the presence of the patient and then having the patient speak directly with them to arrange for a concrete date and time to begin treatment.

More intensive or active strategies are more effective. In an observational study of women entering outpatient alcohol or other drug treatment, those who received a "high-intensity referral" were more likely to complete treatment than those who received a "low-intensity referral"; the "high-intensity referrals" included coerced referrals and interventions in which members of the subject's social network confronted them [1]. A recent randomized controlled trial found improved outcomes among substance dependent subjects who received an intensive referral to self-help groups as opposed to a standard referral [2]. In this study, subjects in the standard treatment arm received a list of self-help groups and were encouraged to attend. In the intensive referral group, a counselor helped subjects select a specific group and then arranged for a meeting between the patient and a member of that group; the counselors then followed up with the subjects to see if they had attended.

Choosing the Appropriate Level of Treatment

The decision on where to refer a patient will depend on a number of factors, the most important of which is the severity of the problem, but must also take into account other factors, including the availability of resources, insurance coverage, patient preference, and even location.

The American Society of Addiction Medicine (ASAM) has developed patient placement criteria to help guide this decision [3]. There are some data to support the utility of these criteria. One observational study of alcoholics admitted to different levels of care reported that those who were *undertreated* (i.e., were placed at a lower level of care than would be recommended by placement criteria) did worse than those who were appropriately matched; moreover, *overtreatment* was not associated with better outcomes [4]. However, another observational study reported that outcomes between "matched" and "mismatched" patients were not significantly different [5]. Nevertheless, these criteria are widely used and many insurers use them to determine medical necessity.

The ASAM placement criteria for adults divide patients into four general treatment levels: (I) outpatient treatment, (II) intensive outpatient treatment or partial hospitalization, (III) medically-monitored inpatient treatment, and (IV) medically-managed intensive inpatient treatment; levels (II) and (III) are respectively sub-divided into two and four further levels. The appropriate level is determined by the patients' status in six dimensions:

1. Acute intoxication and/or withdrawal potential,
2. Biomedical conditions and complications,
3. Emotional and behavioral conditions and complications,
4. Treatment acceptance and resistance,
5. Relapse potential, and
6. Recovery environment.

The criteria can be summarized thus:

Level IV (medically managed inpatient services). This level is analogous to a hospital or psychiatric ward with 24-h nursing and physician coverage. This level of care is appropriate for patients who: (1) have a severe withdrawal risk, or (2/3) require 24-h medical or psychiatric and nursing care for medical or emotional conditions (dimensions 4 through 6 have no impact on determining this level).

Level III (inpatient treatment). This level of care provides inpatient care, but not at a hospital level; there may be some clinical staff, including nurses and physicians, but not around the clock. Some patients may receive medications and monitoring for withdrawal. This level of care is appropriate for patients who: (1) have severe risk of withdrawal, but can be managed at this level, (2/3) have medical or emotional conditions that require monitoring and structure (but not intensive treatment), (4) are resistant to treatment, (5) are unable to control their use despite less-intensive treatment, and (6) are in an environment that is dangerous for recovery. Level (III) is further sub-divided into Level (III.1) (clinically-managed low-intensity residential), (III.3) (medium-intensity residential), (III.5) (medium/high-intensity residential) and (III.7) (medically monitored intensive inpatient).

Level II (intensive outpatient or partial hospitalization). At this level of care, patients are residing at home or in a recovery house and receive outpatient services for most of the day; these services may include medical or psychiatric evaluation and medications. This level is appropriate for patients who: (1) have minimal risk of severe withdrawal, (2/3) mild or manageable biomedical or emotional conditions, (4) are somewhat resistant to change, (5) have a high risk of relapse without close monitoring and support, and (6) are in an unsupportive environment (but can cope with structure and support). Level (II) is further subdivided into level (II.1) (intensive outpatient) and (II.5) (partial hospitalization).

Level I (outpatient treatment). This level of care provides outpatient counseling and support services, but generally does not include medical or psychiatric evaluation or dispensing of medications. It is appropriate for patients who: (1) have no risk of severe withdrawal, (2/3) have no unstable biomedical or emotional conditions, (4) are cooperative, (5) have adequate coping skills and (6) are in a supportive environment.

In general, patients should be referred to the least restrictive or intensive treatment level that would be appropriate for their situation. However, availability of resources often plays a significant role in this decision. For example, a patient who would be appropriate for level (III) treatment may need to be referred to a level (IV) program if there are no level (III) treatment programs available. Or, a patient may be appropriate for intensive outpatient treatment but it is not available, or the patient is unwilling to commit to it, so they end up in outpatient treatment (level I). The medical and mental health needs might be taken care of as part of a comprehensive plan delivered by different clinicians (including the primary care clinician) if they are not all available in one program.

Primary care clinicians can help facilitate referral to these resources. Involving family members and friends in the process (with the patient's permission) is a useful strategy [6]. Typically, patients do not need a formal referral and can contact the resources themselves, but as noted earlier, a "warm hand-off" where the primary care clinician facilitates this process may improve follow-through. Being turned away from a program because the patient is not determined to be appropriate for the level of care offered, or for insurance reasons, when the patient has finally decided to seek treatment can be damaging and efforts should be made to avoid that situation. For patients with insurance, contacting the mental health or substance abuse services section is therefore a reasonable first step (the phone number can often be found on the patient's insurance card). Some communities—particularly large urban centers—have hotlines to help patients connect with resources. In smaller communities, the local health department or the staff at a regional drug treatment center may be able to provide advice and guidance over the phone. If a referral is made to a specific program, it is often helpful to obtain written consent for release of information from the patient to facilitate coordination of care by allowing the program to communicate with the primary care clinician; federal guidelines prohibit drug and alcohol treatment programs from releasing information without the patient's consent (with the exception of emergencies).

We will briefly cover the different types of specialty treatment, beginning with the more intensive treatments.

Inpatient Detoxification

Alcohol detoxification is an important tool in the treatment of patients with alcohol dependence. However, it is also important to remember that most patients with alcohol dependence do not require inpatient detoxification and that this is not a "cure" and is merely the first step in the process of recovery.

Inpatient detoxification is appropriate for patients with severe withdrawal symptoms or prior severe withdrawal (particularly seizures or alcohol withdrawal delirium), as well as patients who have failed outpatient attempts and those with a co-existing medical or psychiatric problem that requires hospitalization. Some hospitals have dedicated units for detoxification, while at other institutions these patients may be treated on medical or psychiatric units. Patients typically spend 3–5 days in the hospital and are then referred to other resources for aftercare. Dedicated detoxification units tend to provide more guidance and assistance to patients in finding aftercare (treatment for the underlying disorder, alcohol dependence), while medical units may not have staff with the necessary expertise to help patients with this process.

Primary care clinicians can help patients, making sure that they are engaged in ongoing treatment. Ideally, coordination of care would begin prior to discharge and primary care clinicians can help by making sure there is an aftercare plan in place and that the patient has a follow-up appointment shortly after discharge. Some residential treatment programs may require a patient to have completed detoxification before they will accept them; in this situation, it may be best to begin the process of referral to aftercare before inpatient detoxification and to coordinate the two in order to ensure a seamless transfer from one level of care to the next. For patients who are entering outpatient treatment after detoxification, the primary practitioner can help by assessing them to see if they may benefit from pharmacotherapy to help them maintain abstinence (see Chap. 5).

Outpatient Detoxification

Many alcoholics can be safely and effectively detoxified as outpatients. Outpatient treatment is best for those at low risk of severe withdrawal who have a stable living situation that is supportive of their recovery. Outpatient detoxification can be done through a doctor's office, though dedicated programs can generally provide more services and closer supervision. Outpatient detoxification programs typically see patients on a daily basis for 5 or more days, though for many, the main physical symptoms of withdrawal may be gone by the second day. The patients are evaluated daily and receive medications along with counseling, meetings and other activities while they are at the program and are generally given a few doses of medication to take home for the rest of the day. As with inpatient detoxification, it is important that the patients have an aftercare plan in place for ongoing treatment after detoxification.

Residential Treatment

Residential programs are a heterogeneous treatment modality that can range from recovery houses that are little more than a place to stay, to more intensive treatment facilities. These programs are particularly valuable for patients who are homeless or who live in environments that are not conducive to their recovery. In general, observational data suggest that many who enter this type of treatment do not complete it, but those who stay tend to have better outcomes. Patients who have severe withdrawal symptoms or are at risk for severe withdrawal are typically referred to these programs after inpatient detoxification, while patients with less severe dependence can enter them from the community.

Therapeutic communities are a variant of residential treatment, which are typically organized and led by recovering addicts, though many employ professional staff, who are also often in recovery themselves. In these communities, the focus is on members' behaviors and their lives are often tightly controlled and monitored by the group; in general, contact outside of the community is very limited. Older members serve as role models and undesirable behaviors are sanctioned, often through peer confrontation. These types of programs are probably more effective than their less-structured counterparts, but they typically have high attrition rates.

Modified therapeutic communities are a more recently developed model of care. They are less intense, more flexible and focus more on individualized treatment. These programs emphasize positive reinforcement and conflict resolution instead of confrontation and sanctions. There is some research that supports their effectiveness, particularly for those with a co-existing psychiatric problem.

Recovery houses or halfway houses are homes where a small number of patients in recovery live; they are generally led or supervised by a house manager who is someone in recovery. Patients typically enter these houses after detoxification or more intensive residential treatment and pay a weekly fee to stay. These houses may have 12-step meetings and residents may be monitored through urine drug testing or breathalyzer, but there often is little structure beyond this. Some of these houses are affiliated with treatment programs that provide counseling and other treatment on an outpatient basis.

Outpatient Treatment

Self-help Groups

Self-help groups (also known as "mutual help groups") are one of the oldest and most commonly used forms of treatment. Alcoholics Anonymous (AA) is perhaps the best known example of this approach. These groups are organized and led by recovering alcoholics, not treatment professionals, and many use a "12-step" approach. These meetings are often open to all-comers. The involvement of participants may range from dropping in occasionally, to regular participation in a "home group", to having a "sponsor" or being a sponsor for others; finally, there are some who organize and lead these groups. The data on the effectiveness of these groups (primarily from observational studies) is limited, but suggest that participation is associated with better outcomes [7]. Not surprisingly, those who are more active in these groups tend to do better than those who are less committed [8].

Outpatient Counseling

After self-help groups, outpatient counseling is probably the most commonly used treatment modality; this can be done in a group or individual setting. In contrast to self-help groups, group counseling sessions are typically led by trained counselors. However, the philosophy and approach of these groups are often quite similar, with a focus on the stages of recovery and providing a supportive atmosphere for maintaining abstinence and making lifestyle changes. Counselors are sometimes recovering alcoholics or addicts themselves.

Individual counseling is a more intensive one-on-one treatment led by a trained counselor; like group counseling, it often focuses on stages of recovery and the development of tasks and goals based on the 12-step philosophy. Counselors often assist individuals with social, family and legal problems. A number of studies suggest that both of these modalities are modestly effective in the short term (i.e., while individuals participate), but there are limited data on long-term effectiveness.

Behavioral Therapy

Less commonly, outpatient counseling employs specific evidence-based behavioral therapies. There are a wide variety of behavioral approaches that appear to be effective for treating alcohol dependence. In general, behavioral therapy focuses on particular behaviors that affect an individual's functioning (e.g., alcohol consumption); the therapist works with the patient to find effective strategies to reduce these "target behaviors". A distorted perception of self and the world is thought to lead to negative thoughts and hopelessness that contribute to alcohol use. One strategy is to examine the thought process that underlies specific behaviors in order to help the individual recognize these "dysfunctional" patterns of thinking, and develop strategies to counter them—this is referred to as *cognitive behavioral therapy*. A variant of this approach is referred to as *coping skills therapy*, which tries to foster coping skills to reduce the risk of use; these include assertiveness training, focusing on the consequences of use, finding alternative behaviors, and learning ways to avoid or escape situations that lead to use. Another similar approach is sometimes referred to as *relapse prevention therapy*; this uses a variety of cognitive and coping strategies to deal with high-risk situations and early signs of impending relapse. Patients are encouraged to find healthy activities that decrease their need for alcohol and to prepare for possible lapses in abstinence in order to prevent these from developing into a full-blown relapse. *Network therapy* utilizes behavioral techniques and enlists family members and friends to reinforce compliance and undermine denial.

Yet another behavioral strategy is to provide rewards for desirable behaviors or punishment for undesirable ones—this is often referred to as *contingency management*. Most studies of contingency management use vouchers as a reward for drug-free urine in drug screens, often in the setting of methadone maintenance programs. Another treatment modality attempts to promote "alternate reinforcers" and a healthier lifestyle by combining cognitive behavior therapy with vocational rehabilitation, as well as contingency management and other behavioral modalities—this is sometimes referred to as *community reinforcement*. These approaches appear to be modestly effective while in place, but the effect seems to dissipate once the rewards and other external factors are removed.

Medication

Although medications are covered elsewhere in this book (Chap. 5), they are clearly a part of alcohol detoxification programs. In addition, medications for treating alcohol dependence (naltrexone, acamprosate, disulfiram, and others) can and should be a part of the treatment plan in any of the above specialty treatment settings although many programs do not routinely prescribe them or have prescribers available. The primary care clinician can play a crucial role filling the gap to assure that all available evidence-based treatments are considered for their patient.

Follow up

The coordination of follow up after referral to specialty services is as important as the coordination that goes into the referral itself. Ideally, there should be a seamless hand-off back to the primary care clinician. This can be planned ahead of time (e.g., an appointment made prior to referral) or begin while the patient is still engaged in treatment, particularly once they have completed the initial phase of treatment and are stabilized. Since the privacy laws with regard to alcohol and drug treatment are more restrictive than for other medical problems, it is generally helpful to have the patient sign a release of information form ahead of time to facilitate communication with these programs. One always needs to be prepared for the possibility of relapse, particularly early in recovery and be able to provide help and support to the patient to get back into treatment as soon as possible. Most specialty treatment programs continue to operate as if all patients with alcohol dependence complete treatment, and are seamlessly handed-off back to the medical clinician after discharge. More recently, models have been developed for "continuing care" after a treatment episode. Continuing care recognizes that for some, alcohol dependence is a chronic illness, and in that circumstance the primary care clinician could co-manage the patient along with a specialist clinician providing continuing care. Current releases of information can facilitate such care. Renewed attention to patient-centered medical homes may provide opportunities for continuing care that is well-coordinated.

Summary

Alcohol use disorders are sometimes chronic, and like other chronic illnesses that primary care clinicians manage, require ongoing treatment and monitoring. Like other complex problems, referrals and coordination with specialty care are essential parts of this process. Moreover, like other specialty services, it is important that the primary care practitioner be knowledgeable about the type of services that are available and what happens when patients are referred there.

Key points for making effective referrals include:

- Refer patients to specialty alcohol treatment when they need it, and when they are ready for it, or counsel them to assist with problem recognition.
- Be familiar with local resources and update this information periodically.
- Write a brief letter or make a phone call when referring patients for specialty care.

- Obtain and update bi-directional releases of information to make coordinated clinical care possible.
- Follow up with patients and specialty providers to find out what happened and to facilitate continuing care.

References

1. Loneck B, Garrett J, Banks SM. Engaging and retaining women in outpatient alcohol and other drug treatment: the effect of referral intensity. Health Soc Work 1997;22:38–46.
2. Timko C, DeBenedetti A, Billow R. Intensive referral to 12-step self-help groups and 6-month substance use disorder outcomes. Addiction 2006;101:678–88.
3. Mee-Lee D, Shulman G, Gartner L. ASAM patient placement criteria for the treatment of psychoactive substance-related disorders, 2nd ed. Chevy Chase: American Society of Addiction Medicine; 2001.
4. Magura S, Staines G, Kosanke N, et al. Predictive validity of the ASAM patient placement criteria for naturalistically matched vs. mismatched alcoholism patients. Am J Addict 2003;12:386–97.
5. McKay JR, Cacciola JS, McLellan AT, et al. An initial evaluation of the psychosocial dimensions of the American Society for Addiction Medicine criteria for inpatient versus intensive outpatient substance abuse rehabilitation. J Stud Alcohol 1997;58:239–252.
6. Loneck B, Garrett J, Banks SM. A comparison of the Johnson Intervention with four other methods of referral to outpatient treatment. Am J Drug Alcohol Abuse 1996;22:233–246.
7. Gossop M, Harris J, Best D, et al. Is attendance at alcoholics anonymous meetings after inpatient treatment related to improved outcomes? A 6-month follow-up study. Alcohol Alcohol 2003;38:421–6.
8. Crape BL, Latkin CA, Laris AS, Knowlton AR. The effects of sponsorship in 12-step treatment of injection drug uses. Drug Alcohol Depend 2002;65:291–301.

Chapter 7
Making Effective Referrals to Alcoholics Anonymous and Other 12-step Programs

Maryann Amodeo and Luz Marilis López

This chapter will describe 12-step programs, explain what occurs at meetings, and address common misconceptions. Our central goal is to present practical guidelines to help primary care physicians make referrals to 12-step programs. Effective referrals include introducing patients to these programs, motivating them to attend meetings, having follow-up conversations with them about their experiences at meetings, and encouraging them to consider ongoing affiliation. The guidelines presented here can help you talk with patients who are new to 12-step programs as well as patients who attended in the past but found the experience unhelpful. Since you may wonder whether 12-step programs actually work, we briefly describe the accumulating research evidence for their effectiveness. Perhaps most important, we discuss why your role as a primary care physician is so pivotal.

Although the term 12-step programs refers to a range of mutual help groups such as Narcotics Anonymous, Gamblers Anonymous, Overeaters Anonymous, and Al-Anon Family Groups [1], we focus here on Alcoholics Anonymous (AA) and Narcotics Anonymous (NA) since much of the research on outcomes and many guidelines were written for clinicians referring patients to these groups. It is important to remember, though, that the guidelines can also be helpful in referring patients to other 12-step programs. Note that the term "alcoholic" is used by AA and is equivalent to alcohol dependence. In NA, reference is generally made to "addicts," a term equivalent to those with other drug or substance dependence. In these contexts the labels are not meant pejoratively though some perceive them to be so in other contexts.

M. Amodeo (✉) · L. M. López
Center for Addictions Research and Services,
Boston University School of Social Work,
264 Bay State Road, Boston, MA 02215, USA
e-mail: mamodeo@bu.edu

L. M. López
e-mail: luzlopez@bu.edu

R. Saitz (ed.), *Addressing Unhealthy Alcohol Use in Primary Care,*   73
DOI 10.1007/978-1-4614-4779-5_7, © Springer Science+Business Media New York 2013

What does Research Tell us About Effectiveness?

Program Effectiveness

Rigorously conducted empirical reviews and AA-focused research have shown that AA is helpful for many types of patients with alcohol dependence [2–8]. When AA is used alone, abstinence rates are equal to the abstinence rates for individuals attending formal substance abuse treatment over the long term—3–4 year outcomes [3]. For those using AA or NA as an adjunct to formal treatment, frequent meeting attendance improves abstinence [3] and is associated with significantly higher rates of "successful" treatment completion [9]. In an examination of post-treatment use of 12-step programs compared with formal treatment, researchers conducting a 2-year follow up of a multi-site Veterans Administration study found that patients in 12-step programs had substantially higher rates of abstinence than patients in cognitive-behavioral therapy programs [10].

What are the "active ingredients" contributing to patient recovery? In a recent systematic review of research on AA, Kelly et al. [11] identified three major mechanisms: The program enhances self-efficacy, increases behavioral coping skills, and facilitates adaptive changes in social networks. However, the authors stress that these mechanisms are contingent on the level of patient participation. A finding that echoes throughout the research literature is that longer and more intensive involvement leads to better outcomes. Such involvement includes frequent meeting attendance, speaking at meetings, using the 12 steps, getting a sponsor, sponsoring others, and choosing a home group that provides consistent interaction with the same group of 12-step members who can provide feedback and support.

Effectiveness of Clinician Referrals

Clinician intervention can have a significant impact. There is now good research evidence that professionals can powerfully influence a patient's level of affiliation [1, 12, 13]. Clinicians who perceive that 12-step programs are important and helpful have higher referral rates [14] with patients more engaged in affiliation activities. However, in spite of the fact that clinicians possess the necessary referral skills, many of them have attitudes and beliefs that undermine referral. For example, Humphreys [12] found that clinicians used "matching rules" based on assumptions and hearsay for sending patients to 12-step programs. The rules excluded various kinds of patients (e.g., lower income patients; patients with co-occurring psychiatric and substance use disorders; patients with certain types of spiritual beliefs). However, several studies [12] show program benefits for patients with co-occurring psychiatric disorders. AA and NA have been found to work as well for unemployed, African American, and unmarried addicts as they do for more economically well-off and educated patients [15]. Further, a study of 3,018 male substance abusing patients found that referrals were effective for connecting patients to 12-step programs irrespective of religious background (both, those who believed in God and those who did not benefited) [16].

Humphreys [12] concludes that clinicians need to re-examine their personal attitudes and "matching rules" in view of research evidence.

What are 12-Step Programs and How do they Help People with Alcohol and Other Drug Dependence?

Therapeutic Components

Twelve-step programs offer an array of components that can be thought of as therapeutic in helping members stay clean and sober, learn about addiction, and develop self-awareness. These include: The 12 steps–guidelines for personal growth, necessary for a stable recovery; a meeting environment free of alcohol and drugs; a forum for telling one's story of addiction and recovery without being judged, which helps to reduce shame; the fraternity and mutual support of the group that conveys the message that "you are not alone in your struggle with this condition," and "we are all pulling for your recovery;" the power of example in which members learn how to achieve abstinence and recovery by observing how others do it successfully; and sponsors: members with substantial sobriety who provide advice and support on staying sober. Additional healing factors include the opportunity to sponsor others (as well as have a sponsor for oneself), so members are not stuck in the role of recipients of help but can also guide others; and socializing outside of meetings—when "home groups" become cohesive, members and their families may gather on weekends and other times for social and recreational activities; and slogans—cognitive prompts such as "Live and let live," "First things first," and "Maintain an attitude of gratitude" that help patients prioritize recovery tasks and see their situation as "the glass half full" instead of "half empty." Schenker [17] refers to these slogans as bite size pieces of recovery wisdom that members can summon in times of stress or confusion.

Wide Availability and Accessibility

Twelve-step programs offer a multitude of meetings that are all free-of-charge, convene at neighborhood and community sites, have no requirements for admission (patients need only provide their first name), and no waiting list. A resource with such a low threshold for entry can be invaluable to patients, even if they have many other treatment options. Depending on geographic location, meetings are available daily (including holidays), although they may be more limited in rural areas. Patients can shop around until they find meetings that best fit their needs.

Array of Meetings

There are three types of meeting formats for individuals who are new to the program: Beginners' meetings, Speaker meetings, and Discussion meetings [31]. *Beginners' meetings* are designed for newcomers; program philosophy is explained as are ways in which members can derive the maximum benefit and these are listed in the meeting book. *Speaker meetings* tend to be large (sometimes as many as 100 attendees) with three or four speakers in a lecture style (new attendees can sit in the back and feel relatively inconspicuous). *Discussion meetings* are smaller (10–25); many participants speak and newcomers may be asked to participate by reading a paragraph from program material or discussing a theme. Individuals new to the program must attend "open" meetings (open to the public; these are clearly designated in the meeting book with an O). Closed meetings (designated in the meeting book with a C) are for members only—individuals who have committed themselves to become program members and are working on specific aspects of self-improvement. Individuals who need privacy and strict anonymity (e.g., high-profile public figures, or those who fear job loss if their condition is known) attend closed meetings. If newcomers who are not program members attend closed meetings, they could be asked to leave, so attending open meetings only is very important for newcomers. Meeting books are available from AA's Central Service or patients can also go online and find meetings by zip code.

Considerable Diversity and Inclusivity

A visit to the AA website (www.AA.org) shows specific AA reading material for the following audiences: women, Native Americans, Blacks and African Americans, Jews, gay/lesbian individuals, older adults, members of the Armed Services, and prison inmates. For some years, there have been specialized meetings for women, young people, lesbians and gays, and those with a range of physical disabilities. More recently, especially in urban areas, meetings are offered in languages other than English. AA and NA meetings are often attended by people with both alcohol and other drug problems—the high prevalence of poly-drug abuse has diluted the historical pattern of AA members with only alcohol problems and NA members with only drug problems. More patients with co-occurring psychiatric disorders have become members. In response, AA and NA have published material (see the pamphlet, The AA member: Medications and other drugs) stating that the programs endorse medications for such disorders when prescribed by one's physician.

What is the Best Way for Primary Care Physicians to Learn About These Programs?

Attend AA and NA Meetings

Physicians who attend meetings have greater optimism about the benefits of 12-step programs, which is associated with more favorable referral practices [18]. To be more informed when discussing these programs with your patients, we recommend sampling a variety of meetings in different locations; one meeting provides helpful information but may give a limited view. AA and NA stress that "open" meetings are open to the public, and physicians and healthcare providers are especially welcome. Educating physicians is an important aspect of the public education mission of AA and NA and key to spreading the word to new members. When you attend, use the opportunity to examine your stereotypes about alcoholics, addicts and 12-step programs; introduce yourself at the door to the "greeter" if there is one and explain your purpose in attending—this will help you feel less like an outsider. If asked to introduce yourself, be honest and direct: "I'm Oliver, I'm a physician. I'm here to learn about the program to help my patients."

Be sure to observe the confidentiality of attendees (a primary tenet of the organization) by not disclosing to others the names of people you may see at meetings; no note taking—it is prohibited by the programs; if the meeting closes with the Serenity Prayer or another such brief ceremony, you can stand with the group but you need not participate if it makes you uncomfortable; if you wish, contribute a dollar or two to cover meeting expenses (coffee, refreshments and room rental) when the basket is passed. We recommend meetings in community settings such as churches and schools, rather than in shelters or substance abuse treatment programs, since they are more likely to include a spectrum of individuals with alcohol and drug problems, rather than only those at the severe end of the continuum.

Acquire Program Materials to Educate Patients

As you would when referring patients with other medical conditions to a new treatment or sub-specialist, provide educational materials so they'll understand the nature of the service and possible benefits for them. Some materials can be downloaded from the AA and NA websites and others can be purchased through the mail from the central office (e.g., the AA Big Book, the basic text for AA). However, a more personal and informative way to learn about the program is to drop in to the AA Central Service office, let the volunteers there know you are a physician interested in referring patients, and pick up meeting books and literature to guide you in talking with patients.

Develop AA Contacts

You will find the Central Service office volunteers very willing to help. They can offer tips on motivating patients to attend meetings. They will also let you know the best ways for connecting your patients with AA volunteers who can meet them at meetings, tell them about the program and introduce them to other members. One of your goals should be to acquire a list of contact people whom you can call (or whom your patients can call) with questions. Another option is to ask one of your own patients who has long-term AA or NA recovery if he/she would be available to talk with a new patient who is considering 12-step programs for the first time.

What Should I Keep in Mind when Talking with Patients About Attending?

Discuss Meeting Formats and Options

Help patients find appropriate meetings. (1) Show them a meeting book and how to use it: Recommend they choose a day, then a time that's convenient, and also a comfortable location (e.g., patients may want to avoid their immediate neighborhood to protect their own privacy and that of their neighbors). (2) Encourage them to go with a friend or family member initially. (3) Put them in touch with an AA member who can go with them or meet them at a meeting. Initially, send patients to "open" meetings only, and reassure them that they will not be expected to identify themselves as alcoholics or addicts. This will be a relief because many patients believe this is required and dread the feeling of exposure. Let patients know that you can understand their reluctance to declare themselves in this way at this early stage of trying out a new program. In a similar vein, there is no requirement that attendees be clean and sober when attending meetings, and no requirement that attendees have already made a commitment to abstinence. Program material states that a *desire* to quit is sufficient. Thus, patients should be assured that they can attend meetings without committing themselves to anything ahead of time.

Recommend Meetings that Match Patient Preferences and Needs

Explore patient preferences for meetings. Each local group sponsors a weekly meeting which often reflects the socio-economic level and the racial/ethnic make-up of the local community. Recommend groups that have members with whom the patient is more likely to identify [19–21]. For example, discussing adolescents, Passetti and Godley [22] emphasize that some will prefer adult-attended meetings over youth-attended meetings, and they need meetings at times when they are not in school or at work, and need good access to public transportation since many don't drive.

Exploring what types of meetings would be most comfortable may be especially salient for members of ethnic/racial minority groups as well as other minorities (e.g., by virtue of sexual orientation, physical ability, age). Individuals who live in small ethnic communities or belong to cultural groups where the stigma of substance abuse is very strong (e.g., recently arrived immigrants) will need consistent encouragement to venture out to attend any meetings at all. Neighborhood meetings may feel especially uncomfortable if other attendees already know them or their reputation through the addiction. If language is not a barrier, some will prefer larger, more racially/ethnically diverse meetings where they can have anonymity.

Identify the Specific Benefits for each Patient

For some patients, a benefit may be the daily availability of group support if the patient is surrounded by drinkers and drug users. For others, it may be a sponsor who shares experiences about ways he/she grappled with urges and cravings. For others, it may be the 12 steps that they can use as guidelines for living. Review the list of therapeutic components and ask patients if they think that any of them might be particularly helpful. Let patients know that 12-step programs are helpful for most patients with substance use disorders, but, it is important to acknowledge that there are various routes to recovery.

Let Patients Know that you have Attended Meetings

Tell patients that you have attended meetings to learn about the program and you found the meetings informative. This can reduce the patient's sense of stigma in attending, provide an opportunity to question someone with first-hand knowledge of meetings, and allow a dialogue about how the patient really feels about attending. Acknowledge that attending the first meeting felt awkward. Describe measures you took to reduce your discomfort (e.g., attending with another person, coming early, introducing yourself to the greeter).

Provide a Realistic Assessment of what Might Occur at Meetings

Be forthright with facts and responses to patient concerns (e.g., meeting size, racial/ethnic composition, spiritual themes). Encourage patients to sample a variety of meetings held at different times and locations. Johnson and Chappel [23] recommend that new attendees collect a list (often distributed at meetings) of first names and phone numbers of attendees whom they can contact later if they want more information or just wish to talk. Help patients anticipate what they could say if they encounter an awkward or difficult situation (e.g., ways to introduce themselves– I'm Jay, this is my first time at a meeting, and I'm here to learn more about the program. What to say if a co-worker or neighbor is at the meeting–I've been drinking a little too much recently and thought I would check out a meeting). Help patients brainstorm about accessibility issues (e.g., childcare, transportation). Help patients deal with fears of exposure (both new attendees and long-time members only use their first names) and emotional intimacy (say you just came to see what the program is about–you're a visitor); members will provide you with the "emotional space" that you need.

Anticipate that Patients may have Preconceived Notions

When patients raise objections to trying meetings, view this as an opportunity for dialogue. Discussing what patients have heard about the program, their past experiences in attending, and what worries them about going regularly will decrease the likelihood that they will drop out after attending [24, 25]. Dropouts are also more likely if you pressure patients to attend or if you impose rigid rules (e.g., You must attend now; You must attend 90 meetings in 90 days; I will not continue to treat you if you don't go to AA or NA) [24]. Just taking the time to talk with a patient about these issues is a significant intervention.

Emphasize and support patient choice whenever possible ("AA is one option among several—it is not the only option;" "You can choose a meeting or home group where you feel most comfortable;" "You could try other approaches first, and this one later if the other ones don't work"). Not wanting to go to AA may represent not being ready for any kind of treatment or change, or being ready for treatment but not through AA–you will need to separate this out through exploration and reflective listening (see Chap. 4).

If patients have concerns about the emphasis on spirituality or the concept of a "higher power," you can explain that the program encourages members to interpret the higher power to be whatever the patient believes in, such as the power of the fraternity of the AA program [19, 24, 26]. Nowinski [27, 28] emphasizes the power that comes from the group–"collective identification and bonding and a willingness to trust in the collective wisdom of those who have made the same journey" (p. 342). Concerning the mistaken belief among some Jewish people that 12-step programs are only for Christians, Rabbi Abraham Twerski [29] from the University of Pittsburgh School of Medicine describes the 12-steps as compatible with Judaism, stressing similarities between the steps and the concepts of *musar* (Jewish ethics).

How do I Follow up After the Patient's First Meeting?

During your first appointment after the patient's attendance at meetings, find out what it was like for the patient. Possible questions include: What happened at the meeting? What types of people were there? How did you feel about being there? Any concerns? Did you speak? Did you get a sponsor? Are you thinking of going back to a particular meeting? Are you considering choosing a home group? Was there any information about alcohol or drug problems that was new for you? Did the speakers address issues relevant to your own situation? Don't shy away from listening to the negatives–you can play a crucial role in providing room for the patient to talk about what was surprising, disappointing or alienating. Your goals are to address misconceptions and encourage the patient to maintain an open mind, sample more meetings, read program material, and be vocal with you and program members about questions and concerns.

Help Patients Use Care in Choosing a Sponsor

Choosing a sponsor is an important part of affiliation [17, 24] and patients should be encouraged to choose a temporary sponsor until they know members well enough to choose a permanent one. Sponsors are most useful when they give patients feedback on their participation and challenge them to take responsibility for their actions. Patients should seek sponsors with substantial clean/sober time (i.e., years rather than months); sponsors with less than 10 years may be more helpful than those with more than 10 years because the experience is still fresh and advice is based on proximal rather than remote experiences. Some sponsors have so many people looking to them for support that they are not as available as they need to be for someone newly sober. Sponsors new to the role may be too inexperienced for very needy patients. The quality of the sponsor's recovery is important as well—does the sponsor put his/her own advice into action? Does he/she have a sense of humility about the role of sponsor and about his/her own recovery?

Encourage Ongoing Activities Known to Improve Recovery

A recent randomized clinical trial found that *intensive referral* (counselors linked patients to 12-step volunteers and patients used 12-step journals to report on meeting attendance) was more effective than *standard referral* (patients received a meeting schedule and encouragement to attend) in helping patients become proactive in participating. The intensive-referral patients got a sponsor, read AA literature, engaged in service (e.g., making coffee for meetings, chairing a meeting), and gained self-identity as group members [13]. Using a community sample of alcoholics and addicts who were also in day treatment, Witbrodt and Kaskutas [30] found that the number of 12-step meetings attended and the number of 12-step activities in which patients were engaged predicted abstinence. Having a sponsor and doing service work were highly associated with abstinence at 12 months and after. These studies direct us to educate patients about the benefits of active involvement. We can say with assurance that going to occasional meetings and sitting in the back of the room without interacting with others is likely to have little benefit. However, attending meetings regularly, learning the program philosophy, engaging in service activities, and using the various therapeutic components are likely to meet with success.

References

1. Humphreys K, Wing S, McCarty D, Chappel J, et al. Self-help organizations for alcohol and drug problem: toward evidence-based practice and policy. J Subst Abuse Treat. 2004;26: 151–158.
2. Bond J, Kaskutas LA, Weisner C. The persistent influence of social networks and alcoholics anonymous on abstinence. J Stud Alcohol. 2003;64:579–588.
3. Emrick CD, Tonigan JS, Montgomery H, Little L. Alcoholics Anonymous: what is currently known? In: McCrady BS, Miller WR, editors. Research on alcoholics anonymous: opportunities and alternatives. Piscataway: Rutgers Center of Alcohol Studies; 1993. pp. 41–76.
4. Gossop M, Stewart D, Marsden J. Attendance at narcotics anonymous and alcoholics anonymous meetings, frequency of attendance and substance use outcomes after residential treatment for drug dependence: a 5-year follow-up study. Addiction. 2008;103:119–125.
5. Kelly JF. Mutual help for substance use disorders: history, effectiveness, knowledge gaps and research opportunities. Clini Psychol Rev. 2004;23(5):639–663.
6. McKellar JD, Harris AH, Moos RH. Patients' abstinence status affects the benefits of 12-step self-help group participation on substance use disorder outcomes. Drug Alcohol Dependence. 2009;99(1–3):115–122.
7. Timko C, Moos RH, Finney JW, Lesar MD. Long-term outcomes of alcohol use disorders: comparing untreated individuals with those in alcoholics anonymous and formal treatment. J Stud Alcohol. 2000;61(4):529–540.
8. Tonigan JS, Toscova R, Miller WR. Meta-analysis of the literature on Alcoholics Anonymous: sample and study characteristics moderate findings. J Stud Alcohol. 1996;57(1):65–72.
9. Fiorentine R, Hillhouse MP. Drug treatment and 12-step program participation: the additive effects of integrated recovery activities. J Subst Abuse Treat. 2000;18(1):65–74.
10. Humphreys K, Moos RH. Encouraging post-treatment self-help group involvement to reduce demand for continuing care services: two-year clinical and utilization outcomes. Alcohol: Clin Exp Res. 2007;25(5):711–716.
11. Kelly JF, Magill M, Stout RL. How do people recover from alcohol dependence? A systematic review of the research on mechanisms of behavior change in alcoholics anonymous. Addiction Res Theory. 2009;17(3):236–259.
12. Humphreys K. Professional interventions that facilitate 12-step self-help group involvement. Alcohol Res Health. 1999;23(2):93–98.
13. Timko C, DeBenedetti A. A randomized controlled trial of intensive referral to 12-step self-help groups: one-year outcomes. Drug Alcohol Dependence. 2007;90:270–279.
14. Laudet AB, White WL. An exploratory investigation of the association between clinicians' attitudes toward 12-step groups and referral rates. Alcohol Treat Q. 2005;23(1):31–45.
15. Miller NS, Verinis JS. Treatment outcomes for impoverished alcoholics in an abstinence-based program. Int J Addictions. 1995;30:753–763.
16. Winzelberg A, Humphreys K. Should patients' religiosity influence clinicians' referral to 12-step self-help groups? Evidence from a study of 3,018 male substance abuse patients. J Clin Consult Psychol. 1999;67(5):790–794.
17. Schenker MD. A clinician's guide to 12-step recovery: integrating 12-step programs into psychotherapy. New York: W.W Norton; 2009.
18. Gunderson EW, Levin FR, Smith L. Screening and intervention for alcohol and illicit drug abuse: a survey of internal medicine house-staff. J Addict Dis. 2005;24(2):1–18.
19. Chappel JN, Dupont RL. 12-step and mutual help programs for addictive disorders. Psychiatric Clinics N Am. 1999;22(2):425–446.
20. Riordan RJ, Walsh L. Guidelines for professional referral to alcoholics anonymous and other 12-step groups. J Counsel Dev. 1994;72(4):351–355.
21. Tonigan JS, Ashcroft F, Miller WR. AA groups dynamics and 12-step activity. J Stud Alcohol. 1995;56:616–621.

22. Passetti LL, Godley SH. Adolescent substance abuse treatment clinicians' self-help meeting referral practices and adolescent attendance rates. J Psychoact Drugs. 2008;40(1):29–40.
23. Johnson NP, Chappel JN. Using AA and other 12-step programs more effectively. J Subst Abuse Treat. 1994;11(2):137–142.
24. Caldwell PE. Fostering patient connections with alcoholics anonymous: a framework for social workers in various practice settings. Social Work Health Care. 1999;28(4):45–61.
25. Laudet AB. Substance abuse treatment providers' referral to self-help: review and future empirical directions. Int J Self Help Self Care. 2000;1(3):213–225.
26. Caldwell PE, Cutter HSG. Alcoholics anonymous affiliation during early recovery. J Subst Abuse Treat. 1998;15(3):221–228.
27. Nowinski J. Facilitating 12-step recovery from substance abuse and addiction. In: Rogers F, Keller DS, Morgenstern J. editors. Treating substance abuse: theory and technique. New York: Guilford; 1996. pp. 37–67.
28. Nowinski J. Self-help groups for addictions. In: McCready BS, Epstein EE. editors. Addictions: a comprehensive guidebook. New York: Oxford University Press; 1999. pp. 328–346.
29. Twerski A. Jews & alcoholics anonymous: dispelling the myth that Jews aren't alcoholics and that alcoholics anonymous is only for Christians. *Tablet: A New Read on Jewish Life*. www.TabletMag.com.
30. Witbrodt J, Kaskutas LA. Does diagnosis matter? Differential effects of 12-step participation and social networks on abstinence. Am J Drug Alcohol Abuse. 2005;31(4):685–707.
31. Alcoholics Anonymous website: www.AA.org.

Chapter 8
Management of Patients with Alcohol Dependence in Recovery: Options for Maintenance and Anticipating and Managing Relapse in Primary Care

Thomas J. Doyle, Peter D. Friedmann and William H. Zywiak

In this chapter, we focus our discussion on the challenges primary care clinicians face while identifying those in recovery and facilitating maintenance of sobriety (or at least low risk drinking) in patients with early or longer term recovery from alcohol dependence. We review specific techniques that primary care clinicians can use to help patients with alcohol-related problems and recent studies of technology-based interventions and patient outreach that can be integrated into the primary care patient-centered medical home [1, 2].

Identifying Patients in Recovery

More than 20 % of adults in primary care settings have a past or current substance use disorder, and many physicians are unaware of their patients' substance use histories [3, 4]. Of patients with alcohol or other drug problems, patients in recovery are the

T. J. Doyle (✉)
Primary Care and Hospitalist Services, Providence VA Medical Center, Providence, RI, USA

Warren Alpert Medical School of Brown University, Providence, RI, USA
e-mail: Thomas.doyle@va.gov

P. D. Friedmann
Research Service, Providence VA Medical Center, Providence, RI, USA

Division of General Internal Medicine, Rhode Island Hospital, Providence, RI, USA

Health Services, Policy & Practice, Warren Alpert Medical School of Brown University, Providence, RI, USA
e-mail: pfriedmann@lifespan.org

W. H. Zywiak
Decision Sciences Institute, Pawtucket, RI, USA

Psychiatry & Human Behavior, Warren Alpert Medical School of Brown University, Providence, RI, USA
e-mail: zwiak@pire.org

R. Saitz (ed.), *Addressing Unhealthy Alcohol Use in Primary Care,*
DOI 10.1007/978-1-4614-4779-5_8, © Springer Science+Business Media New York 2013

majority seen in the primary care setting [5, 6]. These patients may have achieved abstinence through completion of an addictions treatment program, attendance at a self-help program, or, as is most common in the general population, on their own [7]. Examination may provide some clues (e.g., spider nevi) as to the history, but it is not a substitute for non-judgmental, direct questioning using validated tools. When asked if they use alcohol or other drugs, recovering patients may say "no," whether they stopped a week or a year ago. It is thus essential to routinely use screening questions that identify lifetime problems, such as the CAGE questionnaire, and ask all patients who do not drink why they do not partake, since drinking is normative behavior [8]. Liver profiles may be a useful monitoring strategy and inroad into discussing the possibility of heavy drinking. Alcohol biomarkers may be useful as well [9]. Kristenson et al. [10] used changes in GGT levels to provide biofeedback, and obtained improved drinking outcomes in a randomized clinical trial.

Establish a Supportive Patient–Physician Relationship

The primary care physician is in a unique position to provide continued care for individuals presenting with a variety of chronic relapsing conditions. A supportive, non-judgmental patient–physician relationship is especially important to the management of persons with substance use disorders. Because of the negative interactions many such patients have had with the healthcare system, they are often guarded and quick to sense disrespect from healthcare providers. Interview *style* may be more important than content. The physician should convey concern, empathy and respect through the use of open-ended questions, listening, and paraphrasing back the patient's words and ideas so the patient knows the physician has listened (reflective listening) [11, 12]. Affirmation of the patient's positive statements and even modest successes (arriving at the appointment, duration of abstinence, challenges overcome, improvements in health, and positive lifestyle changes) will build both the therapeutic relationship and the patient's self-esteem more effectively than directive advice-giving [13]. Even if the patient is uninterested in changing his/her drinking at the present time, by emphasizing rapport, the physician can leave the window open to renew the discussion at a subsequent visit.

The physician should assess and take seriously the patient's agenda [13]. Many addicted patients complain about physicians who focus exclusively on substance use as the source of all their ailments and fail to work-up distressing problems adequately. Not taking complaints seriously or their dismissal as substance-related can be a major barrier to the addicted patient developing trust in the physician. However, a patient-centered approach does not mean the absence of disagreement; on the contrary, it can make confrontation more effective. For example, if the physician believes a behavior or situation places the recovering patient at high-risk for relapse that should be stated directly. If the patient disagrees management should be negotiated with the same concern used in addressing patients with coronary artery disease who resist changing a sedentary lifestyle. In both cases, judgmental approaches produce no clinical benefit and may alienate the patient. In a supportive, ongoing relationship, future meetings hold the possibility of helping the resistant patient to recognize and address their risky behaviors [2].

Most patients in primary care settings are not bothered by inquiries about alcohol use and recovery, and recognize such conversations as appropriate [14]. Indeed, many patients view alcohol counseling as a marker of higher quality primary care [15], and may be favorably impressed by a physician's interest in their recovery and knowledge of recovery-relevant information such as 12-step programs.

Schedule Regular Follow Up

The primary care clinic is the most common clinical setting visited by patients, and is therefore well suited for regular follow-up. Primary care also has a preventive service, longitudinal care orientation. As in other chronic conditions, data to guide visit frequency are limited, but common sense dictates that risk should serve as a guide. The likelihood of relapse is greatest during the first 3 months of abstinence but extends for at least 12 months. The 1 year anniversary has been identified as a specific risky time for having one drink to see what would happen [16].

Assist Recovering Patients to Recognize and to Cope with Relapse Precipitants and Craving

In order to counsel patients to prevent relapse, it is important to have a clear understanding of relapse as a process in which the return to substance use results from a series of maladaptive responses to stressors or stimuli [16]. The initial return to use results when the addicted person inadequately copes with emotions, situations or cues that create craving. Research suggests that there are three main relapse factors that may occur as groups of antecedents. These three broad classes of relapse precipitants include negative affect, craving/cues, and social pressure [17, 18]. Negative affective states include frustration, anger, fatigue, boredom, or family conflict such as marital arguments. Social pressure can be a direct offer of alcohol, or more commonly, a general social function where alcohol is being served. Twelve-step groups use the acronym "HALT: Don't get **H**ungry, **A**ngry, **L**onely, or **T**ired" to warn members about affective triggers, and the expression "People, Places, and Things" to warn about situational triggers [19–21]. For example, handling cash will trigger craving in many cocaine dependent people [22]. Sometimes just being in a particular neighborhood, because of its past associations (e.g., a bar), will cause these feelings. Often the addicted person will end up in "the old neighborhood" and not recall how he or she got there. Such decision chains lead inexorably toward relapse, and the patient should recognize and break them before entering a familiar tavern [23].

Primary care physicians should use their listening, assessment and counseling skills to help recovering patients understand and anticipate their personal affective and situational triggers [24]. For patients with a previous relapse, discussion of its circumstances will illuminate personal triggers. A patient log of craving (and drinking, if any), like the diabetic finger stick glucose log, is another useful tool to help patients recognize their triggers. The log should include times and places where such urges or desires occur, their intensity on a one-to-ten scale, and the coping response [25]. Early in recovery, avoidance of situations associated with craving and prior substance use is a sensible strategy. Tests of personal control should be specifically discouraged. Since exposure to adversity is universal, the recovering patient's ability to cope with risky states and situations will determine the success of recovery [26]. Effective didactic methods are available to addiction specialists to help recovering people develop coping strategies [27, 28]. Thus, the physician should strongly advocate completion of both specialty treatment and "aftercare" (a term that refers to specialty treatment that continues after an initial episode of specialty care).

For patients without access to aftercare, the primary care physician might use counseling, role-play and appropriate mental health referrals to help the patient find constructive ways to express anger and frustration, alleviate boredom, see beyond dysphoria, counter social pressures, and anticipate and manage craving. The recovering patient should understand that craving episodes are an uncomfortable but normal part of recovery, lasting only minutes to hours, and nothing of which to be ashamed. Further, the frequency of craving will diminish as the period of abstinence gets longer, becoming very infrequent after 6 months [18]. After seeing craving for what it is, the patient should talk through it with a sponsor, a supportive family member or friend, the physician or other member of the primary care team, a treatment counselor, or the Alcoholics Anonymous (AA)/Narcotics Anonymous (NA)/Cocaine Anonymous (CA) hotline. Alternatively, the patient could go to an AA/NA/CA meeting or social, or engage in prayer, meditation, exercise, reading, a hobby, or behavioral methods learned in a treatment program [27, 28]. Facilitating involvement in 12-step recovery efforts is a cost-effective way to prevent relapse [29], and is discussed in detail in Chap. 7.

Advise Recovering Patients to Develop a Plan to Manage Lapses

Despite their best efforts, many recovering persons will use again. After initial use (a lapse), the individual may experience guilt, shame, and/or anxiety. These negative feelings can lead to an attitude that "there is nothing more to lose," resulting in a return to heavy substance use to assuage the negative feelings [23]. The patient should be urged to see past the negative feelings brought on by initial use and understand their potential for harm. The physician should remind the recovering person that recovery is a learning process, with a lapse providing valuable lessons.

The patient and clinician should negotiate an individualized contract of premeditated responses to initial use, including limiting use and seeking help after first use. Any return to substance use poses a significant danger to the patient, analogous to suicide risk, and ideally the physician, the physician on-call or a member of the primary care team will be accessible should a crisis arise and the sponsor is unavailable

[30]. Such patients need prompt evaluation and consideration of referral for specialty addictions treatment.

Mobilize Family Support and Facilitate Positive Lifestyle Changes

Talking over problems or feelings with a partner and other family members and developing more leisure activities have been found to predict better treatment outcomes [31]. In addition, drinking episodes that end when someone has intervened are also associated with subsequent better outcomes (as opposed to drinking episodes that end due to the patient feeling physically bad or because of work problems) [31]. The primary care clinician is in a good position to facilitate the support of families for recovery.

Although not guarantees of abstinence, productive roles and leisure activities lower recovering patients' susceptibility to relapse. The physician should encourage productive life steps such as finding a job or going to school, and positive personal habits or activities such as exercise, meditation, hobbies, volunteer work and spending time with family. Aerobic exercise may decrease craving [32]. However, strivings should be tempered by the reality that over-extending can distract from recovery, cause stress, and paradoxically increase relapse risk.

Manage Depression, Anxiety and Other Comorbid Conditions

Psychiatric disorders and symptoms masked by substance use often become evident in early recovery. Furthermore, depression, anxiety and other negative emotional states are common precipitants of relapse [33, 34]. Physicians should screen for and manage these symptoms in their recovering patients [32–35]. Since diagnosis and pharmacotherapy of anxiety disorders can be challenging in recovery, psychiatric or addiction medicine consultation is recommended for most recovering patients with anxiety symptoms [36]. Depression is also difficult to diagnose definitively in early recovery, but treatment of depressive symptoms with antidepressant medication and counseling reduces relapse rates [37, 38]. Coordinated, interdisciplinary referral is often critical, especially for recovering patients with chronic pain or serious psychiatric comorbidity. *Chap.* 11 discusses the management of psychiatric comorbidity in detail.

Consider Adjunctive Pharmacotherapy

In addition to medications to decrease affective symptoms, pharmacotherapy can reduce craving and decrease relapse risk [39]. For example, naltrexone reduces craving and heavy drinking [40, 41]. Chapter 5 addresses the use of pharmacotherapy to reduce alcohol use.

Future Directions

Innovative use of telephone [42] and internet communications has the potential to effectively encourage and maintain sobriety from alcohol abuse and thus assist in interventions to prevent relapse. Aftercare through telephone contact appears to be useful in settings with limited aftercare. For example, only 50 % of patients typically follow-up with alcohol treatment after inpatient detoxification [43] and telephone aftercare has been shown to be a useful addition at this point in the treatment system [44]. In particular, extended telephone monitoring was shown to improve drinking outcomes in a randomized study, especially among female patients and less motivated patients [45]. Given the time constraints in a primary care practice it may be effective to include information on reliable web-based counseling for alcohol relapse. Primary care physicians should be proactive in offering recommendations for reliable internet information geared toward sobriety maintenance including web sites maintained by NIAAA (www.niaaa.nih.gov), and others.

References

1. Friedmann PD, Saitz R, Samet JH. Management of the patient recovering from alcohol or other drug problems. Relapse prevention in primary care. JAMA. 1998;279:1227–1231.
2. Friedmann PD, Charuvastra A, Herman DS, Dube C, DeSantiago S, Freedman S, Stein MD. PRIMECare. Promote recovery in medical care. A guideline for the maintenance care of medical patients in recovery from alcohol abuse or dependence. Providence: Division of General Internal Medicine, Rhode Island Hospital; 2001.
3. Robins LN, Helzer JE, Weissman MM, et al. Lifetime prevalence of specific psychiatric disorders in three sites. Arch Gen Psychiatry. 1984;41:949–958.
4. Buchsbaum DG, Welsh J, Buchanan RG, Elswick RK. Screening for drinking problems by patients self-report. Even "safe" levels may indicate a problem. Arch Intern Med. 1995;155:104–108.
5. O'Connor P, Samet J. Prevalence and assessment of readiness for behavioral change of illicit drug use among primary care patients [Abstract]. J Gen Intern Med. 1996;11 Suppl:53.
6. Samet J, Vega M, Nuciforo S, Williams C. Assessment of readiness for behavioral change of substance abusers in primary care [Abstract]. J Gen Intern Med. 1995;11 Suppl:53.
7. Sobell LC, Cunningham JA, Sobell MB. Recovery from alcohol problems with and without treatment: prevalence in two population surveys. Am J Pub Health. 1996;86:966–972.
8. National Institute on Alcohol Abuse and Alcoholism. The physician's guide to helping patients with alcohol problems. NIH Publication No. 95-3769. Washington, DC: National Institutes of Health; 1995.
9. Allen JP, Anton R. Biomarkers as aids to identification of relapse in alcohol treatments. In: Galanter M, editor. Recent developments in alcoholism: Volume 16 research on alcoholism treatment. New York: Kluwer; 2003.
10. Kristenson H, Ohlin H, Hulten-Nosslin M, Trell E, Hood B. Identification and intervention of heavy drinking in middle-aged men: results and follow-up of 24–60 months of long-term study with randomized controls. Alcohol: Clin Exp Res. 1983;7:203–209.
11. Miller WR, Rollnick S. Motivational interviewing: preparing people to change addictive behavior. New York: Guilford; 1991.
12. Miller WR, Rollnick S. Motivational interviewing: preparing people to change addictive behavior. 2nd ed. New York: Guilford; 2002.

13. Barnes HN. Addiction, psychotherapy, and primary care. Subst Abuse. 1995;16:31–38.
14. Aalto M, Seppa K. Usefulness, length and content of alcohol-related discussions in primary health care: the exit poll survey. Alcohol Alcohol. 2004;39(6):532–535.
15. Saitz R, Horton NJ, Cheng DM, Samet JH. Alcohol counseling reflects higher quality of primary care. JGIM. 2008;23(9):1482–1486.
16. Kirshenbaum AP, Olsen DM, Bickel WK. A quantitative review of the ubiquitous relapse curve. J Subst Abuse Treat. 2009; 36, 8–17.
17. Zywiak WH, Stout RL, Longabaugh R, Dyck I, Connors GJ, Maisto SA. Relapse onset factors in project MATCH: the relapse questionnaire. J Subst Abuse Treat. 2006;31:341–345.
18. Zywiak WH, Westerberg VS, Connors GJ, Maisto SA. Exploratory findings from the reasons for drinking questionnaire. J Subst Abuse Treat 2003;25:287–292.
19. Alcoholics Anonymous. Living sober. New York: Alcoholics Anonymous World Services; 1975.
20. Alcoholics Anonymous. Twelve steps and twelve traditions. New York: Alcoholics Anonymous World Services; 1952.
21. Nowinski J, Baker S, Carroll K. Twelve step facilitation therapy manual: a clinical research guide for therapists treating individuals with alcohol abuse or dependence. National Institute on Alcohol Abuse and Alcoholism Project MATCH monograph series, DHHS publication no. (ADM) 94-3722. Washington, DC: Superintendent of Documents, U.S. Government Printing Office; 1995.
22. Wallace BC. Psychological and environmental determinants of relapse in crack cocaine smokers. J Subst Abuse Treat. 1989;6:95–106.
23. Marlatt GA, Gordon JR, editors. Relapse prevention: maintenance strategies in the treatment of addictive behaviors. New York: Guilford; 1985.
24. Flitcraft AH, Hadley SM, Hendricks-Matthews MK, McLeer SV, Warshaw C. American Medical Association diagnostic and treatment guidelines on domestic violence. Chicago: American Medical Association; 1994.
25. Gorski TT, Miller M. Staying sober workbook. Independence: Independence Press; 1988.
26. Connors GJ, Longabaugh R, Miller WR. Looking forward and back to relapse: implications for research and practice. Addiction. 1996;91 Suppl:S191–S196
27. DeJong W, Finn P, Grand J, Markoff LS. Relapse prevention. Clinical report series. DHHS Pub. No. (ADM)93-3845. Washington, DC: Superintendent of Documents, US Government Printing Office, National Institute on Drug Abuse; 1994.
28. Norcross JC, Koocher GP, Fala NC, Wexler HK. What doesn't work? Expert consensus on discredited treatments in the addictions. J Addict Med. 2011;4:174–180.
29. Hoffmann NG, DeHart SS. Committee on benefits project: working toward clinically effective and cost efficient treatment. Providence: National Council on Alcoholism and Drug Dependence and the Brown University Center for Alcohol and Addiction Studies; 1996.
30. Hirshfeld RMA, Russell JH. Current concepts: assessment and treatment of suicidal patients. N Engl J Med. 1997;337:910–915.
31. Zywiak WH, Stout RL, Connors GJ, Maisto SA, Longabaugh R, Dyck I. Factor analysis and predictive validity of the Relapse Questionnaire in Project MATCH. In: Zywiak WH, Westerberg VS (Chairs), New perspectives on relapse and treatment outcome from the Replication and Extension Project and Project MATCH. Symposium at the Annual Meeting of the Research Society on Alcoholism, Montreal, QB, 2001.
32. Gorski TT. Relapse—issues and answers. Addiction Recovery. 1991;3:17–18.
33. McLellan A, Luborsky L, Woody G, O'Brien C, Druley K. Predicting response to alcohol and drug abuse treatments. Role of psychiatric severity. Arch Gen Psychiatry. 1983;40:620–625.
34. Rounsaville BJ, Dolinsky Z, Babor T, Meyer R. Psychopathology as a predictor of treatment outcome in alcoholics. Arch Gen Psychiatry. 1987;44:505–513.
35. Connors GJ, Maisto SA, Zywiak WH. Understanding relapse in the broader context of post-treatment functioning. Addiction. 1996;91 Suppl:S173–S19.
36. Ziedonis D, Brady K. Dual diagnosis in primary care. Detecting and treating both the addiction and mental illness. Med Clin N America. 1997;81:1017–1036.

37. Mason BJ, Kocsis JH, Ritvo EC, Cutler RB. A double-blind, placebo-controlled trial of desipramine for primary alcohol dependence stratified on the presence or absence of major depression. JAMA. 1996;275:761–767.
38. Ziedonis DM, Kosten TR. Depression as a prognostic factor for pharmacological treatment of cocaine dependence. Psychopharm Bull. 1991;27:337–343.
39. Saitz R, O'Malley SS. Pharmacotherapies for alcohol abuse. Med Clin N America. 1997;81:881–907.
40. Anton RF, et al. Combined pharmacotherapies and behavioral interventions for alcohol dependence: the COMBINE study: a randomized controlled trial. JAMA. 2003;295(17):2003–2017.
41. Monti PM, Kadden RM, Rohsenow DJ, Cooney NL, Abrams DB. Treating alcohol dependence: A coping skills training guide. 2nd ed. New York: Guilford; 2002.
42. McKay JR. Treating substance use disorders with adaptive continuing care. Washington, DC: American Psychological Association; 2009.
43. Mark TL, Dilonardo JD, Chalk M, Coffey RM. Factors associated with receipt of treatment following detoxification. J Subst Abuse Treat. 2003;24: 299–304.
44. Zywiak WH, Stout RL., Schneider R., Shepard D, Swift RM. Case monitoring following detoxification: 1-year clinical outcomes. [Abstract]. Alcohol: Clin Exp Res 2007;31(6) Suppl:271A.
45. Lynch, KG, Van Horn D, Drapkin M, et al. Moderators of response to telephone continuing care for alcoholism. Am J Health Behav. 2010:34(6):788–800.

Chapter 9
Managing Pain in the Context of Unhealthy Alcohol Use

Erik W. Gunderson and Daniel P. Alford

Introduction

For the primary care clinician treating patients with unhealthy alcohol use, pain syndromes are frequently clinical issues that pose unique challenges relative to the management of low risk or non-alcohol users with pain. Unhealthy alcohol use and its consequences may impact both the assessment and management of pain. Such considerations are particularly important when prescribing medications that can interact with alcohol or alcohol-related comorbidities, such as acetaminophen, nonsteroidal anti-inflammatory drugs (NSAIDs), and opioid medications. Rather than a comprehensive review of general pain management (e.g., Ballantyne, 2005) [1], this chapter provides recommendations on how to approach the patient with unhealthy alcohol use and pain. Special attention is devoted to the safe and effective use of opioid analgesics, given the inherent risks of interactions and misuse, and that observational studies demonstrate that patients with current or past alcohol use disorders are at higher risk for subsequent prescription opioid misuse [2].

E. W. Gunderson (✉)
Department Psychiatry & Neurobehavioral Sciences and Department of Medicine,
University of Virginia, Charlottesville, VA 800623, USA
e-mail: erikgunderson@virginia.edu

Director and Founder, Center for Wellness and Change LLC, Charlottescille, VA, USA

D. P. Alford
Boston University School of Medicine, Section of General Internal Medicine,
Clinical Addiction Research and Education (CARE) Unit, Boston Medical Center,
801 Massachusetts Avenue, 2nd Floor, Boston, MA 02118, USA
e-mail: dan.alford@bmc.org

R. Saitz (ed.), *Addressing Unhealthy Alcohol Use in Primary Care,*
DOI 10.1007/978-1-4614-4779-5_9, © Springer Science+Business Media New York 2013

Pain Prevalence in Patients with Unhealthy Alcohol Use

Chronic pain affects over 100 million Americans [3] and significantly afflicts over 20 % of primary care patients [4], many of whom drink alcohol [5]. Data are limited in which the prevalence or characterization of various pain syndromes have been ascertained specifically in primary care patients with unhealthy alcohol use. However, national survey data along with findings from smaller primary care alcohol intervention studies suggest that patients with unhealthy alcohol use (including those with alcohol use disorders) are at increased risk for deterioration in general physical functioning relative to the general population. For example, elderly at-risk alcohol users identified in primary care exhibited decreased general physical function on the Medical Outcomes Study (MOS) SF-36 [6, 7] relative to similarly aged adults across the United States. [8]. The 560 patient sample was a mean 72 years old and drank a mean 17.9 drinks per week, and had a mean 21.1 binge episodes in the past 3 months [7]. Although specific pain levels were not reported, the MOS SF-36 physical function measurement assesses limitations in important activities of daily living (ADLs) potentially impacted by chronic pain, including lifting, carrying groceries, and climbing stairs. National survey data indicate similar deterioration in physical health among drinkers aged $\geq$ 60 at high risk for DSM-IV alcohol use disorders [9]. Patients with unhealthy alcohol use will present with a similar constellation of pain syndromes as the general primary care population, such as back pain, the most common pain reported by U.S. adults [10]. Excessive alcohol consumption itself may contribute to certain painful medical conditions, including acute and chronic pain syndromes due to: (1) traumatic injuries suffered while intoxicated; (2) painful medical co-morbidities related to acute alcohol use (e.g., hepatitis) or chronic alcohol dependence such as pancreatitis, neuropathies and myopathies; and (3) nutritional deficiencies resulting in neuropathies.

General Approach to Managing Pain

The general approach to managing pain begins with a complete pain and functional assessment, followed by realistic goal setting and determination of the treatment plan. Both pain and functional status should be assessed and documented on initial and subsequent evaluations. Therapy should be evaluated based on pain relief and functional improvement. A variety of pain scales can be used, including numeric and visual analog intensity scales. One quick approach is to ask patients on a scale of 0 (no pain) to 10 (most severe pain), what is their pain now, what was the best, and what was the worst pain they experienced in the past 24 h? Functional assessments should include inquiry about how pain interferes with daily activities. The PEG (pain, enjoyment, and general activity) questionnaire is a validated three-question assessment tool that can be used in primary care settings [11]. The three questions are: (1) What number best describes your *pain on average* in the past week? (0 = no pain, 10 = pain as bad as you can imagine); (2) what number best describes how, during the past week, pain has interfered with your *enjoyment of life*? (0 = does not interfere,

10 = completely interferes); and (3) what number best describes how, during the past week, pain has interfered with your *general activity*? (0 = does not interfere, 10 = completely interferes). Setting goals is a critical part of managing pain. Primary care clinicians and patients should discuss realistic expectations regarding pain control and functional improvement prior to initiating therapies.

Improvement of both quality of life and functionality are as important as pain relief. In patients with unhealthy alcohol use, avoidance of adverse medication interactions with alcohol is another important goal. Hence, non-pharmacologic approaches in managing pain should be considered. Non-pharmacological therapies that are evidence based include physical therapy, pain psychology (e.g., cognitive behavioral therapy), massage therapy, spinal manipulation, and acupuncture [12]. Recommendations for these therapies are not altered for patients with unhealthy alcohol use.

Non-opioid Pharmacotherapies

Non-opioid pharmacotherapies should be first line analgesics for patients suffering with chronic pain. However, patients with chronic alcohol dependence and chronic liver dysfunction are at high risk for adverse reactions to many commonly used non-opioid (prescribed and over-the-counter) analgesics. Some of the more concerning complications include gastrointestinal bleeding, hepatic injury, and renal failure.

Nonsteroidal Anti-inflammatory Drugs

Nonsteroidal anti-inflammatory drugs (NSAIDs) exert their analgesic effect by inhibiting the cyclooxygenase 2 (COX 2) enzyme. Upper gastrointestinal bleeding (UGIB) is a major complication of NSAID use that is exacerbated by unhealthy alcohol use. In one study, the risk of UGIB was highest among patients using NSAIDs along with heavy alcohol use (> 21 drinks per week) with a relative risk of 2.8 compared to those who drank less than 1 drink per week [13]. The severity of UGIB will also increase in patients with alcohol-associated liver disease due to synthetic dysfunction (i.e., coagulopathy) and splenic sequestration of platelets (i.e., thrombocytopenia). Since NSAIDs are mostly hepatic metabolized, patients with liver dysfunction will have increased serum levels potentially increasing risk for renal impairment due to inhibition of prostaglandins with marked reduction in GFR.

Acetaminophen

Acetaminophen is a mild-to-moderate analgesic that can be used on a short- or long-term basis with similar efficacy as NSAIDs. Since acetaminophen can cause hepatotoxicity and the half-life is prolonged in patients with liver dysfunction, use of this medication raises concern and requires careful monitoring in patients with unhealthy alcohol use. Although there are no long-term prospective studies assessing the safety of long-term acetaminophen in patients with unhealthy alcohol use, retrospective data indicate chronic alcohol abuse is an independent risk factor for acetaminophen-induced hepatotoxicity [14], including accidental toxicity among individuals taking acetaminophen for chronic pain [15]. While up to 3 g/day of acetaminophen is generally safe, patients with underlying liver disease should limit their acetaminophen daily dose to less than 2 g/day [16], and no safe dosing threshold has been established for patients with unhealthy alcohol use.

Adjuvant Analgesics

Adjuvant analgesics such as antidepressants and anticonvulsants are commonly used to manage chronic pain. All these medications have primary FDA indications for non-pain diagnoses and require weeks to achieve an analgesic effect. Tricyclic antidepressants (TCAs) are some of the most commonly prescribed adjuvant analgesics for neuropathic pain. Because of their reliance on hepatic biotransformation and tendency to cause sedation, patients with liver dysfunction may become overly sedated on TCAs. In addition, the intestinal anticholinergic effects (constipation) may worsen a patient's hepatic encephalopathy. Selective-serotonin reuptake inhibitor (SSRI) antidepressants may be well tolerated but only have a weak analgesic effect. Serotonin–norepinephrine reuptake inhibitors (SNRI) such as duloxetine and venlafaxine are also well tolerated and may have more analgesic efficacy than SSRIs. The anticonvulsant gabapentin has efficacy in treating neuropathic pain and is not metabolized by the liver. However, gabapentin can be sedating, which may be more pronounced in patients with unhealthy alcohol use.

Topical Agents

An advantage of topical (non-opioid) agents is the lack of systemic side effects. Topical agents include lidocaine and capsaicin. Lidocaine is a local anesthetic agent that comes in patches. Capsaicin, an active ingredient in hot chili peppers, has been used with some success in patients with neuropathic pain. However, it must be applied 3–4 times a day to be effective and causes a burning sensation prior to anesthesia. Pain relief is usually modest and can take several weeks to take effect.

Skeletal Muscle Relaxants

Skeletal muscle relaxants (e.g., baclofen, cyclobenzaprine, tizanidine) have efficacy in treating acute pain with associated spasticity but have a limited to no role in treating chronic pain. Use of these medications is limited by excess sedation and may be too risky to use in patients with unhealthy alcohol use. Carisoprodol should be avoided as it is metabolized into a barbiturate, meprobamate, which is a highly addictive sedative.

Opioid Medication Prescription

Opioids are among the most commonly prescribed medication class in the United States. Whether for acute or chronic pain management, there is great concern about potential interaction between the sedating effects of alcohol and opioids. When combined, the substances may synergistically suppress respiration centers and maintenance of airway tone, potentially leading to overdose. Such events could occur when opioids are taken as prescribed, or if in the setting of alcohol intoxication, the patient inadvertently consumes more than intended. In addition, unhealthy alcohol use and particularly long-standing alcohol dependence may result in hepatic dysfunction, which will alter drug metabolism [17, 18]. When selecting an appropriate opioid regimen, factors to consider include the medication duration of action, amount dispensed, and chronicity of prescribing. Of note, tramadol is unscheduled by the Drug Enforcement Agency (DEA), yet it exerts its analgesic effects via opioid agonism and weak norepinephrine/serotonin reuptake inhibition. Tramadol has been shown to have potential for abuse and addiction, and should be used with the same caution as other opioids when managing pain among patients with unhealthy alcohol use.

Given potential concerns about opioid misuse and adverse interactions in individuals with unhealthy alcohol use, prescribing should target the minimally effective dose and length of treatment. The treatment goal is to decrease pain to tolerable levels and improve function while minimizing adverse effects, such as with hepatic impairment and prescription opioid misuse.

Hepatic Impairment

Patients with asymptomatic chronic liver disease without cirrhosis metabolize analgesics similar to the general population. However, drug metabolism may be slowed in those with severe disease such as hepatitis or cirrhosis, even if synthetic function is near normal [16]. Opioids are largely metabolized by the liver via cytochrome P450 (CYP) system (CYP2D6 and 3A4) or glucuronidation [16]. Impairment in these mechanisms leads to increased bio-availability and decreased clearance of the parent drug and metabolites, thus increasing potential toxicity. In the setting of cirrhosis, a reduction serum protein and albumin may lead to greater free drug availability, and increased adverse effects from opioids that are highly protein bound, such as meperidine, which should be avoided also because of its toxic metabolite [19]. With hepatic impairment, opioid dose and/or prescribing interval should be reduced [17]. Close monitoring for sedation is particularly important for longer acting preparations such as methadone, given that levels can build up in the system with repeated dosing.

Establishing Risk of Opioid Misuse

Primary care physicians face a tremendous challenge balancing safe and effective pain treatment with the need to recognize and hopefully prevent problems associated with opioid medications. Not surprisingly, many primary care physicians and house-staff are uncomfortable managing chronic pain and express concern about prescription opioid abuse [20–24], which is understandable given that approximately one-third of primary care patients receiving chronic opioid pharmacotherapy demonstrate aberrant medication taking or other substance misuse [5, 25].

For patients with unhealthy alcohol use, the risk for prescription opioid misuse may be higher than low-risk or non-drinkers [26, 27]. Once a patient has progressed to an alcohol use disorder, the risk for prescription opioid misuse is even more concerning based on pain clinic [28, 29] and primary care data [30, 31]. In a one-year prospective study of a primary care, chronic pain, disease management program, those with current or past alcohol abuse had over 2.5 times the odds of opioid misuse during one year of monitoring [30]. Forty-four percent of patients with current or past alcohol abuse exhibited evidence of prescription opioid misuse compared to 23 % without, an association which persisted even after adjusting for other potential predictors [30]. One study of patients with chronic pain on long-term opioids found that a diagnosis of opioid dependence was significantly associated with lifetime alcohol dependence [31].

Other factors common among patients with unhealthy alcohol use have been found to be associated with increased risk of opioid misuse including a personal or family history of a substance use disorder, younger age, legal problems, tobacco dependence, and psychiatric comorbidity [25, 28, 29]. These and other factors have been incorporated into clinical prediction tools to stratify risk for those who may go on to exhibit aberrant opioid medication taking. Two brief patient self-report instruments that are easily integrated in practice include the five question version of the Screener and Opioid Assessment for Patients with Pain (SOAPP) [32] and the Opioid Risk Tool (ORT) [33]. The tools help predict the likelihood that a patient initiating opioids will display aberrant medication taking behaviors in the future, rather than measuring risk of current diversion or opioid use disorders. Survey items ask about mood swings and psychological disease, personal and family history of substance use, legal problems, medication misuse, pre-adolescent sexual abuse, and smoking a cigarette < 60 min after awakening [32, 33]. Based on the patient's score, risk is stratified in advance, allowing the clinician to counsel the patient and structure prescribing and monitoring accordingly. Identification of higher risk profile may warrant early consultation with an addiction, pain management, or psychiatric specialist, such as with active substance use disorders or untreated psychiatric conditions [34].

Table 9.1 Universal precautions during opioid prescribing

Establish the diagnosis and necessity for opioids
Determine risk for opioid misuse
Opioid informed consent about treatment interactions and risks including physical dependence, addiction, and tolerance
Opioid treatment agreement, written or verbal
Determine appropriate opioid and non-opioid pharmacologic and non-pharmacologic treatment
Pre- and regular post-treatment pain and functional assessment
Adherence monitoring: prescription monitoring programs (PMPs), urine drug testing, pill counts
Careful documentation at all stages

Structuring Care During Opioid Prescribing

Universal Precautions

When initiating acute or chronic opioid therapy for primary care patients with unhealthy alcohol use, particular care should be taken to structure treatment in order to effectively manage pain and improve function, yet also promote prevention and recognition of problems associated with opioids or other substances. Calls have been made to institute "universal precautions" when prescribing chronic opioid medication, an approach adapted from the infectious disease field in which routine prevention strategies are implemented for all patients, regardless of perceived risk, to reduce stigma and improve outcomes [34]. Universal precautions necessitate a standardized approach for *all* patients receiving opioid medication, encompassing assessment and diagnostic formulation, informed consent, patient monitoring, and documentation (Table 9.1).

Though described primarily for chronic opioid prescribing, aspects of universal precautions should be applied during both acute and chronic pain management through conservative prescribing of the minimally effective dose in terms of number of pills and medication strength. For acute pain, the anticipated length of the pain syndrome must be considered with prescription of an appropriate time-limited supply. Left-over medication is a concerning source for misuse, not only for the patient, but for others in the household and community [35]. A time-limited opioid trial when initiating treatment of chronic pain can help establish expectations with the patient that opioids may not be necessary or appropriate life long, especially given a lack of long-term efficacy data beyond several months [36]. In addition, the time-limited trial allows monitoring of potential concerning behaviors that could indicate misuse. All patients should be counseled to store opioid medication in a secure location and discard extra medication after resolution of the pain syndrome. Lastly, regarding conservative prescribing, the lowest effective medication strength also should be used for both acute and chronic pain, given that higher doses are associated with increased consequences such as overdose [37].

Informed Consent and Opioid Treatment Agreements

After an appropriate assessment and decision to prescribe opioid treatment, informed consent should take place to review the limitations and potential risks of opioid analgesics. Potential risks include interactions and adverse effects outlined above and development of physiologic dependence [38], which includes tolerance (analgesic effect is diminished at the same opioid dose) and/or opioid withdrawal if medication is decreased or stopped. The patient should be informed about potential for addiction and hyperalgesia, a paradoxical increased pain sensitivity resulting from neuroadaptive changes during chronic opioid use [39].

Completion of a written signed opioid treatment agreement, previously called a pain or opioid contract [40] enables the clinician and patient to review treatment and behavioral expectations, including: visit frequency, medication storage, avoidance of opioid, and other substance misuse, dosing as prescribed without unsanctioned increases, use of one pharmacy and one prescriber, and the adherence monitoring plan. Opioid treatment agreement use is gaining traction in primary care despite a notable lack of clinical outcome data [2] and potential concern about legal limitations and stigma of written agreement use [41]. Opioid treatment agreements may help improve primary care physician confidence in managing pain [42, 43], and even without a signed document, agreement components should be discussed with the patient and documented in the medical record to clarify expectations and help structure care.

Adherence Monitoring

Urine drug testing is a mainstay of patient risk assessment and monitoring during prescription opioid treatment to confirm use of the prescribed opioid as well as detect use of non-prescribed medications and illicit drugs. Tests can include point-of-service immunoassay dip tests that provide an immediate result in the office, or laboratory testing that confirms parent drug or metabolite via gas chromatography/mass spectrometry (GC/MS), either with or without quantitative levels. A rapid result during in-office testing is particularly useful to inform treatment decision-making "in the moment" and provides an opportunity for discussion with the patient. Familiarity with the substances being tested in the office or laboratory test is crucial to differentiate, for example, an opiate test that assesses morphine levels at a certain cut-off (e.g., 300 ng/mL) from an opioid-specific test such as oxycodone (e.g., 100 ng/mL). Opiate tests will detect recent use of opiate poppy-plant derivatives (e.g., codeine, morphine, and diacetylmorphine or heroin), whereas synthetics such as fentanyl or methadone will be undetected on opiate tests. Semi-synthetics such as hydrocodone or oxycodone are unreliably detected on opiate dip tests, necessitating the use of opioid-specific tests for confirmation. Other recent substances that can be tested for include benzodiazepines and barbiturates, which may interact with alcohol and opioids, as well as stimulants such as cocaine, which is associated prescription opioid misuse [44]. Clinical guidelines on urine testing in primary care are available and highly recommended for further review [45]. The general approach for integration of urine drug screening in practice is to test for the medication prescribed along with commonly used illicit drugs and other controlled medications. Positive detection of the prescribed opioid or its metabolite supports medication adherence, although false negative results can occur such as with low dose regimens taken intermittently on an as-needed basis. Positive findings of non-prescribed opioid or illicit drug use provides an opportunity for discussion about the substance use patterns and problems, and may necessitate greater treatment structure with increased monitoring or outside referral for addiction evaluation.

Adherence monitoring may also incorporate pill counts at patient visits or random call backs to examine compliance with medication dosing and to detect evidence of diversion. Writing a 28-day supply rather than "one month" or 30-days is recommended to limit the accumulation of extra days' medication if the patient returns on 4-week intervals (on the same day of the week) and also to avoid running out of medication on a weekend. Missing medication during pill counts could indicate use above recommended levels due to inadequate pain relief at the currently prescribed dose, misuse, or diversion. Family member or significant other corroboration with patient consent may be useful to monitor medication taking.

There is growing availability of prescription monitoring programs (PMPs) across the United States, which is a major advance in adherence monitoring to verify the validity of prescriptions and monitor use of controlled substances. PMPs are online state databases that can be rapidly searched even while the patient is in the office to track receipt of scheduled medication prescriptions from pharmacies. PMP use is favorably rated by physicians and strongly recommended by the Federal government to reduce doctor shopping and help confirm medication utilization [46]. Limitations include a potential two-week or more delay for posting of recent prescription pick-up and a lack of information sharing between states, which is a particular limitation for practices near state borders. Primary care clinicians can find out more information about their state's PMP by going to the Alliance of States with Prescription Monitoring Programs website at http://www.pmpalliance.org/. Registration is generally brief and free.

Adherence monitoring can be tailored for patients deemed higher risk with increased frequency of visits and fewer days of medication prescribed. Structure could include 24-hour call back to the clinic for pill counts and urine drug testing, both of which can be instituted at every visit, randomly, or in response to concerning behaviors. Non-physician clinical staff can be engaged in the primary care setting to assist with adherence monitoring. Utilization of structured approaches is intended to deter and identify early prescription opioid misuse [44, 47–49].

Opioid Misuse and Opioid Use Disorders

Opioid misuse refers to use that is not consistent with medical guidelines. It can include any of the following: *non-medical use, substance abuse or dependence, addiction, or diversion.* Non-medical use is defined as the use of prescription medication without a prescription or the use of a prescription medication for purposes other than those for which it is prescribed (e.g., for the feelings it produces or to get high). Opioid use disorders, including abuse, dependence or addiction, are a cluster of cognitive, behavioral and physiological symptoms indicating that the individual continues use of the substance despite significant substance-related problems. Finally diversion is defined as diverting opioids from therapeutic channels to share or sell them for recreational use, treatment of untreated pain in others, or for financial gain.

It is important to monitor patients for benefit (i.e., analgesia, function) and harm (i.e., misuse) by frequent face-to-face follow-up visits especially when initiating opioids and at times of dose adjustment. Opioid misuse can be detected by patients exhibiting "aberrant medication taking behaviors" such as running out of medications early, losing medications, and nonadherence with other recommended therapies. It is also important to try to distinguish when these behaviors represent misuse versus inadequate pain control. The clinician's level of concern and action should be based on the pattern and severity of these behaviors. If a patient takes more opioids than prescribed, the intervention might be to reeducate the patient about the dangers of overusing opioids, while if the behavior is more severe such as altering a prescription (e.g., altering the number of pills to be dispensed) then the appropriate response will be to stop prescribing opioids and refer the patient to specialty addiction treatment.

The diagnosis of an opioid use disorder can be made using standardized Diagnostic and Statistical Manual, Fourth Edition, (DSM-IV) [38] abuse and dependence criteria as outlined for alcohol use disorders in Chap. 3. Among patients on chronic opioids, however, it is essential to understand the discrepancy between physiological dependence vs. DSM-IV dependence, the latter of which is often used interchangeably with addiction. Physiological dependence is due to a compensatory neuroadaptive response to opioid treatment whereby the patient develops tolerance or experiences signs and symptoms of opioid withdrawal when the opioid dose is reduced or stopped. Physiological dependence alone is neither necessary nor sufficient for an addiction diagnosis, which includes components of uncontrolled, compulsive and continued use despite harm. Among patients diagnosed with opioid addiction, medication treatment with the partial opioid agonist buprenorphine is effective and available in office settings, which may be preferable to patients and help expand access beyond specialty program-based settings [50]. However, for primary care patients with chronic pain and unhealthy alcohol use, addiction referral may be more appropriate.

In most instances, no single factor from patient history or monitoring will definitively indicate an opioid or other substance problem. Furthermore, the diagnosis will rarely be clear at an initial office visit, but rather will require longitudinal monitoring and assessment of treatment response. Over time, clinicians often will have to weigh various factors for and against the benefit of continued opioid prescribing. In addition to patient-related factors, such decision is necessarily based on clinician comfort and experience with pain management and substance treatment, as well as system-based factors, including the ability of the practice setting to feasibly enhance structure if needed. If the decision is made to discontinue opioids, the process should include gradual opioid tapering, non-opioid based approaches to control pain, and ancillary medications to treat emergent withdrawal symptoms. To the extent that hyperalgesia may be present, pain potentially could improve off opioid medication for some patients [39]. For patients discontinued off prescribed opioids because of opioid, alcohol, or other substance use disorders, an addiction treatment referral is essential due to morbidity and mortality when the diseases are untreated.

References

1. Ballantyne JC. The Massachusetts General Hospital handbook of pain management. 3rd ed. Philadelphia: Lippincott Williams & Wilkins; 2005.
2. Chou R, Fanciullo GJ, Fine PG, et al. Clinical guidelines for the use of chronic opioid therapy in chronic noncancer pain. J Pain. 2009;10:113–130.
3. Institute of Medicine. Relieving pain in America: A blueprint for transforming prevention, care, education, and research. 2011. http://www.iom.edu/~/media/Files/Report%20Files/2011/Relieving-Pain-in-America-A-Blueprint-for-Transforming-Prevention-Care-Education-Research/Pain%20Research%202011%20Report%20Brief.pdf. Accessed 29 July 2011.
4. Gureje O, Von Korff M, Simon GE, Gater R. Persistent pain and well-being: a World Health Organization Study in primary care. JAMA. 1998;280(2):147–151.
5. Chelminski PR, Ives TJ, Felix KM, et al. A primary care, multi-disciplinary disease management program for opioid-treated patients with chronic non-cancer pain and a high burden of psychiatric comorbidity. BMC Health Serv Res. 2005;5:3.
6. McHorney CA, Ware JE, Lu JFR, et al. The MOS 36-item short-from health survey (SF-36): III. tests of data quality, scaling assumptions, and reliability across diverse patient groups. Med Care. 1994;32:40–66.
7. Oslin DW, Grantham S, Coakly E, et al. PRISM-E: comparison of integrated care and enhanced specialty referral in managing at-risk alcohol use. Psychiatr Serv. 2006;57:954–958.
8. Hays RD, Sherbourne CD, Mazel RM. User's manual for the medical outcomes study (MOS) core measures of health-related quality of life. Santa Monica: RAND Corporation. 1995. http://www.rand.org/content/dam/rand/pubs/monograph_reports/2008/MR162.pdf. Accessed 29 July 2011.
9. Sacco P, Bucholz KK, Spitznagal EL. Alcohol use among older adults in the National Epidemiologic Survey on alcohol and related conditions: A latent class analysis. J Stud Alcohol Drugs. 2009;70:829–838.
10. Deyo RA, Mirza SK, Martin BI. Back pain prevalence and visit rates: estimates from the U.S. national surveys, 2002. Spine. 2006;31(23):2724–2727.
11. Krebs EE, Lorenz KA, Bair JM, et al. Development and initial validation of the PEG, a three-item scale assessing pain intensity and interference. J Gen Intern Med. 2009;24(6):733–738.
12. Chou R, Huffman LH. Nonpharmacologic therapies for acute and chronic low back pain: a review of the evidence for an American Pain Society/American College of Physicians Clinical Practice Guideline. Ann Intern Med. 2007;147:492–504.
13. Kaufman DW, Kelly JP, Wiholm BE et al. The risk of acute major upper gastrointestinal bleeding among users of aspirin and ibuprofen at various levels of alcohol consumption. Am J Gastroenterol. 1999;94:3189–3196.
14. Schmidt LE, Dalhoff K, Poulsen HE. Acute versus chronic alcohol consumption in acetaminophen-induced hepatotoxicity. Hepatology. 2002;35(4):876–882.
15. Schiødt FV, Rochling FA, Casey DL, Lee WM. Acetaminophen toxicity in an urban county hospital. N Engl J Med. 1997;337:1112–1118.
16. Chandok N, Watt KDS. Pain management in the cirrhotic patient: the clinical challenge. Mayo Clin Proc. 2010;85:451–458.

17. Verbeeck RK. Pharmacokinetics and dosage adjustment in patients with hepatic dysfunction. Eur J Clin Pharmacol. 2008;64:1147–1161.
18. Elbekai R, Korashy H, El-Kadi A. The effect of liver cirrhosis on the regulation and expression of drug metabolizing enzymes. Curr Drug Metab. 2004;5:157–167.
19. Smith HS. Opioid metabolism. Mayo Clin Proc. 2009;84:613–624.
20. Bhamb B, Brown D, Hariharan J, et al. Survey of select practice behaviors by primary care physicians on the use of opioids for chronic pain. Curr Med Res Opin. 2006;22(9):1859–1865.
21. Upshur CC, Luckmann RS, Savageau JA. Primary care provider concerns about management of chronic pain in community clinic populations. J Gen Intern Med. 2006;21:652–655.
22. O'Rorke JE, Chen I, Genao I, Panda M, Cykert S. Physicians' comfort in caring for patients with chronic nonmalignant pain. Am J Med Sci. 2007;333(2):93–100.
23. Chen I, Goodman B, Galicia-Castillo M, et al. The EVMS pain education initiative: a multifaceted approach to resident education. J Pain. 2007;8:152–160.
24. Gunderson EW, Coffin PO, Chang N, Polydorou S, Levin FR. The interface between substance abuse and chronic pain management in primary care: a curriculum for medical residents. Substance Abuse. 2009;30(3):253–260.
25. Reid MC, Engles-Horton LL, Weber MB, et al. Use of opioid medications for chronic noncancer pain syndromes in primary care. J Gen Intern Med. 2002;17:173–179.
26. Blazer DG, Wu Li-Tzy. The epidemiology of at-risk and binge drinking among middle-aged and elderly community adults: National Survey on Drug Use and Health. Am J Psychiatry. 2009;166:1162–1169.
27. Caamao-Isorna F, Mota N, Crego A, et al. Consumption of medicines, alcohol, tobacco and cannabis among university students: a 2-year follow-up. Int J Public Health. 2011;56(3):247–252.
28. Michna E, Ross EL, Hynes WL, et al. Predicting aberrant drug behavior in patients treated for chronic pain: importance of abuse history. J Pain Symptom Manage. 2004;28:250–258.
29. Michna E, Jamison RN, Pharm LD, et al. Urine toxicology screening among chronic pain patients on opioid therapy: frequency and predictability of abnormal finding. Clin J Pain. 2007;23:173–179.
30. Ives TJ, Chelminski PR, Hammett-Stabler CA, et al. Predictors of opioid misuse in patients with chronic pain: a prospective cohort study. BMC Health Serv Res. 2006;6:46.
31. Boscarino JA, Rukstalis M, Hoffman SN, et al. Risk factors for drug dependence among out-patients on opioid therapy in a large US health-care system. Addiction. 2010;105(10):1776–1782.
32. Akbik H, Butler SF, Budman SH, et al. Validation and clinical application of the screener and opioid assessment for patients with pain (SOAPP). J Pain Symptom Manage. 2006;32(3):287–293.
33. Webster LR, Webster RM. Predicting aberrant behaviors in opioid-treated patients: preliminary validation of the opioid risk tool. Pain Med. 2005;6(6):432–442.
34. Gourlay DL, Heit HA, Almahrezi A. Universal precautions in pain medicine: a rational approach to the treatment of chronic pain. Pain Med. 2005;6:107–112.
35. The National Center on Addiction and Substance Abuse (CASA) at Columbia University. Under the counter: The diversion and abuse of controlled prescription drugs in the U.S. New York, NY. July 2007
36. Chou R, Huffman LH. Medications for acute and chronic low back pain: a review of the evidence for an American Pain Society/American College of Physicians clinical practice guideline. Ann Intern Med. 2007;147:505–514.
37. Dunn KM, Saunders KW, Rutter CM, et al., Opioid prescriptions for chronic pain and overdose: a cohort study. Ann Int Med. 2010;152(2):85–92.
38. American Psychiatric Association (APA). Diagnostic and statistical manual, fourth edition (text revision) (DSM-IV-TR). July 2000.
39. Tompkins DA, Campbell CM. Opioid-induced hyperalgesia: clinically relevant or extraneous research phenomenon? Curr Pain Headache Rep. 2011;15(2):129–136.

40. Fishman SM, Bandman TB, Edwards A, Borsook D. The opioid contract in the management of chronic pain. J Pain Symptom Manage. 1999;18:27–37.
41. Gitlin MC. Contracts for opioid administration for the management of chronic pain: a reappraisal. J Pain Symptom Manage. 1999;18(1):6–8.
42. Touchet BK, Yates WR, Coon KA. Opioid contract use is associated with physician training level and practice specialty. J Opioid Manag. 2005;1(4):195–200.
43. Fagan MJ, Chen JT, Diaz JA, Reinert SE, Stein MD. Do internal medicine residents find pain medication agreements useful? Clin J Pain. 2008;24:35–38.
44. Meghani SH, Wiedemer NL, Becker WC, et al. Predictors of resolution of aberrant drug behavior in chronic pain patients treated in a structured opioid risk management program. Pain Med. 2009;10:858–865.
45. Christo PJ, Manchikanti L, Ruan X, et al. Urine drug testing in chronic pain. Pain Physician. 2011;14:123–143.
46. Office of National Drug Control Policy (ONDCP). Fact sheet: prescription drug monitoring programs. 2011.http://www.whitehousedrugpolicy.gov/publications/html/pdmp.html. Accessed 29 July 2011.
47. Goldberg KC, Simel DL, Oddone EZ. Effect of an opioid management system on opioid prescribing and unscheduled visits in a large primary care clinic. J Clin Outcomes Manage. 2005;12(12):621–628.
48. Manchikanti L, Manchukonda R, Damron KS, et al. Does adherence monitoring reduce controlled substance abuse in chronic pain patients? Pain physician. 2006;9(1):57–60.
49. Wiedemer NL, Harden PS, Arndt IO, Gallagher RM. The opioid renewal clinic: a primary care, managed approach to opioid therapy in chronic pain patients at risk for substance abuse. Pain Med. 2007;8(7):573–584.
50. Gunderson EW, Fiellin DA. Office-based maintenance treatment of opioid dependence: how does it compare with traditional approaches? CNS Drugs. 2008;22(2):99–111.

Chapter 10
Medical Consequences of Unhealthy Alcohol

Adam J. Gordon, Joanne M. Gordon and Lauren Matukaitis Broyles

> *There is this to be said in favor of drinking, that it takes the*
> *drunkard first out of society, then out of the world.*

Ralph Waldo Emerson.

Alcohol consumption may increase the risk of causing a myriad of medical and mental health conditions and contributing to the morbidity of these conditions (Fig. 10.1). Risky alcohol use (consumption amounts that place a person at risk for health consequences) may also complicate medical treatment by reducing adherence to medication and attention to treatment plans. Unhealthy behaviors, including un-protected sex, illicit drug use, drinking while driving, often occur with alcohol consumption and additionally contribute to medical diseases and trauma. Further-more, co-existing health conditions, use of tobacco and other abused substances, and genetic and environmental factors can also influence development of specific disease in alcohol users. Alcohol use is the third leading cause of preventable death in the United States.

Risky alcohol use is a pattern of alcohol consumption that increases someone's *risk* of harm associated with medical and mental health conditions. In this chapter we include risky alcohol use in our definition of *unhealthy alcohol use* as an amount or pattern of alcohol consumption that places a person *at risk for*, or *is causing,* physical health damage. The pattern and amount of alcohol consumed by an individual that is unhealthy may vary based on the individual characteristics (e.g., sex, race, and

A. J. Gordon (✉) · L. M. Broyles
University of Pittsburgh School of Medicine and VA Pittsburgh Healthcare System,
Pittsburgh, PA, USA
e-mail: adam.gordon@va.gov

J. M. Gordon
Missouri State University, Springfield, MO, USA
e-mail: joannemgordon@gmail.com

L. M. Broyles
e-mail: lauren.broyles@va.gov

R. Saitz (ed.), *Addressing Unhealthy Alcohol Use in Primary Care,*
DOI 10.1007/978-1-4614-4779-5_10, © Springer Science+Business Media New York 2013

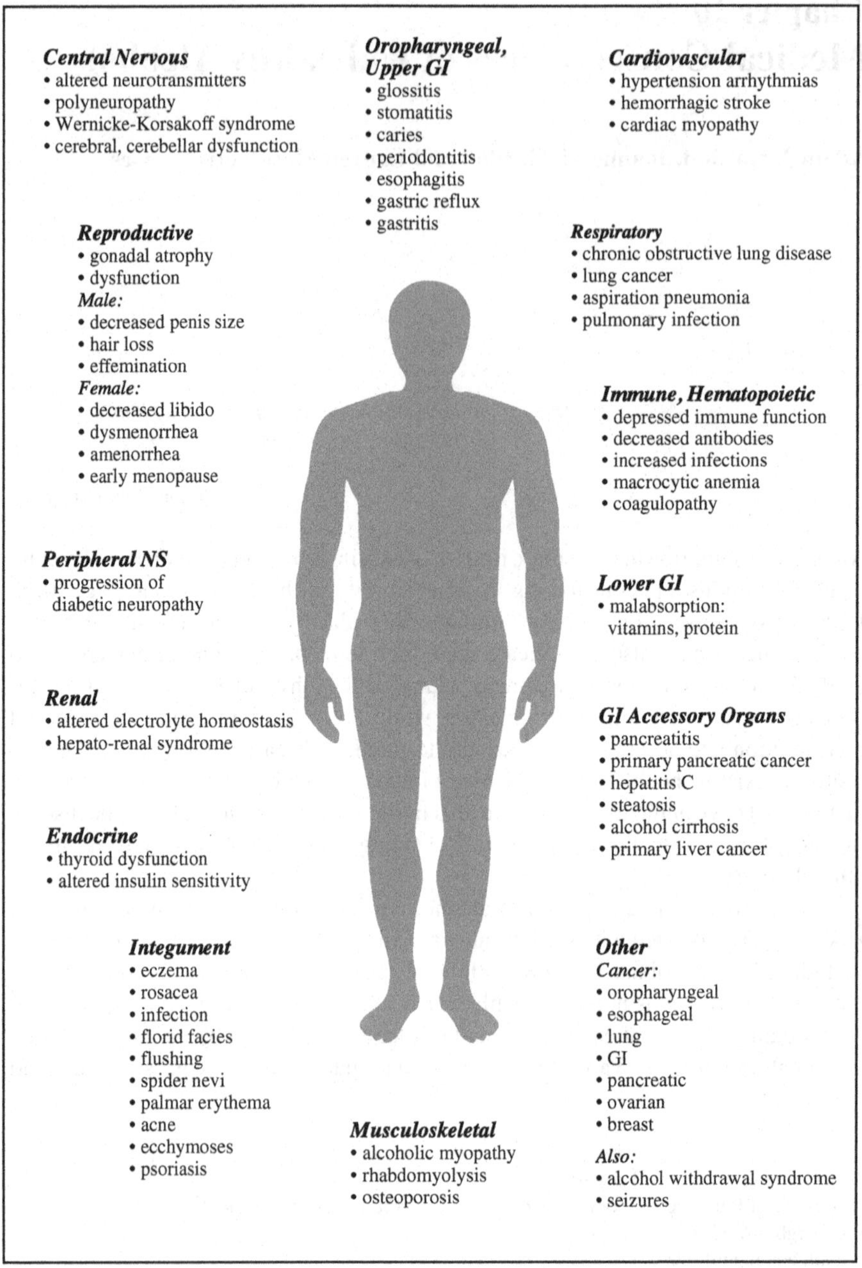

Central Nervous
- altered neurotransmitters
- polyneuropathy
- Wernicke-Korsakoff syndrome
- cerebral, cerebellar dysfunction

Reproductive
- gonadal atrophy
- dysfunction

Male:
- decreased penis size
- hair loss
- effemination

Female:
- decreased libido
- dysmenorrhea
- amenorrhea
- early menopause

Peripheral NS
- progression of diabetic neuropathy

Renal
- altered electrolyte homeostasis
- hepato-renal syndrome

Endocrine
- thyroid dysfunction
- altered insulin sensitivity

Integument
- eczema
- rosacea
- infection
- florid facies
- flushing
- spider nevi
- palmar erythema
- acne
- ecchymoses
- psoriasis

Oropharyngeal, Upper GI
- glossitis
- stomatitis
- caries
- periodontitis
- esophagitis
- gastric reflux
- gastritis

Musculoskeletal
- alcoholic myopathy
- rhabdomyolysis
- osteoporosis

Cardiovascular
- hypertension arrhythmias
- hemorrhagic stroke
- cardiac myopathy

Respiratory
- chronic obstructive lung disease
- lung cancer
- aspiration pneumonia
- pulmonary infection

Immune, Hematopoietic
- depressed immune function
- decreased antibodies
- increased infections
- macrocytic anemia
- coagulopathy

Lower GI
- malabsorption: vitamins, protein

GI Accessory Organs
- pancreatitis
- primary pancreatic cancer
- hepatitis C
- steatosis
- alcohol cirrhosis
- primary liver cancer

Other
Cancer:
- oropharyngeal
- esophageal
- lung
- GI
- pancreatic
- ovarian
- breast

Also:
- alcohol withdrawal syndrome
- seizures

Fig. 10.1 Organ systems affected by excessive alcohol intake

age), the pattern of alcohol use (e.g., binge drinking, daily drinking, drinking episod-ically), or the amount of consumption (e.g., amount of consumption per day, week, or year; lifetime alcohol exposure). Acute alcohol intake is associated with some conditions (e.g., acute alcohol poisoning, aspiration pneumonia, hypoglycemia), chronic alcohol intake is associated with others (e.g., brain damage, esophagitis, and malabsorption), and both acute and chronic alcohol consumption is associated with others (e.g., gastritis, pancreatitis, cerebrovascular accidents). Simply put, spe-cific medical diseases, disease symptoms, or medical complaints may occur based on different levels of alcohol drinking patterns and amount of alcohol consumed. Alcohol withdrawal syndrome can also cause medical consequences and is covered in another chapter of this book. It is important to note that while unhealthy alcohol use amounts have been generally defined as greater than 14 standard drinks per week or more than 4 on an occasion for males and greater than 7 standard drinks per week or more than 3 on an occasion for females and everyone over 65 years of age, alco-hol consumption below (or above) these limits can result in medical consequences. Although many people who experience some of the more serious consequences of unhealthy alcohol use (e.g., alcoholic cirrhosis, head and neck cancers) report long-term heavy (e.g., >4 drinks) daily drinking, exact thresholds, where risks increase, have been difficult to define. In other words, risk curves for the incidence of alcohol consequences generally begin at any drinking. For example, the risk for breast cancer appears to be associated with drinking 3–6 drinks per week [2].

Practitioners should be aware of the incident and co-occurring medical illnesses that are influenced by alcohol consumption (and patterns of that consumption) and be aware of preventive health strategies to reduce the risk of harms associated with unhealthy alcohol use. In this chapter, we summarize the major medical illnesses caused by or associated with unhealthy alcohol use and relate preventive strategies for mitigating these harms.

Circulatory System

Two recent reviews found that alcohol consumption, compared to no alcohol con-sumption, can reduce cardiovascular disease, coronary heart disease, and enhance favorable levels of high-density lipoprotein, apolipoprotein A1, adiponectin, and fibrinogen. Higher levels of alcohol consumption (variably defined) have been asso-ciated with [1, 5] hypertension and other cardiovascular disease, although the exact amount of alcohol that significantly increases blood pressure is a source of contro-versy. Prospective studies have found a relationship between alcohol intake and blood pressure [7] and it appears this is a J-shaped association; some alcohol consumption may be beneficial on blood pressure. About 30 % of cardiomyopathies (dilated and ischemic) can be attributable to alcohol. Supraventricular tachycardias, including atrial arrhythmias, are known to occur with alcohol intake. Recently, researchers have reviewed the existing evidence and examined in a meta-analysis whether this risk is dependent on the amount of alcohol consumed. It appears that patients who drink at least 1.5 drinks a day have a 1.5 times greater risk for atrial fibrillation compared to lowest alcohol consumption amounts (variably defined) and that the risk of atrial fibrillation appears to increase, in patients who drink 4–86 g/day by 8 % for each additional 10 g of alcohol consumed per day. In "holiday heart syndrome," acute cardiac dysrhythmias (classically atrial fibrillation) occur in heavy drinkers without known cardiac disease. A risk of hemorrhagic stroke (and ischemic stroke) is increased in heavy alcohol drinkers. In a recent study, there was a significant association between ischemic stroke and alcohol [3] consumption (greater than 40 g or about 3 standard drinks in the preceding 24 h (odds ratio [OR], 2.66) or >150 g (one or two standard drinks a day) in the previous week (OR, 2.47).

Altered immune responses, often found in patients with unhealthy alcohol use, may exacerbate existing cardiac conditions. Alcohol may be the causative factor for hypertension in as many as 33 % of men and 8 % of women. Alcohol-induced hypertension can place patients at-risk for dysrhythmias and cardiomyopathy. Reduction of alcohol consumption reduces blood pressure in normotensive and hypertensive patients.

Gastrointestinal, Hepatic, and Metabolic Systems

Excessive alcohol consumption is known to exacerbate several problems in the mouth and oropharynx. Due to vitamin deficiencies and direct toxic effects of alcohol, glossitis, stomatitis, caries, and periodontitis are attributable to unhealthy alcohol consumption. Vitamin deficiencies may occur due to dietary or economic factors among people who consume alcohol. Alcohol consumption impairs the absorption of folic acid, vitamin B12, thiamine, and vitamin A, as well as other nutrients in the small and large intestines. Furthermore, zinc deficiency can occur with chronic alcohol consumption, causing impairment in taste and appetite reduction. Alcohol reduces esophageal peristalsis and decreases esophageal sphincter tone, leading to esophagitis and gastric acid reflux. Alcohol consumption also reduces individuals' gastric emptying and increases gastric secretion, which can cause erosive gastritis. Emesis stimulated by alcohol use can exacerbate gastric and esophageal pathology.

Although some alcohol consumption may prevent or inhibit cholelithiasis, alcohol use is detrimental to the accessory organs associated with the digestive system. Unhealthy alcohol use promotes development of acute and chronic pancreatitis, a risk factor for pancreatic cancer [6]. Recently, research has found a dose-response association between the amount of spirits consumed on a single occasion and the risk of acute pancreatitis; the multivariable adjusted risk ratio (RR) was 1.52 for every increment of 5 standard drinks (12 g of ethanol in this study) of spirits consumed on a single occasion. Recent research also found that there exists a risk for pancreatic cancer death which was higher among participants who drank three or more drinks per day (relative risk [RR], 1.31) and four or more drinks per day (RR, 1.14), compared to non-drinkers. Interestingly, the increased risk at greater than or equal to three drinks per day was primarily seen with liquor use and not with beer or wine use. Alcohol use is the leading cause of pancreatitis. Ethanol-induced pancreatitis is thought to be secondary to direct toxicity to pancreatic acinar cells, leading to release of proteolytic enzymes.

The liver is the most frequently damaged organ in persons misusing alcohol and alcohol-related liver disease is a frequent outcome of long-term alcohol consumption. Alcohol impairs the hepatic system through several pathophysiological mechanisms: production of acetaldehyde, free radicals, and cytokines; passage of bacterial endotoxins through the alcohol-damaged intestinal wall; and direct alcohol-induced inflammation and cell death. Acetaldehyde can lead to the formation of neoantigens by binding with protein and resulting in the formation of auto-antibodies. These autoantibodies can cause tissue damage and inflammation throughout the body, including the liver, heart, gastrointestinal tract, nervous tissue, and muscle.

Cirrhosis can occur in as many as one third of lifetime alcohol drinkers. In 90 % of long-term alcohol drinkers, hepatic steatosis (fatty liver) occurs and can lead to alcoholic hepatitis and alcohol cirrhosis. Fortunately, hepatic steatosis is reversible. Unfortunately, many patients with this condition progress to irreversible fibrosis and cirrhosis. In pre-cirrhotic alcohol-related liver disease, the ratio of aspartate aminotransferase to alanine aminotransferase is often elevated and can be as high as 5:1. Hepatitis associated with alcohol disorders often causes anorexia, nausea, emesis, fevers, chills, and pain—and may be associated with other conditions including varices, bleeding diatheses, ascites, and secondary malnutrition. Primary hepatocellular carcinoma is also associated with alcohol consumption, particularly in those who develop cirrhosis. For unknown reasons, women seem to have a higher incidence of alcohol-induced hepatic pathology than men.

Based in part on malabsorption, maldigestion, suppression of appetite and accompanying reduced dietary intake in the presence of alcohol-induced hepatic, gastric, or pancreatic disease, patients who drink heavily are susceptible to numerous nutritional deficiencies. These deficiencies may include thiamine, folic acid, B vitamins, and ascorbic acid. Regular heavy drinking also leads to negative nitrogen imbalance, increased protein turnover, and inhibition of lipolysis, thus increasing adiposity and risk for other diseases associated with obesity.

Patients who drink heavily are also more likely than non-drinkers to have increased iron stores and ferritin deposits without concomitant vitamin B12 or folic acid deficiencies. Some studies have found a positive correlation between serum Vitamin B12 and several liver enzymes [4]. As alcohol and its metabolites begin to damage liver cells, stored B12 can be released into the circulation, along with liver enzymes. Thus, serum B12 levels may be within normal range, but liver stores are being depleted. Liver enzyme tests may be helpful in determining early hepatic disease in malnourished alcohol-users with normal B12 values.

Endocrine System

Alcohol influences the homeostasis of several endocrine systems. Testosterone and leuteotropins are abnormally secreted in the presence of alcohol. Gonad function is impaired. This impairment can lead to testicular atrophy, low testosterone levels, impaired sperm production and function, and loss of libido. Shrinkage of the penis and loss of hair has also been noted in patients who drink. For alcohol drinkers who are male, effemination may occur. Females may suffer from ovarian atrophy and masculinization leading to decrease in libido, amenorrhea, dysmenorrhea, sterility, and early menopause.

Thyroid function can be impaired by alcohol and reduced thyroxine is common in patients who drink unhealthy amounts of alcohol. Excessive alcohol intake may further activate the hypothalamic-pituitary axis causing elevated glucocorticoid levels. There is some evidence that premature aging occurs with life-long alcohol consumption. Interestingly, compared to non-drinkers, the incidence of diabetes mellitus is decreased in patients who consume moderate amounts of alcohol. This may be due to increased insulin sensitivity and lower plasma insulin levels. Unfortunately, excessive alcohol consumption may worsen diabetic neuropathy and cause hypoglycemia in diabetic patients.

Immune, Lymphatic, and Hematopoietic Systems

Unhealthy alcohol consumption leads to impairment of immune regulation, immune deficiency, and increased autoimmunity, thus increasing the risk of widespread tissue damage by the formation of acetaldehyde-protein antibodies, and increasing the susceptibility to infections. Alcohol reduces the ability of antigen-presenting cells to present pathogens to the immune system and decreases the production of immunoglobulins. Coupled with risky sexual and substance use behaviors prevalent among those who consume unhealthy amounts of alcohol, increases in serious infections, including viral hepatitis, skin infections, and human immunodeficiency syndrome are more common in patients who drink alcohol. Hepatitis C replication is increased with any alcohol consumption and this consumption may inhibit the effects of alpha-interferon activity. Current recommendations are that patients with hepatitis C should abstain from any alcohol consumption. The prevalence of hepatitis C is as much as 10-fold higher in persons with alcohol dependence compared to others, likely secondary to increased risky behaviors associated with alcohol consumption (e.g., intravenous drug use, risky sexual practices) and reduced immune system reactivity to viruses. Autoimmunity, including increased circulating autoantibodies, may directly lead to liver disease and liver failure. For patients with HIV, alcohol may specifically lead to development of HIV-related cerebral disease.

Approximately 50 % of chronic, unhealthy alcohol users have anemia, particularly macrocytic anemia, that either may be associated with vitamin B12 and folic acid deficiencies, or by iron overload. Unhealthy alcohol consumption may result in gastritis and subsequent chronic blood loss. Macrocytic anemia is also found in many individuals with alcoholic cirrhosis. Elevated MCV and RDW are often associated with chronic heavy alcohol use and liver disease. Abnormal platelets, and associated increased risk of bleeding, and abnormal leukocytes are often found in chronic alcoholism. In sum, for patients consuming unhealthy amounts of alcohol, anemia is likely multi-factorial due to red cell production problems (toxicity to the bone marrow), liver disease, iron deficiency, other vitamin deficiencies (including B vitamins), sequestration problems (e.g., hepatomegaly and splenomegaly), and blood loss (mainly through gastrointestinal losses).

Integumentary System

Skin pathologies are common in patients who drink unhealthy amounts of alcohol. These include discoid eczema, rosacea, skin infections, florid facies, rashes from pellagra (niacin deficiency), and flushing. Chronic alcohol use can predispose users to spider nevi and palmar erythema, bruises, and acne generated from multi-system and organ disease processes. Patients who consume alcohol appear to be more at risk for developing psoriasis, and alcohol use may impair the ability to effectively treat this disease.

Musculoskeletal and Nervous Systems

Excessive alcohol intake predisposes patients to hip fractures due to osteoporosis and falls. Alcohol directly impairs osteoblasts leading to decreased bone remodeling and delayed fracture healing. This bone loss appears to be more common in men than in women. When alcohol drinkers drink to excess, unconsciousness and prolonged, sustained body positions may cause muscle damage and rhabdomyolysis. Chronic alcohol consumption can lead to myopathy, by altering myocyte synthesis and function in both skeletal and cardiac muscle. Myocyte damage may be related to direct toxicity of ethanol and its metabolites. Concurrent polyneuropathy may stimulate the development of progressive, but painless, muscle weakness and wasting, although cramps and myalgia also may occur. Alcohol myopathy, and subsequent weakness may occur in as many as half of patients with excessive alcohol consumption, contributing to unsteady gait, falls, and osteopenia. Unfortunately, myopathy may not be reversible once alcohol consumption ceases.

Several neurotransmitter systems are influenced by alcohol, including the gamma-aminobutyric acid (GABA), glutamate, methyl-D aspartate (NMDA), norepinephrine, beta-endorphin, and serotonin systems. Alcohol promotes nutritional polyneuropathy and cerebellar degeneration and widespread damage in the cerebral cortex. Wernicke-Korsakoff syndrome, neuropathy, subarachnoid hemorrhage, and seizures can occur in patients with long-standing alcohol consumption. Wernicke's encephalopathy, caused by vitamin B1 (thiamine) deficiency, is characterized by global confusion, ataxia, and ophthalmoplegia. It can be treated successfully with thiamine with concurrent magnesium replacement. Korsakoff's psychosis or syndrome involves neuronal loss and irreversible damage to the medial thalamic nuclei and mammillary bodies, and is characterized by antegrade and retrograde amnesia, confabulation, apathy, lack of insight, and reduction of conversation. However, there is some evidence from observational studies that compared to non-drinkers, low-risk alcohol use may reduce the risk of dementia. Two types of alcohol neuropathy can occur either independently or concomitantly. One type of neuropathy is primarily due to thiamine deficiency and is associated with motor nerve dysfunction and a rapid onset. Alcohol neuropathy may also occur because of the direct toxic effect of alcohol and is manifested primarily by progressive distorted sensory perception (e.g., pain, burning sensation). Alcoholic neuropathy may also be found in patients with normal thiamine levels but with a decrease in B12. Slow, progressive sensory symptoms may be associated with small fiber axonal loss, and is thought to be related to the toxic effect of acetaldehyde on neurons. B12 neuropathy can be associated with thiamine deficiency or can be independent of thiamine. Those with both thiamine and B12 deficiency may have more varied signs and symptoms; in contrast, B12 deficiency is primarily sensory.

Respiratory System

Patients who drink to excess are at risk for emesis and aspiration pneumonia. A large proportion of patients who have alcohol abuse and dependence also smoke cigarettes. Patients who drink and smoke have high rates of lung cancer and chronic obstructive lung disease, particularly emphysema. Tuberculosis and other pulmonary infections are also associated with excessive, unhealthy alcohol consumption likely due, in part, to living circumstances.

Renal System

Alcohol intake can induce acute and chronic changes in renal function and the ability of the kidneys to regulate electrolyte homeostasis. For example, beer potomania syndrome, associated with large consumption of beer, is secondary to ingestion of large loads of free water (beer) with corresponding low salt and protein intake. This leads to hyponatremia and hypokalemia and failure of the kidney to excrete very dilute urine. Other electrolyte balances that can be impaired include potassium (hypokalemia), magnesium (hypomagnesemia), calcium (hypocalcemia), and phosphate (hypophosphatemia). Alcohol ketoacidosis can occur after alcohol-induced emesis, and other anion gap acidoses can occur after seizures (lactic), and ingestions of toxic alcohols (e.g., methanol or ethylene glycol). Hepato-renal syndrome may occur in patients with concurrent alcohol-induced liver disease.

Neoplasm Risks across Organ Systems

Across multiple organ systems, alcohol has been associated with risk for several types of cancer. For example, many of the cancers associated with alcohol are also associated with smoking. Whether alcohol increases smoking carcinogenic effects, or is synergistic in causing cancer in that circumstance is unknown. However, it is known that alcohol itself is a carcinogen. The US Department of Health and Human Services and the World Health Organization both classify alcohol as a definite carcinogen and some of the cancers it increases are not associated with concurrent smoking (breast cancer).

Cancers of the oral cavity, pharynx, larynx, and esophagus are associated with heavy alcohol consumption. Furthermore, there is an increased risk of gastric, colon, rectal, hepatocellular, endometrial, breast, and ovarian cancers occur with excessive alcohol consumption. Some cancers such as colon cancer are associated with alcohol consumption at levels less than considered typically hazardous; any alcohol consumption may place a person at risk for cancer. Dose-dependent increases in cancers of the upper digestive tract have been consistently associated with alcohol use even after controlling for age, sex, smoking, and educational levels. Risks of cancer related deaths may increase in patients who smoke. Over 40 studies have examined the association of breast cancer with alcohol use. This relationship appears to be a dose-dependent effect starting at low amounts of alcohol and may be associated with increased estrogen and androgens, sensitivity of breast tissue to carcinogens, direct DNA damage, and/or an inability to repair DNA damage. There is some evidence that overweight and obese breast cancer survivors who drink more than three or four standard drinks a week are at an increased risk of recurrence of breast cancer.

Mortality and Alcohol Consumption

While much of this chapter has indicated that some and excessive alcohol consumption (variably defined) can result in medical consequences, it should be noted that any alcohol consumption appears to impart a protective effect on some patients. A linear relationship exists between alcohol consumption and total mortality. However, a J-shaped relationship is observed in certain populations. For example, those persons with high risk of coronary heart disease, [8] some alcohol consumption may be better than none. Despite these findings, there is no consensus whether alcohol use may be protective or that a certain type of alcohol is more protective than others. The reason for the controversy is that there have been no randomized trials testing the effect of drinking alcohol on heart disease or mortality, and although observational studies are generally consistent, results could be explained by methodological problems, particularly the inability to distinguish the effects of alcohol from the effects of other health practices and behaviors.

There is no "ideal" level of alcohol use; for some people, no alcohol consumption is the safest. Regardless, the preponderance of the evidence suggests that if any benefit to alcohol consumption does exist, the consumption should be minimal (less than 1/2–1 standard drink a day)—much less than currently recommended daily or weekly suggested alcohol consumption limits, but also levels at which some harms are seen (e.g., breast cancer risk). In sum, while alcohol consumption at certain levels of consumption may impart medical consequences, alcohol intake may also benefit other physiologic processes. In general, consumption amounts in guidelines that define risky alcohol consumption are at levels where the risks of medical consequences supersede any potential protective effects of alcohol. Careful discussions with patients discussing the risks and benefits of consumption should occur, and abstinence may not be the end goal. Some patients (e.g., those pregnant, with previous hemorrhagic stroke, with hepatic or pancreatic diseases) should abstain from any alcohol consumption as the risks of harm supersede any benefit.

Patients with alcohol abuse and dependence have higher mortality rates than those matched controls who do not have these conditions, but with abstinence, these populations have similar mortality rates. The most common cause of deaths for persons with alcohol abuse and dependence are liver disease, cancer, accidents, suicide, and ischemic heart disease.

Prevention Strategies

Preventive care strategies are best employed based on targeted evaluations based on risk factors and demographic characteristics (e.g., age, sex). For those patients drinking too much alcohol, several preventive health care interventions may reduce subsequent risk of alcohol-related harm, incident disease, and complications of co-occurring diseases. It is reasonable to assess patients who consume unhealthy amounts of alcohol with a complete blood count (including mean corpuscular volume), blood sugar, liver and renal chemistries, and urinalysis. Because alcohol influences serum lipids and cardiovascular risk, these patients should be assessed with a fasting lipid profile. Those patients with co-occurring illicit drug use, particularly injection drug use, should have serum evaluation for viral hepatitis and human immunodeficiency virus (HIV) testing. In the United States, the Centers for Disease Control suggest HIV screening for all patients. Patients who engage in risky sexual behaviors should be considered to be tested for Chlamydia, syphilis, and gonococcal diseases. In addition, *mycobacterium* diseases (e.g., tuberculosis) may be asymptomatic in the patient with unhealthy amounts of alcohol consumption; screening for mycobacterial diseases should particularly occur in persons in endemic regions. Age-appropriate screening tests such as mammography (breast cancer), Papanicolau smears (cervical cancer), and fecal occult blood testing or sigmoidoscopy/colonoscopy (colorectal cancer) should always occur in every patient; because unhealthy alcohol consumption may increase the risk of cancers, screening may be more imperative in this population.

Prevention of diseases associated with excessive alcohol use can occur with preventive counseling to reduce use, immunizations, and chemoprophylaxis. Interventions to reduce alcohol consumption to safer levels of consumption may reduce risk for alcohol-related pathology. Furthermore, for patients with existing-alcohol related pathology, reduction in alcohol intake may reduce alcohol-related disease progression and improve treatment response. Preventive counseling should provide individualized feedback, related to conditions the patient already has. Health care practitioners should counsel risky alcohol drinkers to improve their health habits including nutrition and dietary practices. Because of the incidence of nutritional deficits in patients with risky alcohol use, practitioners should consider offering a daily multivitamin, including 400 IU vitamin D, 100 mg thiamine, and 1 mg of folic acid. If magnesium and 25-hydroxyvitamin D serum levels are low, patients should be offered these supplements. Patients should be offered standard recommended vaccines for adults (e.g., tetanus, diphtheria, pertussis) but because of alcohol-related immune suppression, risky alcohol drinkers should be offered immunizations for pneumococcus, and influenza. Hepatitis A and B immunizations should be offered to those with alcohol-related liver disease, hepatitis C, or injection drug use.

Summary

In summary, alcohol is a toxic substance that affects every organ system of the human body. Clinicians should be aware that drinking alcohol, particularly unhealthy amounts, may place the patient at risk for a myriad of diseases and may complicate treatment of many others. With attention to alcohol as a causative agent of disease and counseling for risky alcohol consumption, health care practitioners may be able to mitigate the effects of alcohol on health harms.

References

1. Brien SE, Ronksley PE, Turner BJ, Mukamal KJ, Ghali WA. Effect of alcohol consumption on biological markers associated with risk of coronary heart disease: systematic review and meta-analysis of interventional studies. Br Med J. 2011;342:d636.
2. Chen WY, Rosner B, Hankinson SE, et al. Moderate alcohol consumption during adult life, drinking patterns, and breast cancer risk. JAMA. 2011;306(17):1884–1890.
3. Guiraud V, Amor MB, Mas JL, Touze E. Triggers of ischemic stroke: a systematic review. Stroke. 2010;41(11):2669–2677.
4. Himmerich H, Anghelescu I, Klawe C, Szegedi A. Vitamin B12 and hepatic enzyme serum levels correlate in male alcohol-dependent patients. Alcohol Alcohol. 2001;36(1):26–28.
5. Ronksley PE, Brien SE, Turner BJ, Mukamal KJ, Ghali WA. Association of alcohol consumption with selected cardiovascular disease outcomes: a systematic review and meta-analysis. Br Med J. 2011;342:d671.
6. Sadr Azodi O, Orsini N, Andrén-Sandberg A, Wolk A. Effect of type of alcoholic beverage in causing acute pancreatitis. Br J Surg. 2011;98(11):1609–1616.
7. Thomson J, Lip G. Alcohol and hypertension: an old relationship revisited. Alcohol Alcohol. 2006;41(1):3–4.
8. White I, Altmann D, Nanchahal K. Alcohol consumption and mortality: modelling risks for men and women at different ages. Br Med J. 2002;325:191–194.

Further Readings

1. Brick J. Medical consequences of acute and chronic alcohol abuse. In: Handbook of the medical consequences of alcohol and drug abuse. 2nd ed. New York: Haworth; 2008.
2. Campbell NRC, Ashley MJ, Carruthers SG, Lacourciere Y, McKay DW. Recommendations on alcohol consumption. CMAJ. 1999;160 Suppl 9:S13–20.
3. Gordon AJ, Gordon JM, Carl K, Hilton MT, Striebel J, Maher M. Physical illness and drugs of abuse. In: Gordon AJ, editor, New York: Cambridge University Press; 2010.
4. Mukamal KJ. In: Basow DS, editor. Overview of the risks and benefits of alcohol consumption. Waltham: UpToDate; 2011.
5. Nace EP. Alcohol. In: Frances RJ, Miller SI, Mack AH, editors. Clinical textbook of addictive disorders. 3rd ed. New York: Guilford; 2005.
6. Patussi V, Mezzani L, Scafato E. An overview of pathologies occurring in alcohol abusers. In: Preedy VR, Watson RR, editors. Comprehensive handbook of alcohol related pathology. Vol. 1. San Diego: Elsevier Academic; 2005. pp. 253–259.
7. Rastegar DA, Fingerhood MI. Alcohol. In: Addiction medicine: an evidence-based handbook. Philadelphia: Lippincott Williams & Wilkins; 2005.
8. Saitz R. Medical and surgical complications of addiction. In: Ries RK, Fiellin DA, Miller SC, Saitz R, editors. Principles of addiction medicine. 4th ed. Philadelphia: Lippincott Williams & Wilkins; 2009.
9. Royal College of Physicians. Alcohol use disorders: diagnosis and clinical management of alcohol-related physical complications (NICE Clinical Guideline 100). London: National Institute for Health and Clinical Evidence, National Clinical Guideline Centre for Acute and Chronic Conditions; 2010.

Chapter 11
Psychiatric Comorbidity

Amy Harrington

When a primary care clinician identifies a patient with an alcohol use disorder, there is a high likelihood that this patient has a psychiatric comorbidity. In the National Epidemiologic Survey on Alcoholism and Related Conditions (NESARC), a study representative of the US population, 40.7 % of people who sought treatment for alcohol dependence had at least one mood disorder and 33 % had at least one anxiety disorder [1]. People who are at-risk drinkers, though they do not meet criteria for dependence or abuse, have higher rates of psychiatric comorbidity than lower risk drinkers or those who abstain from alcohol [2]. If left untreated, mood, anxiety and other psychiatric disorders can interfere with successful treatment and recovery from alcohol dependence, increase the chance of relapse and lead to overall poorer health outcomes. In the worst-case scenario, these conditions can be fatal, as alcohol use is a significant risk factor for suicide. When treating a patient with an alcohol-related illness, it is important to detect and treat comorbid psychiatric illnesses. It is also important to be able to do an appropriate safety assessment so that a patient can be referred to a higher level of psychiatric care (e.g., psychiatrist, hospital), when necessary.

Affective Disorders

Patients with alcohol dependence often have symptoms of depression or erratic mood. Many times, these symptoms will remit as the alcohol use remits. On the other hand, primary affective disorders (i.e., those not caused by alcohol) are a common co-morbidity in this population. In the Epidemiologic Catchment Area Study, 16.5 % of patients with major depressive disorder also had an alcohol use disorder [3]. In the NESARC, 40 % of patients with major depressive disorder also had a lifetime diagnosis of an alcohol use disorder [4]. In both studies, bipolar disorder was the

A. Harrington (✉)
Department of Psychiatry, Division of Addiction Psychiatry,
University of Massachusetts Medical School, Worcester, MA, USA
e-mail: Amy.harrington@umassmemorial.org

R. Saitz (ed.), *Addressing Unhealthy Alcohol Use in Primary Care,*
DOI 10.1007/978-1-4614-4779-5_11, © Springer Science+Business Media New York 2013

psychiatric disorder in which patients were most likely to also have a co-occurring substance use disorder.

Major depressive disorder (MDD) and bipolar disorder (BD) are both characterized by remitting and recurring episodes of symptoms followed by periods of return to baseline. These episodes cause marked impairment in a patient's ability to function. In order to make a diagnosis of a depressive episode, a patient must report either depressed mood or decreased interest in activities for at least two weeks. They have to endorse at least five total symptoms from a set of possible symptoms that include, in addition to the two symptoms already mentioned, changes in sleep, appetite, energy or concentration, feelings of guilt or worthlessness, and recurrent thoughts of death. Patients with BD have hypomanic or manic episodes in addition to depressive episodes. A manic episode is defined as a marked elevated or irritable mood lasting at least 7 days with at least 3 of the following symptoms co-occurring: increased self-esteem, decreased need for sleep, increased rate of talking, the perception of racing thoughts, difficulty maintaining attention, increased goal-directed activity, and excessively participating in pleasurable activities that can have negative consequences. Hypomanic episodes are diagnosed based on the same criteria, though they only need to last 4 days, but are not severe enough to impair functioning or warrant hospitalization.

Screening tests can be helpful for primary care physicians (PCPs) to detect a co-morbid psychiatric disorder such as depression. The Beck Depression Inventory (BDI) has been shown to be valid for detecting depression in patients hospitalized for the treatment of alcohol dependence [5]. The Patient Health Questionniare-9 (PHQ-9) is a measure that provides some guidance as to the level of symptoms a patient is experiencing. It is both sensitive and specific for depression, and it is widely used in primary care settings. In addition to detecting depression, the clinician can get some insight into the level of severity of symptoms. An additional benefit is that it can be self-administered by the patient during time periods when they are waiting to do other things [6]. The PHQ-2, on the other hand, is a brief, two-question screen that can alert a PCP that there is a need to assess further. The questions are: 'Over the last 2 weeks, how often have you been bothered by any of the following problems? "little interest or pleasure in doing things," and "feeling down, depressed or hopeless."' Responses are scored 0–3 each and include "not at all, "several days," "more than half the days," and "nearly every day." A score of 3 or more (sum of both items) is considered a positive screen. Given the rates of depression in patients with alcohol dependence and at-risk drinking are higher as compared with the general population, the PHQ-2 should be administered to any patient who has been identified as having unhealthy alcohol use.

Previous studies, as well as folklore, had suggested that treating symptoms of depression in someone who is drinking excessive amounts of alcohol is ineffective. Clinicians were taught to wait until a sustained period of abstinence before initiating pharmacologic management of depression or anxiety. The predictable result in many clinical settings for patients was that alcohol disorders did not improve as quickly or as much as they might have had depression been addressed, and vice versa. More recent studies, however, suggest that treatment of depression or anxiety in patients with alcohol dependence should not be delayed while awaiting abstinence or while

Table 11.1 Dosing guidelines for several medications for depression or anxiety often prescribed in the primary care setting

Medication	Starting dose	Increase by increment of:	Maximum dose
Citalopram	10–20 mg daily	10–20 mg	40 mg daily
Escitalopram	10 mg daily	5 mg	20 mg daily
Sertraline	25–50 mg daily	25–50 mg	200 mg daily
Fluoxetine	10–20 mg daily	10–20 mg	60 mg daily
Paroxetine (immediate release)	20 mg daily, can dose BID if side effects	10–20 mg total per day	60 mg total per day
Paroxetine (controlled release)	12.5–25 mg daily	12.5–25 mg total per day	75 mg total per day
Bupropion (immediate release or SR formulation)	100–150 mg BID	100–150 mg BID	450 mg in divided doses
Bupropion (XL formulation)	150 mg daily	150 mg daily	300 mg daily

trying to sort out whether the disorder is "primary." Though formal diagnosis of a psychiatric disorder requires the symptoms not be the result of alcohol or another substance of abuse, making this distinction is not immediately relevant if psychiatric symptoms are noted on exam. Treatment should be started without delay, and more formal diagnosis can be sorted out later on in the course of treatment. Not only have recent data suggested that there can be improvement in symptoms of depression when someone is still drinking, the treatment of depression can have a positive effect on drinking outcomes. In a meta-analysis, Nunes and Levin found that while rates of complete remission of depression were low, patients in whom depressive symptoms were adequately treated with antidepressants had significant reductions in the quantity of alcohol consumed [7].

Selective serotonin reuptake inhibitors (SSRIs) are first-line treatment for depressive disorders. If a patient has significant problems with low energy or hypersomnolence, bupropion would be reasonable to try first. This medication is a norepinephrine-dopamine reuptake inhibitor (NDRI) that can address neurovegetative symptoms. A PCP should become familiar with dosing one or two of these medications so that they can initiate treatment in mild-to-moderate cases (Table 11.1). Since alcohol is a depressant, it is reasonable to advise patients to abstain from alcohol if their depression is severe enough to warrant the need for medication. If the symptoms do not respond or if the PCP feels that there are safety concerns, a referral to a mental health provider is indicated. If a patient develops manic or hypomanic symptoms after initiating antidepressant treatment, this could indicate an underlying bipolar illness. Again, referral to a mental health specialist is warranted in order to better clarify the diagnosis.

Sometimes a patient may not meet full criteria for a diagnosis of major depressive disorder, but targetable symptoms may be noted on exam. For example, a patient may have a subjective sense of depressed mood that is distressing but they might not have four of the other criteria needed to make a diagnosis. Given the relatively safe side effect profile of SSRI's, a trial of medication is reasonable. In these cases, both the prescriber as well as the patient should keep in mind exactly what the target symptoms are, and weigh the benefits of potentially relieving these symptoms with the potential side effects. These medications are safe for people who are actively drinking. The one possible exception is the use of bupropion in patients who have physiologic dependence and have experienced withdrawal symptoms. Bupropion can lower the seizure threshold and increase the potential for alcohol withdrawal-related seizures.

Patients with bipolar disorder require treatment with mood stabilizers. There have been several studies suggesting that mood stabilizing medications with anti-convulsant properties are particularly effective for treating bipolar disorder with co-occurring alcohol use disorders. One study found that patients treated with depakote and lithium together did better with regards to drinking outcomes than patients treated with lithium and placebo [8]. Other studies suggest that lamotrigine may be effective in reducing craving for alcohol while simultaneously improving mood symptoms [9].

Anxiety Disorders

In the NESARC, 18 % of individuals with any substance use disorder (alcohol is by far the most common) had at least one anxiety disorder. A diagnosis of panic disorder, social phobia, and generalized anxiety disorder increased the odds of having alcohol dependence within the same 12 months of 3.6, 2.5 and 3.1, respectively [1]. One of the challenges in treating patients who have both alcohol use disorders and anxiety disorders is that some of the medications used by psychiatrists to treat anxiety are contraindicated in someone who is drinking alcohol. Since benzodiazepines and alcohol both work via the same receptor in the brain, concomitant use can be synergistic and lead to greater disinhibition, blackouts, respiratory depression, and potentially death. Alcohol use is essentially a contraindication for prescribing benzodiazepines unless the goal is the treatment of alcohol withdrawal (during which time alcohol use is not continuing). Fortunately a number of alternate agents are available, and are first line treatments for anxiety in primary care settings, including SSRI's and buspirone for daily treatment, and medications like hydrozyxine and clonidine for as-needed treatment.

There is a growing body of evidence on the co-occurrence of post-traumatic stress disorder (PTSD) and substance use disorders, particularly in female patients. While the prevalence of PTSD among people seeking treatment for substance dependence is higher than it is among the general population, for women with substance use disorders the prevalence of PTSD is as high as 30–59 % [10]. Symptoms of PTSD develop after a traumatic stressor in which someone either directly experiences or witnesses an event that threatens death or serious injury. Symptoms fall into several categories, including re-experiencing symptoms like flashbacks and nightmares, avoidance symptoms, such as efforts to avoid thoughts about the trauma or things that remind one of the trauma, and hyperarousal symptoms, such as increased startle response or angry outbursts. Treatment of PTSD that co-occurs with alcoholism involves both psychotherapeutic as well as psychopharmacologic approaches. SSRI's are first-line treatment for PTSD, and there is evidence to suggest that there are certain sub-types of alcohol dependent patients whose drinking outcomes improve on medications like sertraline [11]. In addition, cognitive behavioral therapy and related therapies like Seeking Safety have been shown to be effective for both drinking outcomes as well PTSD-related symptoms. Seeking Safety is a manualized psychotherapy that focuses on exchanging substance use for other more healthy coping skills specifically aimed at the symptoms experienced in PTSD [12].

As with affective disorders, there are both self-administered as well as clinician administered tools that can assess for the presence of an anxiety disorder or quantify the severity of the symptoms. The Beck Anxiety Inventory is a 21-item self-report measure that can also give an indication of severity [13]. The GAD-7 is a newer screen that can be quickly administered to detect the presence of an anxiety disorder [14]. Like the PHQ, The GAD has the same response options and there is a short version that is considered positive with a score of 3 or greater. The question is "Over the last 2 weeks, how often have you been bothered by the following problems?" and the 2 problems in the GAD are "feeling nervous, anxious or on edge" and "not being able to stop or control worrying."

The Primary Care Post Traumatic Stress Disorder (PC-PTSD) is a 4-item screen that has been shown to be equally effective in detecting PTSD as compared with the longer and more in-depth Clinician Administered PTSD Scale (CAPS) [15]. The PC-PTSD is considered positive when there are three affirmative responses to any of the four items which are: "In your life, have you ever had any experience that was so frightening, horrible, or upsetting that, in the past month, you—(1) Have had nightmares about it or thought about it when you did not want to? (2) Tried hard not to think about it or went out of your way to avoid situations that reminded you of it? (3) Were constantly on guard, watchful, or easily startled? (4) Felt numb or detached from others, activities, or your surroundings?"

Psychotic Disorders

Psychotic symptoms include delusions, which are fixed, false beliefs that are firmly maintained despite not being accepted by other people within the culture, and hallucinations, which are the perception of a sensory experience in the absence of an external stimulus. When a patient presents because of their alcohol use and they are also observed to have psychotic symptoms, it is important to take a careful history to get a timeline about the symptoms. A long-time history of these symptoms suggests a primary psychotic disorder like schizophrenia. Delusions or hallucinations that occur solely in the context of a manic or depressive episode suggest a severe mood disorder, which is also common in this patient population. Acute onset of symptoms following a recent cessation or decrease in alcohol use, however, suggests, alcohol withdrawal is the cause. Accurate diagnosis is important in determining treatment as well as the level of urgency of the situation.

Substance abuse and dependence are common among patients with schizophrenia; the prevalence of alcohol dependence is as high as 47 % [16]. Patients who have schizophrenia often come to the attention of mental health professionals early on in life, but some may first present in a primary care setting, and that presentation may be related to an alcohol-related problem.

In general, primary care clinicians should refer a patient who has both active psychotic symptoms as well as unhealthy alcohol use to a mental health or addiction specialist. These patients can be challenging diagnostically. In addition, clinicians often have to navigate a complex algorithm before finding a suitable pharmacologic regimen. Someone with more familiarity with working with psychotic patients might have an easier time with clinical decision-making.

Treatment of psychotic symptoms usually begins with an atypical antipsychotic, such as risperidone, olanzapine, quetiapine, ziprasidone, or aripirazole. While there is no specific interaction between these medications and alcohol, psychotic patients who are actively drinking may have problems with adherence with medications. This should be taken into consideration when deciding on an antipsychotic. For example, clozapine, another atypical antipsychotic, requires intense monitoring and consistent dosing because of its side-effect profile, which includes agranulocytosis. Though very effective, particularly in treatment refractory cases of psychosis, this may not be an appropriate medication in a patient who cannot followthrough with the necessary monitoring or who forgets to take their medications correctly. Other atypical antipsychotics have a preferable side effect profile. There is increasing evidence to suggest that some of the medications in this class may be helpful in reducing craving for drugs of abuse (including alcohol). In a prospective study of patients with schizophrenia and dependence on a variety of substances, those treated with clozapine were less likely to relapse than those treated with other antipsychotics [17]. An open-label study of aripiprazole in cocaine dependent patients with schizophrenia demonstrated a potential role for this medication in reducing craving for alcohol [18]. Further research, in both the area of psychopharmacology as well as in the use of psychotherapeutic interventions such as motivational interviewing and contingency management specifically in this patient population, is needed.

Personality Disorders

Personality disorders are common in patients with alcohol use disorders. Unlike other psychiatric illnesses, which will have episodic flares interspersed with periods of baseline functioning, patients with personality disorders have enduring and inflexible behavior patterns that can make them difficult to form a therapeutic alliance with. They are often preoccupied with their own needs, and as a result, can be manipulative and stir up strong reactions in a practitioner, PCP and psychiatrist alike. It is important to keep in mind that this is a predictable phenomenon in patients with these illnesses, and they can be managed effectively if the clinician knows what to look for.

Two personality disorders in particular that clinicians come across in patients with alcohol use disorders are antisocial personality disorder (APD) and borderline personality disorder (BPD). The predominant feature of APD is a disregard for and violation of the rights of others. Most people with alcohol dependence do not have APD, although they may act in antisocial ways as a result of their addiction. Antisocial behavior secondary to addiction will remit as the addiction does, whereas primary APD, deceitfulness, inability to conform behavior to social norms, aggressiveness and lack of remorse, will persist after the alcoholism goes into remission. Patients with BPD have unstable relationships and affect. Like patients with APD, they can be markedly impulsive, which often results in polysubstance use and heavy episodic drinking.

Treatment primarily focuses on behavioral and psychotherapeutic techniques. Often group therapy is effective for the symptoms of both the personality disorder as well as the alcohol use, because other patients can help hold them accountable for their actions and apply the social pressure that leads to modification of their behavior. The clinician should set firm limits, but be aware of his countertransference (a clinician's personal emotions and attitudes toward a patient that can be based on past relationships or conflicts that clinician has had in his own life) so that he can maintain objectivity in the therapeutic relationship. Psychopharmacologic treatment focuses on symptom reduction, such as treatment of depression or anxiety symptoms that often arise in these patients. It is also important to assess for danger to both self and others regularly.

Attention Deficit/Hyperactivity Disorder (AD/HD)

In recent years, greater attention has been given to the high prevalence of AD/HD in adults with substance abuse or dependence. Approximately one third of adults with AD/HD have either past or current alcohol abuse or dependence [19]. Left untreated, inattention and hyperactivity can make it more difficult for these patients to engage in the psychotherapeutic aspects of addiction treatment. Like anxiety disorders, there is a challenge in treating these patients, as many of the effective treatments are also potentially addicting. Unlike anxiety disorders, however, the stimulant medications that are potentially addictive work on a different substrate from alcohol, and are therefore somewhat safer to use in this patient population (though some risk factors for addictions are not specific to the drug of abuse and patients with alcohol disorders are often at risk for other substance disorders). Studies in children suggest that treating their symptoms with stimulant medications such as methylphenidate does not lead to a higher incidence of substance abuse or dependence later in life [20]. Using long-acting formulations of these medications can decrease the potential for misuse. There are also a variety of non-stimulant medications that have been shown to be effective in treating AD/HD (e.g. atomoxetine).

Suicide

Alcohol use disorders have been associated with increases in suicidal behavior, attempts and completion [21, 22]. Having an alcohol-related diagnosis has been associated with an increased risk of suicide completion, even if the patient does not have another psychiatric diagnosis [22], suggesting alcoholism alone is an independent risk factor for self-harm. In one epidemiologic study, affective disorders and psychotic disorders were associated with a lifetime suicide risk of 6 and 4 % respectively, while alcohol use disorders were associated with a lifetime risk of 7 % for completed suicide [23].

Alcohol use can increase the suicide risk as compared with abstinent individuals independent of whether or not they have major depressive disorder because it leads to disinhibition and increased impulsive behavior. For example, a psychotic patient who is not depressed may be less able to cope with or ignore command auditory hallucinations telling him to kill himself if he is cognitively impaired by or disinhibited by alcohol. It can also have long-term effects that lead to an increased likelihood of self-injury. People who drink heavily are at greater risk for head injury, and traumatic brain injury can lead to decreased inhibition and hypofrontality. Hypofrontality, or decreased neuronal activity of the frontal lobes, can result in specific personality changes including impulsivity, poor judgment, and difficulty in making decisions. Social stressors such as legal problems, marital difficulties, or poor performance at work can contribute to poor social supports and hopelessness. Patients with alcohol use disorders have both short- and long-term stressors that can contribute to increased suicidality. It is important to do a proper safety assessment on patients with alcohol use disorders, regardless of whether or not they have a known mood, anxiety or psychotic disorder.

All patients should be asked a brief screen, such as "do you ever feel so down that you feel like hurting yourself or taking your own life?" A proper safety assessment, however, requires an estimation of risk based on a variety of static and dynamic risks factors and protective factors. Factors associated with an increased tendency for suicide include current suicidal ideation or past attempts, comorbid psychiatric illness, worsening physical illness, a family history of suicide or mental illness, and recent loss of supports or change in socioeconomic status. Certain demographic factors can increase risk, such as male gender, Caucasian race, and either the elderly or adolescent age group. Protective factors include having dependent children, religiosity, and having a good therapeutic relationship with a provider.

Patients with safety issues create a sense of anxiety in clinicians for a variety of reasons, including the concern about liability, should there be a bad outcome. Proper documentation in the medical record is important in these situations so that the clinical reasoning that a provider used to make a decision is recorded. Simply stating that a patient "contracts for safety" is insufficient. One potential way of documenting a safety assessment is as follows:

> Though this patient is at moderate risk of danger to himself given his past suicide attempts, his male gender and his recent substance abuse, he is appropriate for continued out-patient treatment at this time because he reports no current suicidal ideation, he has no access to weapons and he has a good therapeutic alliance with his therapist.

Summary and Recommendations

- Mood disorders are common in this population. SSRIs are safe for use in depressed patients who are actively drinking. Although abstinence from alcohol is recommended, there is no reason to withhold these medications from patients who drink any quantity of alcohol or who are in early sobriety.
- Anxiety disorders such as post-traumatic stress disorder are common in people seeking treatment for substance use, particularly women.
- It is important to get an accurate timeline in a patient reporting psychotic symptoms to determine if these symptoms are alcohol induced (from acute withdrawal, alcoholic hallucinosis, etc.) or if they are due to a primary psychotic disorder.
- Personality disorders are enduring patterns of behavior that can make forming a therapeutic alliance with a patient very difficult. These disorders require behavioral and therapeutic interventions in order to be managed properly.
- AD/HD symptoms in adults with alcohol use disorders can be treated safely with non-stimulant medications or in long-acting formulations of stimulant medication.
- Alcohol use increases the risk for suicide. A proper safety assessment should be documented, and patients should be referred to a mental health professional if on-going safety issues are present.

References

1. Grant BF, Stinson FS, Dawson DA, et al. Prevalence and Co-occurrence of substance use disorders and independent mood and anxiety disorders. Arch Gen Psychiatry. 2004;61:807–816.
2. Bott K, Meyer C, Rumpf HJ, et al. Psychiatric disorders among at-risk consumers of alcohol in the general population. J Stud Alcgohol. 2005; 66:246–253.
3. Reiger DA, Farmer ME, Rae DS, et al. Comorbidity of mental disorders with alcohol and other drug abuse:results for the Epidemiologic Catchment Area (ECA) study. JAMA. 1990;264: 2511–2518.
4. Hasin DS, Goodwin RD, Stinson FS, Grant BF. Epidemiology of major depressive disorder: results from the National Epidemiologic Survey on Alcoholism and Related Conditions. Arch Gen Psychiatry. 2005;62:1097–1106.
5. Tamkin AS, Carson MF, Nixon DH, Hyer LA. A comparison among some measures of depression in male alcoholics. J Stud Alcohol. 1987;48(2):176–178.
6. Kroenke K, Spitzer RL, Williams JBW. The PHQ-9: validity of a brief depression severity measure. J Gen Intern Med. 2001;16(9):606–613.
7. Nunes EV, Levin FR. Treatment of depression in patients with alcohol or other drug dependence: A meta-analysis. JAMA. 2004;291(15):1887–1896.
8. Salloum IM, Cornelius JR, Daley DC, et al. Efficacy of valproate maintenance in patients with bipolar disorder and alchohlism: a double-blind, placebo-controlled study. Arch Gen Psychiatry. 2005;62:37–45.
9. Rubio G, Lopez-Munoz F, Alamo C. Effects of lamotrigine in patients with bipolar disorder and alcohol dependence. Bipolar Disorder. 2006;8:289–293.
10. Brown RI, Wolfe J. Substance abuse and post-traumatic stress disorder co-morbidity. Drug Alcohol Depend. 1994;35:51–59.
11. Hien DA, Cohen LR, Miele GM, et al. Promising treatments for women with comorbid PTSD and substance use disorders. Am J Psychiatry. 2004;161:1426–1432.

12. Najavits LM, Weiss RD, Shaw SR, Muenz LR. Seeking Safety: outcome of a new cognitive-behavioral psychotherapy for women with post-traumatic stress disorder and substance dependence. J Traumatic Stress. 1998;11(3):437–456.
13. Beck AT, et al. An inventory for measuring clinical anxiety: psychometric properties. J Consulting Clinical Psychology. 1998;56(6):893–897.
14. Spitzer RL, et al. A brief measure for assessing generalized anxiety disorder: the GAD-7. Arch Int Med. 2006;166(10):1092–1097.
15. Prins A, Ouimette P, Kimerling R, et al. The primary care PTSD screen (PC-PTSD): development and operating characteristics. Prim Care Psychiatry. 2003;9:9–14.
16. Barbee JG, Clark, PD, Crapanzano BS, et al. Alcohol and substance abuse among schizophrenic patients presenting to an emergency psychiatric service. Nervous Mental Dis. 1989;177(7):379–441.
17. Brunette MF, Drake RE, Xie H, et al. Clozapine use and relapses of substance use disorder among patients with co-occurring schizophrenia and substance use disorders. Schizophr Bull. 2006;32:637–643.
18. Beresford TP, Clapp L, Martin B, et al. Aripiprazole in schizophrenia with cocaine dependence: a pilot study. J Clin Psychopharmacol. 2005;25:363–366.
19. Center for Substance Abuse Treatment. Substance abuse treatment for persons with co-occurring disorders. TIP series 42. HHS Publication No. (SMA) 08-3992. Rockville: SAMHSA; 2005.
20. Wilens TE, Faraone SV, Biederman J, Gunawardene S. Does stimulant therapy of attention-deficit/hyperactivity disorder beget later substance abuse? A meta-analytic review of the literature. Pediatrics. 2003;111:179–185.
21. Bernal M, Haron JM, Bernet S, et al. Risk factors for suicidality in Europe: results from the ESEMED study. J Affect Disorders. 2007;101:27–34.
22. Flensbirg-Madsen T, Knop J, Mortensen EL, et al. Alcohol use disorders increase the risk of completed suicide-irrespective of other psychiatric disorders. A longitudinal cohort study. Psych Res. 2009;167:123–130.
23. Inskip HM, Harris EC, Barraclough B. Lifetime risk of suicide for affective disorder, alcoholism, and schizophrenia. Br J Psychiatry. 1998;172:35–37.

Chapter 12
Other Drug Use

Jennifer McNeely, Joshua D. Lee and Ellie Grossman

Tobacco, alcohol, and illicit drug use are among the leading causes of death in the United States, accounting for over 500,000 deaths per year [1–3]. Tobacco alone is responsible for the majority of these deaths, but illicit drug use is also associated with very high morbidity and mortality. Drug overdose is now second only to motor vehicle accidents as a cause of unintentional injury deaths in the United States [4, 5]. Treatment for substance use disorders reduces morbidity and mortality, but only about 11 % of individuals with substance abuse or dependence are engaged in drug treatment [6]. Primary healthcare providers often constitute the only health system contact for individuals with drug problems [7–9].

Unhealthy alcohol users are much more likely to have concurrent tobacco and illicit drug use. One-third of heavy drinkers also use illicit drugs, and over half of them smoke cigarettes [6]. Failure to identify and assist patients with other drug use can lead not only to exacerbation of the direct health consequences of their use, but can also hinder alcohol treatment and efforts to control other psychiatric and medical conditions. The clinical interaction around alcohol use thus offers a prime opportunity to identify and address tobacco and illicit drug use. Clinicians treating alcohol users should be prepared to recognize other drug use and its attendant comorbidities, and to intervene by providing both preventive care and substance use interventions. Integrating care improves health care outcomes, and should be a goal of service delivery [10–13]. This approach is consistent with current views of addiction as a chronic and multifaceted behavioral health condition [14–17].

J. McNeely (✉) · J. D. Lee
Department of Population Health and Department of Medicine, Division of General Internal Medicine, NYU School of Medicine, New York, NY, USA
e-mail: Jennifer.mcneely@nyumc.org

J. D. Lee
e-mail: Joshua.lee@nyumc.org

E. Grossman
Department of Medicine, Division of General Internal Medicine,
NYU School of Medicine, New York, NY, USA
e-mail: Ellie.grossman@nyumc.org

R. Saitz (ed.), *Addressing Unhealthy Alcohol Use in Primary Care,*
DOI 10.1007/978-1-4614-4779-5_12, © Springer Science+Business Media New York 2013

Recognizing Other Drug Use

Most substance users encountered in general medical settings will not have obvious physical signs or symptoms of drug use, and will not be seeking drug treatment. Substance use problems are thus most likely to be uncovered through routine screening. Screening for alcohol and tobacco in primary care settings is recommended by the United States Preventive Services Task Force (USPSTF). No similar recommendation exists for screening for other drugs of abuse, though there is a growing body of evidence to support it. In the patient with known unhealthy alcohol use, screening for tobacco and illicit drug use is a prudent part of any clinical assessment given the high rates of overlap between these conditions. Illicit drug use is defined here to include misuse of prescription medications (opioids, stimulants, sedatives) as well as use of illegal drugs (e.g., heroin, cocaine, and marijuana).

Tobacco screening is already a common practice in many medical settings, and is usually accomplished with a simple question, asked at each visit [18]: "*Have you ever smoked cigarettes or used any other kind of tobacco?*" Those answering yes should be asked about current use (past 30 days) and quantity (i.e., cigarettes per day).

For illicit drugs, screening questions require a greater level of detail. A number of screening and assessment instruments exist to detect illicit drug use, and some have been validated in medical populations. These include a single question screen: "*How many times in the past year have you used an illegal drug or used a prescription medication for non-medical reasons?*" Any positive response (> 0) to this screening question should prompt further assessment for a substance use disorder, as well as for recency of use and particular drugs used [19]. The CAGE-Adapted to Include Drugs (CAGE-AID) is another validated screening tool that identifies both alcohol and drug use (by adding "or drugs"). As is true for the unmodified CAGE, it is not particularly sensitive for risky use [20].

Assessment

As for alcohol, use of illicit drugs may range from low-risk use to abuse or dependence. Any illicit drug use carries some risk of social and legal consequences, (loss of employment, arrest, etc.), but not all use requires the same level of clinical attention. Specific information about what substances are used, and at what level of risk, is needed to guide interventions. That information can be gained through an in-depth diagnostic interview, but this is impractical in most clinical primary care settings. As an alternative, brief structured assessment instruments have been developed that address the degree and severity of drug use. Their use is required by most payors providing reimbursement for "screening, brief intervention and referral to treatment" (SBIRT) services [21]. In some settings, these instruments are used without an initial screen, but in environments with low prevalence of substance use disorders or limited time (as is the case for most primary care settings), it may be more feasible to administer them only to individuals who have a positive response to a brief screening question. The instruments most commonly used, which have been validated in adult populations, are the Alcohol, Smoking, and Substance Involvement Screening Test (ASSIST), Drug Abuse Screening Test (DAST-10), and Drug Use Disorders Identification Test (DUDIT) (see Table 12.1). The CRAFFT is widely used for adolescents [22].

Among these assessment tools, the alcohol, smoking, and substance involvement screening test (ASSIST) provides the most comprehensive and clinically relevant assessment, because it offers a substance-specific risk score that provides guidance for further intervention. For example, a patient may have high-risk alcohol use, moderate risk cocaine use, and low-risk marijuana use. The NIDA-modified (NM) ASSIST adds specific items on misuse of prescription stimulants and prescription opioids, while streamlining the assessment for alcohol and tobacco (an advantage if another tool is used for alcohol/tobacco assessment but a disadvantage otherwise) [23]. The NM-ASSIST has not been validated, though the ASSIST instrument on which it is based has undergone extensive validation testing in diverse populations as a screening test, and in one study, as a guide to intervention [24].

Though these assessments were largely developed with healthcare settings in mind, integrating them into routine medical care can be challenging. The key clinical distinction is whether or not dependence is present, because intervention differs based on this level of severity (i.e., brief intervention vs. referral to specialty treatment and/or pharmacotherapy). Most of these assessments require 5–15 min of face-to-face interaction with the patient to administer, which is far too long for the typical office visit, and they do not necessarily yield a dependence diagnosis, (though high-risk levels identified do correlate with dependence). The ASSIST and NM-ASSIST additionally have complex skip patterns, and require the provider to calculate risk scores using a specific scoring system. However, automation using computer-administered versions of these assessments may significantly streamline and simplify their use, and may make patient self-administered assessment feasible. The ASSIST and NM-ASSIST are currently available in a web-based format [25, 26].

For patients with current moderate- or high-risk drug use, a clinical interview may follow the structured assessment, and guide subsequent interventions. This should ascertain (1) amount, frequency, route of administration, and duration of use for each substance used; and (2) behavioral risks (overdose, sexual risk). Past drug treatment and self-help (Alcoholics Anonymous (AA), Narcotics Anonymous (NA), other) activities may also be relevant, particularly if a treatment referral is being offered.

Urine drug screens are not a substitute for asking patients about drug use. With the exception of marijuana, which may be detected in the urine for a month or more, a positive drug screen usually reflects only recent use (past 1–4 days). Clinicians should also be aware that commonly used urine toxicology assays do not test for all potential drugs of abuse. An expanded drug screen may be required to detect prescription opioid use, and to distinguish between pharmaceutical and illicit opioids. False positives can occur (as can false negatives due to test characteristics and purposeful evasion) and interpretation can be difficult and may require consultation with a clinical pathologist.

Table 12.1 Validated brief instruments for substance use assessment [25]

Instrument	No. of items (time required)	Target population	Measures recent or lifetime use?	Administered by clinician or patient self-administered?	Includes alcohol or tobacco?	Substance specific results?
Alcohol, Smoking, and Substance Involvement Screening Test (ASSIST)[a] [24]	10 initial items, followed by 1–6 additional items for each substance used, and one question on injection drug use (5–15 min)	Adults	Recent (3 mos) and lifetime	Clinician	Yes—both	Yes
Drug abuse screening test (DAST)-10 [19, 85]	10 items (5 min)	Adults	Lifetime	Patient	No	No
Drug Use Disorders Identification Test (DUDIT) [86]	11 items (5 min)	Adults and Adolescents	Recent[b]	Patient	No	No
CRAFFT [22]	6 items (3 min)	Adolescents	Lifetime	Clinician or patient	Yes—alcohol	No

Examples of these instruments can be found in Appendix 1

[a] The NIDA-modified ASSIST is an adapted version of the ASSIST that has not yet been validated. The web-based version can be accessed at: http://www.drugabuse.gov/nidamed/screening/

[b] Two questions do not address lifetime problems related to drug use, but focus of the instrument is recent (current, past year) use

Implications of Comorbid Drug Use

An important reason to identify tobacco and illicit drug use is to address common comorbidities. Medical illness takes a heavy toll among drug users, due to a number of interrelated factors. Direct toxicities of drugs themselves are responsible for a wide variety of medical sequelae, and behaviors associated with drug use (e.g., injection) place drug users at elevated risk for specific conditions (e.g., endocarditis, HIV). Socioeconomic disadvantage and poverty confer environmental risk for infections (e.g., tuberculosis), violence, and accidents. Finally, diminished access to and effective use of care, and disruption of daily routines by active drug use (impeding self-care behaviors such as adherence with medication or appointments) adversely affect clinical outcomes.

The stigma associated with illicit drug use often makes patients reluctant to discuss drug-related problems, out of embarrassment or fear that it will compromise their relationship with the physician [27, 28]. Non-judgmental discussions about drug use in the context of overall health can build effective provider–patient partnerships, and addressing drug use leads to better care of chronic health conditions [10]. The more the physician knows about the patient's drug and alcohol use, the greater the chances that medication interactions or complications from overlapping medical and psychiatric comorbidities will be averted.

Common Comorbidities

Many chronic conditions are more common among people who use drugs than among the general population [29–32].

The litany of medical problems associated with tobacco use is long, and is familiar to most health professionals. Alcohol and tobacco use in combination pose particular health risks. Use of these substances acts synergistically (not just additively) to increase risk of oropharyngeal cancer, laryngeal cancer, and squamous cell carcinoma of the esophagus [33]. Patients with alcohol use disorders who smoke have more structural and functional (cognitive) brain impairment than do those who do not smoke [34]. Alcohol and tobacco act as independent risk factors for other diseases (e.g., liver cancer) [33].

With respect to illicit drug use, most medical providers are aware of infectious diseases (HIV, hepatitis C) that occur at increased rates, particularly among injection drug users. However, illicit drug users are disproportionately affected by a much wider range of chronic conditions (see Table 12.2) [29, 35]. Sexually transmitted infections are common among substance users, often associated with sexual risk incurred in the setting of intoxication and impaired judgment, as well as with exchange of sex for money or drugs. HIV and hepatitis B are transmitted among drug users both sexually and parenterally.

Co-occurring mental health disorders are common among substance users [29, 30]. Among adults with serious psychological distress, rates of illicit drug use

Table 12.2 Medical conditions having increased prevalence among individuals with drug and alcohol abuse or dependence. (Refs. [29, 31, 32])

Pulmonary disease	Chronic obstructive pulmonary disease, asthma, pneumonia, TB
Cardiac disease	Hypertension (alcohol and cocaine); myocardial infarction, accelerated atherosclerosis, dilated cardiomyopathy (cocaine), endocarditis (injection drug use)
Gastrointestinal disease	Cirrhosis, pancreatic disease, acid disorders, gastritis
Musculoskeletal disease	Arthritis, low back pain, sequelae of traumatic injuries
Neurologic disease	Headache, cerebrovascular events (cocaine, amphetamines); seizures (benzodiazepine and alcohol withdrawal, stimulant intoxication)
Psychiatric disease	Mood disorders (depression, bipolar), anxiety disorders, major psychosis, personality disorders
Blood-borne infections	HIV, hepatitis B and C, bacteremia
Sexually transmitted infections	Syphilis, gonorrhea, chlamydia, genital herpes simplex virus, human papilloma virus, trichomoniasis, HIV

(27 %) and smoking (44 %) are approximately double that of the general population [36]. Clinicians should screen for depression, which occurs most commonly, and be attentive to signs and symptoms of mental health disorders such as anxiety, sleep disorders, and post-traumatic stress disorder [37–39]. Individuals with substance use disorders are also more likely to have been victims of violence, to be in abusive relationships, and to have experienced traumatic events [40–42].

Prevention and Harm Reduction

Preventive health care for substance users is an essential part of the clinical interaction, particularly in primary care settings. Regardless of the patient's readiness to change their drug use behaviors, focused screening and interventions for common conditions can significantly improve health, while enhancing the patient–provider relationship (Table 12.3).

Injection drug use (IDU), through the use of shared injection equipment, remains an important driver of the HIV/AIDS and hepatitis C virus (HCV) epidemics. Over one-third (36 %) of AIDS cases, and the vast majority of HCV infections, in the United States can be attributed directly or indirectly to IDU [43, 44]. The majority of these infections can be prevented through the once-only use of syringes and other injection equipment, as recommended by the US Department of Health and Human Services [45]. Though rates of new HIV infections have decreased among IDUs, largely as a result of increased access to sterile syringes, education, and resultant changes in injection behaviors, access to clean injecting equipment remains a challenge for many [46]. For health care and other treatment providers, providing counseling on the importance of once-only use of syringes and on access to sterile syringes, are essential components of preventive care for IDUs, and present opportunities for improved communication and establishment of trust between patient and provider.

Table 12.3 Preventive care for patients who use illicit drugs. (Adapted from McNeely J, Gourevitch MN, Heller D, Paone D, Lee JD. Improving the health of people who use drugs. City Health Information. 2009;28(3):21. http://www.nyc.gov/html/doh/downloads/pdf/chi/chi28-3.pdf)

HIV testing
Hepatitis B and C screening
Tuberculosis (TB) annual screening
Vaccinations
Hepatitis A and B, tetanus, and influenza
Pneumococcal vaccination for all individuals 65 and older, and regardless of age for those with unhealthy alcohol use, HIV and other chronic conditions (including heart, lung, or liver disease; diabetes; sickle cell disease)
Safe sex: Screen for high-risk behavior; counsel on condom use/safe sex practices
Consider STI screening for gonorrhea, Chlamydia, and syphilis
Intimate partner violence screening
Pregnancy: Current and future plans; contraception; counseling on risks to the fetus of smoking, alcohol and other drug use
Injection drug use: Counsel on safe injecting techniques (no sharing of any drugs, paraphernalia or syringes; single use of syringes; availability of sterile syringes)
Overdose prevention: Counsel on risk of overdose, particularly for users combining opioids with alcohol, benzodiazepines, or cocaine

Drug overdose deaths have risen dramatically in recent years [47]. This increase is primarily attributed to deaths caused by use of potent prescription opioid analgesics and secondarily to increasing deaths caused by cocaine and prescription psychotherapeutic drugs, while deaths due to heroin and other illicit drugs have remained essentially stable. Older users, and particularly those with other medical problems, are at greatest risk for fatal overdose, but older users, and particularly those with other medical problems, are also at increased risk [47]. Returning to use after a period of abstinence (and subsequent decreased tolerance), such as following an episode of drug treatment or incarceration, is associated with a significantly increased risk of overdose. Overdose deaths can be prevented, and health care providers working with substance users, particularly opioid users, have important contributions to make toward this goal. Illicit drug users should be educated about overdose risk, particularly that associated with potent or long-acting prescription opioids and using opioids in combination with alcohol, sedatives, and cocaine. In many US cities, service providers distribute naloxone to drug users and teach them how to administer it in case of opioid overdose. Evaluation of the New York City program showed that distribution and administration to IDUs is feasible and safe, and indicated that such programs may be able to reduce overdose deaths on a larger scale [48].

Managing Other Drug Use

In addition to managing medical and psychiatric comorbidities, the clinician can also effectively intervene directly to help patients reduce or stop using tobacco and other drugs.

Tobacco Use

There is strong evidence supporting clinical interventions for smoking cessation, including counseling and pharmacotherapy [49]. Given the high prevalence of tobacco use among patients with alcohol or illicit drug use disorders, the question of *when* to address tobacco cessation is commonly raised. Many clinicians will choose to address more than one substance use disorder simultaneously (e.g., alcohol and tobacco). Despite the high prevalence of comorbid tobacco and other substance-use disorders, we have little evidence about effective strategies for treating both conditions. One meta-analysis indicated that combined treatment for tobacco and other substance-use disorders does not seem to result in long-term smoking cessation (despite short-term positive effects), but does enhance abstinence from alcohol and other drugs [50]. However, other studies have not shown the same impact on alcohol and drug use [51], making it unclear what strategy works best. In general, standard tobacco cessation treatments seem to show efficacy in alcohol-dependent populations, but with lower quit rates than other populations [34]. It is possible that these populations require more intensive treatments over a longer time to optimize success. From a clinical standpoint, it is most practical to intervene on whatever substance use behavior the patient is most ready to address, and to address more than one substance if the patient is ready for that approach.

In general, smoking cessation pharmacotherapy and counseling strategies are both effective to help people quit smoking—but the combination is more effective than either component alone. According to the 2008 US Public Health Service guidelines, there are seven first-line medications available to help smokers quit: nicotine replacement therapy (NRT) in five varieties, bupropion SR, and varenicline. All of these medications are effective, and differences in performance are slight. There may be some evidence pointing to superior effectiveness of combination NRT (i.e., long-acting transdermal form plus short-acting form) or varenicline, but the superiority of these options over the other first-line medications is not clear-cut [52]. For most smokers choosing among these medications, the critical variables involve cost, mode of administration, dosing schedule, and side effect profile. Many smokers try several different medication regimens before finding one that works for them.

Evidence to date suggests that most cessation medications have similar efficacy in alcohol-dependent populations as they do in those without alcohol use disorders [53]. There have been some concerns about the use of bupropion SR and varenicline in psychiatric populations, and both medications have Food and Drug Administration (FDA) black-box warnings regarding possible suicidality. However, for neither medication is it yet clear whether the suicidality is related to a co-existing mood disorder and/or the experience of nicotine withdrawal and smoking cessation, or to the smoking cessation pharmacotherapy itself [54]. There have been case series describing the use of varenicline among psychiatrically stable alcohol-dependent patients with no unusual pattern of adverse effects [55], but there have been no large-scale trials published in this population. For bupropion, the key contraindication to consider in alcohol-dependent populations is the possibility of inducing seizures. Bupropion can

Table 12.4 Commonly prescribed medications to treat tobacco and opioid dependence

Medication	Typical dosage and frequency
Tobacco Treatment [87]	
Nicotine patch	7–21 mg patch/24 h
Short-acting nicotine	
Gum	2 mg or 4 mg (up to 24 pcs/day)
Lozenge	2 mg or 4 mg (up to 20 pcs/day)
Vapor inhaler	6–16 cartridges/day
Nasal spray	1–2 sprays/hour (up to 40 per day)
Bupropion SR	150 mg/day for 3 days, then maintenance dose of 150 mg twice daily
Varenicline	Gradual escalation over first month to maintenance dose of 1 mg twice daily
Opioid Treatment	
Methadone	60–120 mg[a] once daily [67]
Buprenorphine	16–24 mg once daily [79]
Buprenorphine HCl (Subutex™)	
Buprenorphine-naloxone (Suboxone™)	
Naltrexone (XR-NTX, Vivitrol™)	380 mg *IM* once per month [78]

[a]Methadone dose may vary widely between individuals and should be determined by a knowledgeable practitioner, guided by symptoms and treatment response of the patient

lower the seizure threshold for patients who are prone to seizures, so for patients who are actively undergoing alcohol withdrawal or have other predispositions to seizures, bupropion would not be an appropriate medication choice. (See Table 12.4.)

Illicit Drug Use

Resources to help patients reduce or stop use of illicit drugs are similar to those available for alcohol. These include brief interventions and self-help for moderate risk users, and detoxification, pharmacotherapy, mutual help and specialty treatment referrals for dependent users.

Brief interventions for illicit drug use are modeled on the same approach that has demonstrated effectiveness for unhealthy alcohol use. They typically involve a limited number of brief (10–15 min) counseling sessions that focus on helping the patient to reduce or eliminate substance use [56]. The important components of these approaches are discussed in detail in Chap. 4. Specific guidance on providing brief interventions to illicit drug users is available from NIDAMED (http://www.nida.nih.gov/nidamed/screening/), and summarized in Fig. 12.1.

Conducting an assessment of substance use with the ASSIST or NM-ASSIST provides a substance-specific risk stratification (high-moderate-low). This risk assessment can then be used to guide the clinical intervention.

There is good evidence that brief interventions can produce significant and sustained reductions in alcohol consumption [57–59]. A growing body of evidence

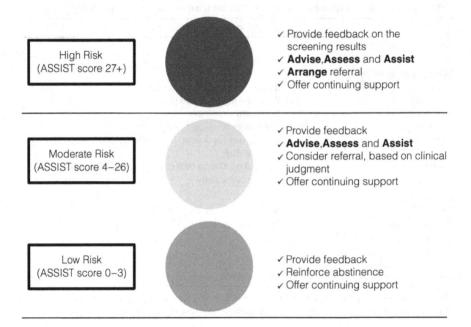

Fig. 12.1 Brief intervention for substance use. (Adapted from NIDA-MED Screening for Drug Use in General Medical Settings: Quick Reference Guide http://www.nida.nih.gov/nidamed/quickref/screening_qr.pdf)

indicates that brief interventions implemented in healthcare settings may also be effective for users of illicit drugs, though the research basis for recommending their widespread use is still being developed [60–63]. In practice, a strong case can be made for addressing illicit drug use in patients with known unhealthy alcohol use, analogous to the multidimensional approach to addressing other health behaviors (i.e., obesity, exercise) in primary care [64, 65].

A critical component of the brief intervention is working with the patient to set goals for behavior change. Some patients will be ready to address alcohol and illicit drugs concurrently, while others will choose to focus on just one substance. Some will not be ready to reduce or cease substance use, but may be receptive to counseling on preventing adverse health consequences of use. For patients who are ready to address illicit drug use, the clinician should be prepared to offer assistance in the form of brief intervention counseling, as well as referral for more intensive treatment for those who are interested in a higher level of care.

Specialty treatment for illicit drug use is based on the same principles as for alcohol, and most programs address these disorders concurrently. These programs vary widely, and may range from brief inpatient rehabilitation programs lasting one month or less, to residential settings with stays of over one year, to outpatient programs offering group counseling on a weekly basis. These programs are described elsewhere

(Chaps. 6 and 7) for treatment of alcohol disorders. Most include psychosocial and behavioral interventions, and include self-help groups such as Alcoholics Anonymous (AA) or Narcotics Anonymous (NA) both during and after formal treatment [56]. Some programs focus specifically on treatment of co-occurring psychiatric and addictive disorders.

An important distinction must be made when treating patients for opioid dependence (heroin or misuse of prescription opioids). For these patients, pharmacotherapy with methadone or buprenorphine is the treatment of choice [66]. Methadone is a long-acting opioid agonist that has been used in the treatment of opioid dependence since the early 1970s. Methadone maintenance treatment has been the most widely researched modality of substance abuse treatment, and has proven effective in reducing illicit drug use and improving health and social functioning [67, 68]. When prescribed for addiction treatment, methadone is provided through specialized methadone maintenance treatment programs (MMTPs). These structured programs dispense methadone on-site and require patients to attend regular counseling sessions.

Buprenorphine, (available as Suboxone or Subutex), is a mixed opioid agonist-antagonist, approved by the US FDA for treatment of opioid dependence in 2002. Buprenorphine carries a lower risk of abuse, dependence, and overdose compared to full opioid agonists [69]. In contrast to methadone, buprenorphine may be prescribed in a diversity of health care settings, including primary care or psychiatry clinics. Qualified physicians can prescribe buprenorphine as part of routine primary medical care, and patients fill their prescriptions at a pharmacy. Similar to methadone, buprenorphine treatment is associated with significant decreases and cessation of opioid use, decreased risk behaviors, and improved health status [70, 71]. Primary care-based buprenorphine treatment is feasible and effective even for populations that are often difficult to engage in care, including homeless patients and those with co-occuring psychiatric disorders [72, 73]. Physicians must complete an 8 hour training (portions of which can be completed online) and then apply for a DEA waiver to prescribe buprenorphine. This process is coordinated through the federal Substance Abuse and Mental Health Services Administration; information for physicians is available on the SAMHSA website (http://buprenorphine.samhsa.gov/waiver_qualifications.html) [74].

Oral and injectable naltrexone are further treatment options for office-based opioid treatment, though use of these agents to date has largely been restricted to specialty treatment settings, research studies, and highly motivated individuals averse to agonist (buprenorphine, methadone) treatment (e.g., physicians, pilots). Naltrexone is a full mu opioid antagonist with superior receptor binding affinity, which 'blocks' the euphoric and hypoventilatory effects of illicit opioids. Oral naltrexone has never gained traction as community opioid treatment, as it must be initiated only after a patient has fully withdrawn from illicit or prescriped opioids and is no longer opioid tolerant, then adhered to daily or multiple times per week, and cannot be easily restarted once relapse to opioid use occurs [75]. Extended-release naltrexone (XR-NTX) is an injectable 'depot' form of naltrexone, recently FDA-approved for alcohol (2006) and opioid (2010) dependence. XR-NTX must only be initiated following opioid detoxification, and following a 'challenge' with either naloxone or several doses of oral naltrexone in order to rule out the possibility of precipitated opioid withdrawal. A standard dose of XR-NTX provides 4 to 5 weeks of mu-opioid antagonism, during which the possibility of sustained opioid relapse and renewed opioid tolerance is thought to be remote [76–78]. It remains to be seen to what extent this long-acting formulation of naltrexone will become part of usual opioid treatment in the United States and how rates of retention and adverse events will compare to agonist medications.

As with alcohol, medically supervised detoxification should precede treatment for patients with opioid and benzodiazepine dependence, since these can cause life-threatening or severely uncomfortable withdrawal symptoms. Patients initiating opioid pharmacotherapy with methadone or buprenorphine do not require opioid detoxification prior to beginning treatment, but may still require detoxification for co-morbid alcohol or benzodiazepine use. Additionally, buprenorphine prescribers must be aware that the first dose of medication is taken when the patient experiences moderate opioid withdrawal symptoms, to avoid a precipitated withdrawal reaction [79].

Conclusion

Providers and patients alike may be reluctant to raise the subject, but putting substance use 'on the table' during the clinical interaction has inherent benefit. Engaging patients in discussions of drug and tobacco use improves patient care by helping the provider to identify and treat medical and psychiatric comorbidities, avoid potentially harmful drug interactions, understand and improve adherence to treatment, and build trust. It can also enhance the patient's ability to reduce unhealthy alcohol use.

It is part of the medical provider's role to motivate and support healthy behavior change. With respect to substance use, this means being prepared to provide the required assistance–which could include everything from nicotine replacement for smoking cessation, to a brief intervention for moderate risk cocaine use, to buprenorphine pharmacotherapy or specialty treatment referral for opioid dependence. It is thus incumbent upon primary care providers to be informed about not only tobacco and alcohol, but also illicit drug use [80]. As medicine rapidly evolves toward patient-centered models of care that integrate treatment of multiple behavioral interventions into primary care services, physicians will have increased resources, but also an increased responsibility, to address the full range of substance use and its health consequences [81–83].

References

1. Mokdad AH, Marks JS, Stroup DF, Gerberding JL. Actual causes of death in the United States, 2000. JAMA. 2004;291:1238–45.
2. Neumark YD, Van Etten ML, Anthony JC. Drug dependence and death: survival analysis of the Baltimore ECA sample from 1981–1995. Sust Use Misuse. 2000;35:313–27.
3. Robert Wood Johnson Foundation and Schneider Institute for Health Policy. Substance abuse: the nation's number one health problem. Princeton: Robert Wood Johnson Foundation; 2001.

http://www.rwjf.org/files/publications/other/SubstanceAbuseChartbook.pdf. Accessed 5 May 2011.

4. Centers for Disease Control and Prevention. Unintentional poisoning deaths–United States, 1999–2004. MMWR Morbid Mortal Wkly Rep. 2007;56:93–6.

5. Center for Substance Abuse Research (CESAR). Unintentional drug overdose deaths continue to increase; now second leading cause of unintentional deaths. CESAR Fax. 2011;20(19).

6. Substance Abuse and Mental Health Services Administration. Results from the 2009 National Survey on Drug Use and Health: National Findings. RockvilleMD: Office of Applied Studies, NSDUH Series H-38 A, HHS Publication No. SMA 10–4856Findings), 2010. http://oas.samhsa.gov/NSDUH/2k9NSDUH/2k9Results.htm #7.3.2. Accessed 5 May 2011.

7. Whitlock EP, Polen MR, Green CA, Orleans T, Klein J. Behavioral counseling interventions in primary care to reduce risky/harmful alcohol use by adults: a summary of the evidence for the U.S. Preventive Services Task Force. Ann Intern Med. 2004;140:557–68.

8. Solberg LI, Maciosek MV, Edwards NM. Primary care intervention to reduce alcohol misuse, ranking its health impact and cost effectiveness. Am J Prev Med. 2008;34:143–52.

9. Madras BK, Compton WM, Avula D, Stegbauer T, Stein JB, Clark HW. Screening, brief interventions, referral to treatment (SBIRT) for illicit drug and alcohol use at multiple healthcare sites: comparison at intake and 6 months later. Drug Alc Depend. 2009;99:280–95.

10. Laine C, Hauck WW, Gourevitch MN, Rothman J, Cohen A, Turner BJ. Regular outpatient medical and drug abuse care and subsequent hospitalization of persons who use illicit drugs. JAMA. 2001;285:2355–62.

11. Weisner C, Mertens J, Parthasarathy S, Moore C, Lu Y. Integrating primary medical care with addiction treatment: a randomized controlled trial. JAMA. 2001;286:1715–23.

12. O'Connor PG, Selwyn PA, Schottenfeld RS. Medical care for injection-drug users with human immunodeficiency virus infection. N Engl J Med. 1994;331:450–9.

13. Samet JH, Friedmann P, Saitz R. Benefits of linking primary medical care and substance abuse services: patient, provider, and societal perspectives. Arch Intern Med. 2001;161(1):85–91.

14. Institute of Medicine. Improving the quality of health care for mental and substance-use conditions. Washington, DC: National Academies Press; 2006.

15. Scott CK, Dennis ML, Laudet A, Funk RR, Simeone RS. Surviving drug addiction: the effect of treatment. Am J Public Health. 2011;737–44.

16. National Institutes of Health, National Institute on drug abuse. Strategic Plan; 2009. http://www.drugabuse.gov/StrategicPlan/StratPlan09/Index.html. Accessed 5 May 2011.

17. Kuehn BM. Treatment given high priority in new white house drug control policy. JAMA. 2010;303:821–22.

18. Agency for Healthcare Research and Quality. Helping smokers quit: a guide for clinicians. http://www.ahrq.gov/clinic/tobacco/clinhlpsmksqt.htm. Accessed 5 May 2011.

19. Smith PC, Schmidt SM, Allensworth-Davies D, Saitz R. A single-question screening test for drug use in primary care. Arch Intern Med. 2010;170:1155–60.

20. Brown RL, Rounds LA. Conjoint screening questionnaires for alcohol and other drug abuse: criterion validity in a primary care practice. Wis Med J. 1995;94:135–40.

21. Substance Abuse and Mental Health Services Administration (SAMHSA). Coding for SBI Reimbursement. http://www.samhsa.gov/prevention/SBIRT/coding.aspx. Accessed 5 May 2011.

22. Knight JR, Shrier LA, Bravender TD, Farrell M, Vander Bilt J, Shaffer HJ. A new brief screen for adolescent substance abuse. Arch Pediatr Adolesc Med. 1999;153:591–6.

23. National Institute on Drug Abuse (NIDA). Screening for drug use in general medical settings: a resource guide for providers. http://www.drugabuse.gov/nidamed/resguide/resourceguide.pdf. Accessed 14 May 2011.

24. Humeniuk R. Validation of the Alcohol, Smoking and substance involvement screening test (ASSIST) and pilot brief intervention: A technical report of phase II findings of the WHO ASSIST Project. World Health Organization; 2008. http://www.who.int/substance_abuse/activities/assist_technicalreport_phase2_final.pdf.) Accessed 14 May 2011.

25. Join Together. Drug screening.org questionnaire. http://www.drugscreening.org/about.aspx. Accessed 14 May 2011.

26. National Institute on Drug Abuse (NIDA). NIDA Quick Screen: Clinician's screening tool for drug use in general medical settings. http://ww1.drugabuse.gov/nmassist/. Accessed 14 May 2011.

27. Merrill JO, Rhodes LA, Deyo RA, Marlatt GA, Bradley KA. Mutual mistrust in the medical care of drug users: the keys to the 'narc' cabinet. J Gen Intern Med. 2002;17:327–33.

28. The National Center on Addiction and Substance Abuse (CASA) at Columbia University. Missed opportunity: National survey of primary care physicians and patients on substance abuse. April 2004. http://www.casacolumbia.org/articlefiles/380-Missed%20Opportunity%20Physicians%20and%20Patients.pdf. Accessed 5 May 2011.

29. Mertens JR, Lu YW, Parthasarathy S, Moore C, Weisner CM. Medical and psychiatric conditions of alcohol and drug treatment patients in an HMO. Arch Intern Med. 2003;163:2511–7.

30. Mertens JR, Weisner C, Ray GT, Fireman B, Walsh K. Hazardous drinkers and drug users in HMO primary care: prevalence, medical conditions, and costs. Alcohol Clin Exp Res. 2005;29:989–98.

31. Devlin RJ, Henry JA. Clinical review: major consequences of illicit drug consumption. Crit Care. 2008;12(1):202. (Epub 8 Jan. 2008)

32. Compton WM, Thomas YF, Stinson FS, et al. Prevalence, correlates, disability, and comorbidity of DSM-IV drug abuse and dependence in the United States: results from the National Epidemiologic Survey on Alcohol and Related Conditions. Arch Gen Psychiatry. 2007;64:566–76.

33. Pelucchi C, et al. Cancer risk associated with alcohol and tobacco use: focus on upper aerodigestive tract and liver. Alcohol Res Health: J Nat Inst Alcohol Abuse Alcohol. 2006;29: 193–8.

34. Kalman D, et al. Addressing tobacco use disorder in smokers in early remission from alcohol dependence: the case for integrating smoking cessation services in substance use disorder treatment programs. Clin Psychol Rev. 2010; 30:12–24.

35. Lee JD, McNeely J, Gourevitch MN. Management of associated medical conditions. In: Ruiz P, Strain E, editors. Substance abuse: a comprehensive textbook. 5th ed. Baltimore: Lippincott Williams & Wilkins; 2011 [in press].

36. Substance Abuse and Mental Health Services Administration. Results from the 2006 National Survey on Drug Use and Health: National Findings. Rockville, MD: Office of Applied Studies, NSDUH Series H-32, HHS Publication No. SMA 07-4293), 2007. http://oas.samhsa.gov/NSDUH/2k6NSDUH/2k6results.cfm#Ch8. Accessed 5 May 2011.

37. Center for Substance Abuse Treatment. Identifying and helping patients with co-occurring substance use and mental disorders: a guide for primary care providers. Subst Abuse Brief Fact Sheet. 2006;4(2). http://kap.samhsa.gov/products/brochures/pdfs/saib_fall06_v4i2.pdf

38. Ziedonis D, Brady K. Dual Diagnosis in primary care: detecting and treating both the addiction and mental illness. Med Clin North Am. 1997;81(4):1017–36.

39. Epstein J, Barker P, Vorburger M, Murtha C. Serious mental illness and its co-occurrence with substance use disorders. 2002. www.oas.samhsa.gov/CoD/Cod.htm. Accessed 14 May 2011.

40. Center for Substance Abuse Treatment. Substance abuse treatment and domestic violence. Treatment Improvement Protocol (TIP) Series 25. Rockville: U.S. Department of Health and Human Services, Substance Abuse and Mental Health Services Administration;1997.

41. McCauley JL, Danielson CK, Arnstadter AB, et al. The role of traumatic event history in non-medical use of prescription drugs among a nationally representative sample of US adolescents. J Child Psychol Psychiatry. 2010;51:84–93.

42. Miller BA, Downs WR, Gondoli DM. Spousal violence among alcoholic women as compared to a random household sample of women. J Stud Alcohol. 1989;50(6):533.

43. Centers for Disease Control and Prevention. Fact sheet: drug-associated HIV transmission continues in the United Centers for States. http://www.cdc.gov/hiv/resources/Factsheets/idu.htm. Accessed 12 August 2009.

44. Armstrong GL, Wasley A, Simard EP, McQuillan GM, Kuhnert WL, Alter MJ. The prevalence of hepatitis C virus infection in the United States, 1999 through 2002. Ann Intern Med. 2006;144:705–14.
45. U.S. Department of Health and Human Services, Public Health Service. HIV Prevention Bulletin: Medical advice for persons who inject illicit drugs. http://www.cdcnpin.org/Reports/MedAdv.pdf. Accessed 14 May 2011.
46. Hall HI, Song R, Rhodes P, et al. Estimation of HIV incidence in the United States. JAMA. 2008;300:520–29.
47. Warner-Smith M, Darke S, Lynskey M, Hall W. Heroin overdose: causes and consequences. Addiction. 2001;96:1113-25.
48. Piper TM, Stancliff S, Rudenstine S, Sherman S, Nandi V, Clear A, Galea S. Evaluation of a naloxone distribution and administration program in New York City. Sub Use Misuse. 2008;43:858–70.
49. Fiore MC, Jaen CR, Baker TB, et al. Treating tobacco use and dependence: 2008 update. Clinical Practice Guideline. Rockville: U.S. Department of Health and Human Services, Public Health Service; 2008. http://www.surgeongeneral.gov/tobacco/treating_tobacco_use08.pdf. Accessed 14 May 2011.
50. Prochaska J, Delucchi K, Hall S. A meta-analysis of smoking cessation interventions with individuals in substance abuse treatment or recovery. J Consult Clin Psychol. 2004;72:1144–56.
51. Joseph A, et al. A randomized trial of concurrent versus delayed smoking intervention for patients in alcohol dependence treatment. J Stud Alcohol. 2004;65:681–91.
52. Fiore MC, JC, Baker TB, et al. Treating tobacco use and dependence: 2008 update. Quick reference guide for clinicians. Rockville: U.S. Department of Health and Human Services, Public Health Service; 2008.
53. Cooney N, et al. Smoking cessation during alcohol treatment: a randomized trial of combination nicotine patch plus nicotine gum. Addiction. 2009;104:1588–96.
54. Gunnell D, Wise L, Davies C, Martin RM. Varenicline and suicidal behaviour: a cohort study based on data from the General Practice Research Database. Br Med J. 2009;339:b3805.
55. Hays JT, et al. Varenicline for tobacco dependence treatment in recovering alcohol-dependent smokers: an open-label pilot study. J Subst Abuse Treatment. 2011;40:102-7.
56. Center for Substance Abuse Treatment. A guide to substance abuse services for primary care clinicians. Treatment Improvement Protocol (TIP) Series 24. Rockville: U.S. Department of Health and Human Services, Substance Abuse and Mental Health Services Administration; 1997. http://www.ncbi.nlm.nih.gov/books/NBK14386/. Accessed 14 May 2011.
57. Whitlock EP, Polen MR, Green CA, Orleans T, Klein J. Behavioral counseling interventions in primary care to reduce risky/harmful alcohol use by adults: a summary of the evidence for the U.S. Preventive Services Task Force. Ann Intern Med. 2004;140:557–68.
58. Solberg LI, Maciosek MV, Edwards NM. Primary care intervention to reduce alcohol misuse, ranking its health impact and cost effectiveness. Am J Prev Med. 2008;34(2):143–52.
59. Kaner EFS, Beyer F, Dickinson HO, et al. Effectiveness of brief alcohol interventions in primary care populations. Cochrane Database Syst Rev. 2007;(2)CD004148.
60. Madras BK, Compton WM, Avula D, Stegbauer T, Stein JB, Clark HW. Screening, brief interventions, referral to treatment (SBIRT) for illicit drug and alcohol use at multiple healthcare sites: comparison at intake and 6 months later. Drug Alc Depend. 2009;99(1–3):280–95.
61. Bernstein J, Bernstein E, Tassiopoulos K, Heeren T, Levenson S, Hingson R. Brief motivational intervention at a clinic visit reduces cocaine and heroin use. Drug Alcohol Depend. 2005;77: 49–59.
62. World Health Organization. The effectiveness of a brief intervention for illicit drugs linked to the alcohol, smoking, and substance involvement screening test (ASSIST) in primary health care settings: a technical report of phase III findings of the WHO ASSIST randomized controlled trial. World Health Organization; 2008. http://www.who.int/substance_abuse/activities/assist_technicalreport_phase3_final.pdf. Accessed 14 May 2011.
63. Saitz R, Alford DP, Bernstein J, Cheng DM, Samet J, Palfai T. Screening and brief intervention for unhealthy drug use in primary care settings: randomized clinical trials are needed. J Addict Med. 2010;4:123–30.

64. Coups EJ, Gaba A, Orleans CT. Physician screening for multiple behavioral health risk factors. Am J Prevent Med. 2004;27(S1):34–41.

65. Institute of Medicine. Primary care: America's health in a new era. Washington, DC: National Academy Press; 1996.

66. National Quality Forum. National voluntary consensus standards for the treatment of substance use conditions: evidence-based treatment practices. Washington, DC: National Quality Forum; 2007.

67. Institute of Medicine. Federal regulation of methadone treatment. In: Rettig RA, Yarmolinsky A, editors. Washington, DC: National Academy Press; 1995.

68. Institute of Medicine. Treating drug problems, Vol. 1. In Gerstein DR, Harwood HJ, editors. Washington, DC: National Academy Press; 1990.

69. Walsh SL, Preston KL, Stitzer ML, Cone EJ, Bigelow GE. Clinical pharmacology of buprenorphine: ceiling effects at high doses. Clin Pharmacol Ther. 1994;55:569–80.

70. O'Connor PG, Oliveto AH, Shi JM, et al. A randomized trial of buprenorphine maintenance for heroin dependence in a primary care clinic for substance users versus a methadone clinic. Am J Med. 1998;105:100–5.

71. Substance Abuse and Mental Health Services Administration. The SAMHSA evaluation of the impact of the DATA Waiver Program: final summary report. Rockville: Center for Substance Abuse Treatment, US Dept. of Health and Human Services; 2006. www.buprenorphine.samhsa. gov/FOR_FINAL_summaryreport_colorized.pdf. Accessed 14 May 2011.

72. Alford DP, LaBelle CT, Richardson JM, et al. Treating homeless opioid dependent patients with buprenorphine in an office-based setting. J Gen Intern Med. 2007;22:171–6.

73. Kosten TR, Morgan C, Kosten TA. Depressive symptoms during buprenorphine treatment of opioid abusers. J Sub Abuse Treatment. 1990;7:51–4.

74. Center for Substance Abuse Treatment (CSAT) Buprenorphine Information Center. http://www.buprenorphine.samhsa.gov/. Accessed 14 May 2011.

75. Minozzi S, Amato L, Vecchi S, Davoli M, Kirchmayer U, Verster A. Oral naltrexone maintenance treatment for opioid dependence. Cochrane Database Syst Rev. 2011;4:CD001333.

76. Sullivan MA, Vosburg SK, Comer SD. Depot naltrexone: antagonism of the reinforcing, subjective, and physiological effects of heroin. Psychopharmacology (Berl). 2006;189:37–46.

77. Comer SD, Sullivan MA, Yu E, Rothenberg JL, Kleber HD, Kampman K, Dackis C, O'Brien CP. Injectable, sustained-release naltrexone for the treatment of opioid dependence: a randomized, placebo-controlled trial. Arch Gen Psychiatry. 2006;63:210–8.

78. Krupitsky E, Nunes EV, Ling W, Illepereuma A, Gastfriend DR, Silverman BL. Injectable extended-release naltrexone for opioid dependence: a double-blind, placebo-controlled, multicentre randomized trial. Lancet. 2011;377:1506–13.

79. Substance Abuse and Mental Health Services Administration Center for Substance Abuse Treatment (CSAT). Clinical guidelines for the use of buprenorphine in the treatment of opioid addiction: substance abuse and mental health services administration; 2004.

80. O'Connor PG, Nyquist JG, McLellan AT. Integrating addiction medicine into graduate medical education in primary care: the time has come. Ann Int Med. 2011;154:56–9.

81. Pincus HA, Spaeth-Rublee B, Watkins KE. The case for measuring quality in mental health and substance abuse care. Health Affairs. 2011;30:730–36.

82. Croghan TW, Brown JD. Integrating mental health treatment into the patient centered medical home. (prepared by Mathematica Policy Research under Contract No. HHSA290200900019ITO2.) AHRQ Publication No. 10–0084-EF. Rockville: Agency for Healthcare Research and Quality; 2010.

83. Institute of Medicine. Improving the quality of health care for mental and substance-use conditions. Washington, DC: National Academies Press; 2006.

84. Lanier D and Ko S. Screening in primary care settings for illicit drug use: assessment of screening instruments—a supplemental evidence update for the U.S. Preventive Services Task Force. Evid Synth. 2008;58(2):1–13 (AHRQ).

85. Skinner HA. The drug abuse screening test. Addict Behav. 1982;7:363–7.

86. Berman AH, Bergman H, Palmstierna T, Schlyter F. Evaluation of the Drug Use Disorders Identification Test (DUDIT) in criminal justice and detoxification settings and in a swedish population sample. Eur Addict Res. 2005;11:22–31.
87. Tran N. Treating tobacco addiction. City Health Inf. 2010;29(suppl 3):1–8. http://www.nyc.gov/html/doh/downloads/pdf/chi/chi29-suppl3.pdf. Accessed 3 June 2011.

Chapter 13
To Drink or Not to Drink? "Moderate" Alcohol Consumption in a Clinical Context

Timothy S. Naimi

Overview

Most of this book is oriented towards identifying and intervening with those who drink risky amounts or in risky ways, and working with them either to reduce or discontinue their drinking. However, the public has become engaged in the controversy surrounding "moderate" drinking. In addition, many health professionals believe that moderate alcohol consumption has health benefits, and some espouse moderate alcohol consumption as a potential preventive or therapeutic agent or as part of a healthy lifestyle. While there are clear risks and potential benefits associated with alcohol consumption, these have been reviewed elsewhere. Instead, this chapter will focus on the narrower clinical context around counseling patients who don't drink at all, or who drink at levels below thresholds used to delineate risky drinking. The topic of "moderate" drinking also has relevance for patients drinking risky amounts who might consider cutting back on their alcohol consumption. In this regard, there are two issues to address: The first is whether a non-drinker should consider beginning to drink for possible health benefits, and the second is what constitutes low-risk drinking for those who already consume alcohol. This approach may also save time and effort for those clinicians who might otherwise try to weigh complex, individualized decisions with their patients when that time might be better invested on other important aspects of patient care.

Definitional and Contextual Issues

What, exactly, is "moderate" drinking? For clinicians, the joke goes that moderate drinking is defined as alcohol consumption in a patient that does not exceed that of the physician. There is some truth to this in that no single definition of moderate

T. S. Naimi (✉)
Clinical Addictions Research Unit, Section of General Internal Medicine,
Boston Medical Center, Boston, MA, USA

Boston University Schools of Medicine and Public Health, Boston, MA, USA
e-mail: Timothy.naimi@bmc.org

R. Saitz (ed.), *Addressing Unhealthy Alcohol Use in Primary Care,*
DOI 10.1007/978-1-4614-4779-5_13, © Springer Science+Business Media New York 2013

drinking is widely recognized, and thus the term exists largely as a colloquial—rather than medical—term for patients and physicians alike. This lack of a standardized definition is reflected in the panoply of additional terms used to circumscribe this concept, including "social" drinking, "light" drinking, "responsible drinking," or "occasional" drinking. It is not clear how most clinicians define moderate drinking, but many may think of it as the absence of drinking at levels delineating clearly risky consumption, or as an absence of any adverse consequences of alcohol consumption, or simply as a lack of a diagnosable alcohol use disorder (i.e., alcohol abuse or alcohol dependence) among those who drink. Researchers often define moderate drinking on the basis of daily 1 or 2 drink thresholds, but these levels may pertain to *average* consumption, or to *per-occasion* or *consumption during drinking days* (i.e., days when people actually drink). While there is little research on the subject, members of the general public are unfamiliar with low-risk drinking guidelines.

The lack of a clear, quantitative definition of moderate drinking is less than ideal since it permits alcohol-related relativism and renders the term inordinately value-laden. In other words, few patients would choose to believe or acknowledge that they drink immoderately or irresponsibly (i.e., other than moderately or responsibly). In addition, the lack of a clear definition may hinder physicians when communicating with patients about alcohol consumption levels that constitute low-risk drinking. By contrast, there is less ambiguity when it comes to physicians knowing optimal blood pressure or blood glucose levels. In an encouraging development, the recently updated U.S. Dietary Guidelines defined moderate drinking as consuming "up to 1 drink per day for women and up to 2 drinks per day for men [1]". It is important to note that the 1/2 thresholds in the Dietary Guidelines *refer to consumption during drinking days, and not average alcohol consumption*. Previously, the 2005 Dietary Guidelines described these levels of consumption as drinking "in moderation". Nonetheless, this seems likely to be promulgated as the standard definition of moderate or low-risk drinking in the future.

But what are we after conceptually? In a clinical context, we should be communicating in terms of risk, and among those who already drink, we should recommend drinking that minimizes harms (or maximizes benefits, depending on one's perspective). In this light, the term "low-risk" drinking, rather than moderate drinking, seems a more appropriate term for clinicians and public health professionals. This would keep the focus on risk, and would be implicitly aligned with quantitative levels of alcohol consumption that are evidence-based rather than value-laden. The low-risk drinking term is also a reminder that any alcohol consumption (even amounts thought by some to be beneficial) is associated with some risk. For example, even drinking a few drinks on a per-occasion basis increases the risk of motor vehicle crashes, unintentional injuries, and other adverse outcomes [2–5]. Furthermore, compared with no alcohol consumption there is a positive linear relationship between average alcohol consumption and the death risk among those aged 40 years old and younger, and there are some patient populations in which any alcohol consumption is considered risky, such as those with current or past alcohol dependence, those on multiple medications, pregnant women, and youth. In addition, ethanol is a recognized human carcinogen that increases the risk for a number of cancers, even at low levels of consumption [6–9]. Finally, people who do not drink at risky levels subsequently may progress to risky drinking or develop an alcohol use disorder [10].

Should Clinicians Recommend Drinking to Their Patients Who Don't?

Recommending that clinicians talk to their patients about alcohol consumption has become a common recommendation arising from epidemiological studies about associations between alcohol consumption and selected health outcomes. Should a physician recommend that a non-drinker consider drinking for health-related reasons? In a clinical context, this is tantamount to prescribing alcohol as a therapeutic or chemoprophylactic agent (like isoniazid or aspirin). So from a pharmacologic perspective, would low-dose alcohol qualify as a preventative therapeutic agent? Would it meet US Food and Drug Administration approval based on randomized trials delineating efficacy and harms to appropriately evaluate the risks and benefits? The answer to both questions is no, and the US Dietary Guidelines explicitly discourage anyone from initiating alcohol consumption or drinking more frequently on the basis of health considerations [1].

To date, there have been no (zero) randomized trials about alcohol consumption and any morbidity or mortality outcome. Furthermore, alcohol might not qualify as a study drug, given its adverse safety profile: Alcohol has a high potential for abuse and dependence, is a recognized human carcinogen, and is a leading preventable cause of death and disability worldwide [6, 11, 12]. In the US alcohol is a leading preventable cause of death [13] and accounts for approximately 80,000 deaths annually, with an average of 29 years of life lost per alcohol-attributable death. Even assuming cardiovascular health benefits for low-dose alcohol based on associations found in observational studies, alcohol consumption causes many more deaths and years of potential life lost that it "prevents" in the United States and Canada [14, 15].

Although, most observational studies have found a J-shaped curve in which low average alcohol consumption is associated with lower mortality than not drinking at all, it is important to remember that reams of consistent observational studies can be consistently wrong. Indeed, findings from even well done observational studies with plausible biologic hypotheses may differ from those of randomized controlled trials, and these differences are believed to be partly due to residual or unmeasured confounding (factors that explain the relation with health outcome besides alcohol that are associated with both alcohol use and the health outcome). For example, observational studies suggested that increased beta carotene intake might be associated with reductions in cardiovascular disease (CVD) and cancer, and that hormone replacement therapy and vitamin E supplementation were associated with reductions in CVD and dementia, and that *Chlamydia* infection was associated with atherosclerotic heart disease. However, beta-carotene, vitamin E, hormone replacement therapy, and antimicrobial treatment for *Chlamydia* were found to be ineffective or harmful when subjected to randomized trials [16–20]. Hormone replacement therapy offers a particularly striking example, since dozens well-done observational studies by the world's leading epidemiologists suggested 40 % reductions in coronary heart disease.

While confounding (i.e., when the relationship between exposure and outcome is influenced by one or more factors associated with both exposure and outcome, but is unrelated to potential causal mechanisms between the two) is an important theoretical consideration in any observational study. Evidence suggests that confounding is a serious problem in alcohol studies conducted among Western populations. First, most traditional coronary heart disease risk factors are more prevalent and intense among non-drinkers [21, 22], and most analyses attempt to account for these differences statistically. Even in well-controlled studies, however, residual confounding (i.e., effects of these risk factors that are insufficiently eliminated by statistical tools) would likely bias studies in favor of moderate drinkers compared with non-drinkers. Furthermore, those with more risk factors have more possible combinations of risk factors that could be synergistic. To the extent that synergistic risks (i.e., independent effects of interactions between multiple factors) are not captured in observational studies, this would further bias studies in favor of moderate drinkers. Finally, because coronary heart disease risk factors tend to cluster in certain individuals and populations, it seems plausible that unknown or unmeasured confounders may also be more prevalent among non-drinkers than those with low average alcohol consumption, again biasing studies in favor of moderate drinkers.

In addition to the distribution of traditional cardiac risk factors, moderate average alcohol consumption appears to be a marker of affluence, leisure, education, social advantage, good mental health, healthy behaviors (such as healthy diets and physical activity) and having nice teeth (literally) [21, 23], and none of these factors or favorable circumstances is plausibly caused by alcohol consumption itself. These psycho-socio-economic markers, many of which are also considered "nontraditional" risk factors, are, in turn, major determinants of mortality [24]. Since there are no likely causal relationships between, for example, drinking alcohol and having previously achieved higher educational attainment, it seems particularly likely that moderate drinking is merely a reflection or result of prosperity and wellness, rather than its genesis. This observation makes non-traditional risk factors a rich source of potential confounding that could distort or explain the apparent relationship between alcohol consumption and favorable health outcomes. Unfortunately, unlike traditional risk factors, few surveys that include alcohol consumption also include questions about many (if any) of these non-traditional risk factors, which makes it difficult or impossible to account for them statistically.

As with confounding, selection bias (i.e., when there is a systematic error in the selection or enrollment of study subjects that distorts the relationship between alcohol and outcomes) is more than a theoretical problem with existing observational studies of low-dose alcohol. Established moderate drinkers enrolled in observational studies or participating in surveys are a select group different than non-drinkers who might be randomized to drink in a trial: They themselves elected to drink alcohol; they probably tolerated or enjoyed its effects since they did not stop drinking prior to the survey or inception of the study cohort (otherwise they would have been classified as non-drinkers or former drinkers); they did not become heavy drinkers (otherwise they would have not have been classified as moderate drinkers); they did not die from alcohol (otherwise they would have been unavailable to participate); and they were of sufficient physical and mental capacity to be study respondents or survey participants.

The "sick quitter" issue is another type of selection bias based on the fact that those who are ill or frail often stop drinking and become non-drinkers [25]. In some studies, former drinkers, which include sick quitters, are combined with the non-drinking group, thus contaminating non-drinking study groups with unhealthy persons who were previously exposed to alcohol [26]. This is inevitable when information is obtained only about current but not prior alcohol consumption, as is often the case. When information about previous drinking status is available, however, many researchers mitigate the sick quitter bias by excluding former drinkers from their analyses. However, this still biases results against nondrinkers, since it selectively removes a frail population whose poor health outcomes attributable to alcohol consumption would otherwise have accrued to the drinking group in a randomized trial with an intention-to-treat protocol (the type of evidence required for medication approval) [27].

Rates of alcohol-related problems and binge drinking are lower among study participants compared with the general population [28, 29], and approximately one-quarter of US adults who consume moderately, based on average consumption, also binge drink (i.e., consumed 5 or more drinks on ≥ 1 occasions during the past 30 days) [30]. Since binge drinking is associated with a loss of any protective association between alcohol consumption and coronary heart disease [31–34], the associations between moderate alcohol consumption and disease outcomes observed in studies may overestimate benefits (or underestimate the risks) of moderate drinking compared to what would be observed among the general population.

Many of the limitations discussed above could be addressed by conducting randomized controlled trials of low-dose alcohol; such trials are feasible and can and have been conducted [35]. However, were randomized trials to demonstrate that moderate drinking reduced CVD or all-cause mortality in supervised trial populations, there are additional considerations to be addressed before recommending drinking to any segment of the general population. In real world scenarios, for example, how many people with contraindications to alcohol consumption might begin to drink? How many who might benefit from low-dose ethanol would begin to drink but at higher doses, or develop an alcohol-related problem or an alcohol use disorder? Finally, to what extent would risky drinkers or youth use any health recommendation promoting any amount of alcohol consumption to justify their drinking or resist the notion that their drinking is problematic?

These questions are particularly important since members of the general public would not receive the careful screening and follow-up provided to clinical trial participants. Many Americans don't routinely visit health providers at all. Among those who do, relatively few are screened about their use of alcohol, despite the fact that such screening is recommended by the U.S. Preventive Services Task Force [36]. As it is, most Americans overestimate the number of drinks that constitute "moderate" drinking [37], approximately half of current drinkers in the United States consume alcohol in excess of U.S. Dietary Guidelines limits, and approximately 30 % of current drinkers report past month binge drinking.

For Patients Who Consume Alcohol, How Much Should they Drink?

For those who already drink alcohol and have no contraindications to drinking, the U.S. Dietary Guidelines limits are up to 1 drink per day for women and up to 2 drinks per day for men. As mentioned earlier, these levels refer to consumption during drinking days, and not to average daily consumption [1]. Generally speaking, this means that drinking less alcohol when one drinks will result in better health outcomes than drinking more [38]. Some clinicians feel uncomfortable with the perceived stringency of these recommended limits. This is partly due to the fact that per-occasion consumption among many drinkers (including health professionals) exceeds these levels, and there may be an assumption that drinking above these thresholds is associated with the health effects and stigma associated with an alcohol use disorder. While this concern is understandable, the mere absence of clearly risky drinking does not necessarily constitute low-risk drinking. From a guidelines perspective, risky drinking is defined as consuming 4 or more drinks for women or 5 or more drinks for men in a day, or the consumption of > 7 drinks per week for women or > 14 drinks per week for men, or an average consumption of > 1 drinks per day for women and > 2 drinks per day for men. Assuming one does not exceed the weekly (i.e., average) guideline, in terms of *consumption during drinking days* there is a "gray area" of alcohol consumption between the low-risk limits in the U.S. Dietary Guidelines (1/2 drinks in a day for women and men, respectively) and the thresholds just below risky drinking (3/4 drinks in a day for women and men, respectively).

Recently, a study demonstrated that drinking in the gray area of daily consumption was associated with increased risk of prevalent and incident alcohol dependence, incident alcohol-related interpersonal problems, and prevalent job loss compared with those who drank within the Dietary Guidelines recommendation [10]. In addition, evidence suggests that drinking in excess of the 1/2 daily limits for women and men is associated with an increased risk of the metabolic syndrome and hypertension [39]. Furthermore, the risk of unintentional injuries and motor vehicle crashes is increased when drinking 3 or 4 drinks or when one attains blood alcohol concentrations associated with drinking at those levels compared with not drinking at all [2, 5]. And finally, although drinking 3/4 drinks for women or men falls just short of levels defining binge drinking, a number of studies have demonstrated that binge drinking nullifies the protective associations between low average alcohol consumption and coronary heart disease in observational studies.

Because average alcohol consumption is a mathematical calculation that does not necessarily capture discrepant patterns about how people actually drink within groups circumscribed by fixed levels of average consumption, and because drinking patterns are increasingly recognized as crucial determinants for alcohol-related outcomes [40, 41], average alcohol consumption is poorly suited as a sole metric on which to base recommendations about low-risk drinking. In fact, however, the vast majority of studies about alcohol-related mortality and chronic disease outcomes are based on studies of average alcohol consumption (and often about consumption reported for a very brief time period decades before the outcome of interest). Despite this limitation, the nadir for mortality risk based on average alcohol consumption is only approximately one-half of a standard U.S. drink per day for men and approximately one-third of a drink per day for women [42], which is even less than the "one a day that [purportedly] keeps the doctor away." Importantly, these meager levels of average alcohol consumption are considerably less than the U.S. Dietary Guidelines' limits for daily consumption. In addition, there is generally no protective association with low-risk alcohol consumption and reduced mortality in those less than 40 years of age.

Given competing mortality risks from alcohol, it seems especially important to consider all-cause mortality as the metric of interest when assessing its health effects. Existing studies endorse the idea that various levels of average alcohol consumption have variable effects for different health outcomes [43, 44]. As with studies about total mortality, these conclusions are based on non-randomized studies. Most studies find that low average alcohol consumption is associated with small-to-moderate reductions in CVD outcomes including myocardial infarction and ischemic stroke, but an increased risk at higher average consumption levels [45]. Most studies find an increased risk of cancer death associated with alcohol consumption; while most of this excess risk is due to relatively high levels of average consumption, certain cancers are more common even at low levels of ethanol consumption, including breast cancer [9, 46]. The risk of injury increases with increasing amounts of average alcohol consumption; this increase is observed with consumption of 2 drinks per day, and increases dramatically at higher levels of alcohol consumption [47].

The Bottom Line

The controversy around moderate alcohol consumption has become a distraction for patients and physicians, and can detract from efforts to implement effective clinical and policy interventions to reduce risky drinking. While it is possible that low-dose alcohol consumption may be beneficial for some health outcomes, the appeal of possible health panaceas generally, and of alcohol in particular (because many enjoy drinking), may have resulted in a reduced scientific standard when considering low-dose alcohol as a potential therapeutic agent. To date, there has not been a single randomized controlled trial of low-dose alcohol consumption and any morbidity or mortality outcome, and existing observational studies are limited by confounding and selection bias. Furthermore, alcohol is a leading preventable cause of death and social problems in the United States and elsewhere. Therefore, absent evidence from randomized trials and weighing the real-world implications of any public health or clinical guidelines promoting alcohol consumption, we think clinicians should follow current clinical and public health recommendations which focus on reducing excessive drinking among those who already drink, and which discourage the initiation of alcohol consumption or more frequent drinking for health reasons. Among all drinkers, reducing alcohol consumption to low-risk levels outlined in the U.S. Dietary Guidelines (reducing consumption to no more than 2 drinks in a day for men or 1 drink in a day for women) would yield enormous clinical, public health and social benefits. Were there health benefits from low-dose ethanol consumption, such reductions in consumption would have the salutary side-effect of increasing the number of persons to whom such benefits might accrue.

References

1. U.S. Department of Health and Human Services and U.S. Department of Agriculture. Dietary Guidelines for Americans, 2010. http://www.health.gov/dietaryguidelines/dga2010/DietaryGuidelines2010. pdf. Accessed 5 Nov 2011.
2. Vinson DC, MacLure M, Reidinger C, et al. A population-based case-crossover and case-control study of alcohol and the risk of injury. J Stud Alcohol. 2003;64:358–366.
3. Wechsler H, Nelson TF. Relationship between level of consumption and harms in assessing drink cut-points for alcohol research: commentary on Many college freshmen drink at levels far beyond the binge threshold by White et al. Alc Clin Exp Res. 2006;30:922–927.
4. Weitzman ER, Nelson TF. College student binge drinking and the prevention paradox: implications for prevention and harm reduction. J Drug Education. 2004;34:247–266.
5. Zador PL, Krawchuk SA, Voas RB. Alcohol-related relative risk of driver fatalities and driver involvement in fatal crashes in relation to driver age and gender: an update using 1996 data. J Stud Alcohol. 2000;61:387–395.
6. National Toxicology Program, U.S. Department of Health and Human Services. Report on Carcinogens, 12th ed. 2011. http://ntp.niehs.nih.gov/ntp/roc/twelfth/roc12.pdf. Accessed 10 Nov 2011.
7. Allen NE, Beral V, Casabonne D, et al. Moderate alcohol intake and cancer incidence in women. J Natl Cancer Inst. 2009;101:296–305.
8. Baan R, Straif K, Secretan B, et al. World Health Organization International Agency for Research no Cancer Monograph Working Group. Carcinogenicity of alcoholic beverages. Lancet Oncology. 2007;8:292–293.
9. Bagnardi V, Blangiardo M, La Vecchia C, et al. A meta-analysis of alcohol drinking and cancer risk. Br J Cancer. 2001;85:1700–1705.
10. Dawson DA, Grant BE. The gray area of consumption between moderate and risk drinking. J Stud Alc Drugs. 2011;72:453–458.
11. Ezzati M, Lopez AD, Rodgers A, et al. Selected major risk factors and global and regional burden of disease. Lancet. 2002;360:1347–1360.
12. National Institute on Alcohol Abuse and Alcoholism. Tenth Special Report to the U.S. Congress on Alcohol and Health. Bethesda: National Institutes of Health; 2000.
13. Mokdad AH, Stroup D, Marks JS, et al. Actual causes of death in the United States, 2000. JAMA. 2004;291:1238–1245.
14. Centers for Disease Control and Prevention. Alcohol-Related Disease Impact (ARDI). http://www.cdc.gov/alcohol/ardi.htm. Accessed 28 March 2008.
15. Rehm J, Mathess C, Popova S, et al. Global Burden of Disease and Injury and Economic cost Attributable to Alcohol use and Alcohol use Disorder, Lancet. 2009;373:2223–2233.

16. Anderson JL. Infection, antibiotics, and atherothrombosis—end of the road or new beginnings? N Eng J Med. 2005;352:1706–1709.
17. Blacker D. Mild cognitive impairment—no benefit from vitamin E, little from donepezil. N Eng J Med. 2005;352:2439–2441.
18. Greenberg ER. Antioxidant vitamins, cancer, and cardiovascular disease. N Eng J Med. 1996;334:1189–1190.
19. Women's Health Initiative Investigators. Risks and benefits of estrogen plus progestin in healthy postmenopausal women—principal results from the Women's Health Initiative randomized controlled trial. JAMA. 2002;288:321–333.
20. Yaffe K. Hormone therapy and the brain—deja vu all over again? JAMA. 2003;289:2717–2719.
21. Naimi TS, Brown DW, Brewer RD, et al. Cardiovascular risk factors and confounders among nondrinking and moderate-drinking U.S. adults. Am J Prev Med. 2005;28:369–373.
22. Wannamethee G, Shaper AG. Men who do not drink: a report from the British Regional Heart Study. Intl J Epidemiol. 1988;17:307–316.
23. Hansel B, Thomas F, Pannier B, et al. Relationship between alcohol intake, health and social status and cardiovascular risk factors in the urban Paris-Ile-De-France Cohort: is the cardioprotective action of alcohol a myth? European J Clin Nutr. 2010;64:561–568.
24. Marmot M. Social determinants of health inequalities. Lancet. 2005;365:1005–1006.
25. Liang W, Chkritzhs T. Reduction in alcohol consumption and health status. Addiction. 2011;106:75–81.
26. Fillmore KM, Kerr WC, Stockwell T, et al. Moderate alcohol use and reduced mortality risk: systematic error in prospective studies. Addiction Research and Theory. 2006;14:101–132.
27. Shaper AG. Alcohol consumption decreases with the development of disease. Addiction. 2011;106:123–125.
28. Jousilahti P, Veikko S, Kuulasmaa K, et al. Total and cause-specific mortality among participants and non-participants of population-based health surveys: a comprehensive followup of 54,372 Finnish men and women. J Epidemiol and Community Health. 2005;59:310–315.
29. Rosengren A, Wilhelmsen L, Berglund G, et al. Non-participants in a general population study of men, with special reference to social and alcoholic problems. Acta Med Scand. 1987;221:243–251.
30. Naimi TS, Brewer RD, Mokdad AH, Denny C, Serdula M, Marks JS. Binge drinking among U.S. adults. JAMA. 2003;289:70–75.
31. McElduff P, Dobson AJ. How much alcohol and how often? Population based case-control study of alcohol consumption and risk of a major coronary event. British Medical Journal. 1997;314:1159–1164.
32. Roerecke M, Rehm J. Irregular heavy drinking occasions and risk of ishcemic heart disease: a systematic review and meta-analysis. Am J Epidemiol. 2010. doi: 10.1093/aje/kwp1451.
33. Kauhanen H, Kaplan GA, Goldberg DE, Salonen JT. Beer binging and mortality: results from the Kuopio ischaemic heart disease risk factor study, a prospective population-based study. British Medical Journal. 1997;315:846–851.
34. Mukamal KJ, Maclure M, Muller JE, et al. Binge drinking and mortality after acute myocardial infarction. Circulation. 2005;112:3839–3845.
35. Freiberg MS, Samet JH. Alcohol and coronary heart disease: the answer awaits a randomized controlled trial. Circulation. 2005;112:1379–1381.
36. U.S. Preventive Services Task Force. Screening and behavioral counseling interventions in primary care to reduce alcohol misuse. http://www.uspreventiveservicestaskforce.org/uspstf/uspsdrin.htm. Accessed 11 Nov 2011.
37. Abel EL, Kruger ML. Hon v. Stroh Brewery Company: what do we mean by moderate and heavy drinking? Alcohol Clin Exp Res. 1995;19:1024–1031.
38. Kloner RA, Shereif RH. To drink or not to drink? That is the question. Circulation. 2007;116:1306–1317.
39. Fan AZ, Russell M, Naimi TS, et al. Patterns of alcohol consumption and the metabolic syndrome. J Clin Endocrinol Metab. 2008;93:3833–3838.

40. Rehm J, Stempos CT, Trevisan M. Alcohol and cardiovascular disease—more than one paradox to consider. Average volumes of alcohol consumption, patterns of drinking and risk of coronary heart disease—a review. J Cardiovasc Risk. 2003;10:15–20.
41. Rehm J, Baliunas D, Borges G, et al. The relationship between different dimensions of alcohol consumption adn burden of disease: an overview. Addiction. 2010;105:817–843.
42. DiCastelnuovo A, Costanzo S, Bagnardi V, et al. Alcohol dosing and total mortality in men and women: an updated meta-analysis of 34 prospective studies. Arch Intern Med. 2006;166:2437–2445.
43. Rehm J, Room R, Graham K, et al. The relationship of average volume of alcohol consumption and patterns of drinking to burden of disease: an overview. Addiction. 2003;98:1209–1228.
44. Carrao G, Bagnardi V, Zambon A. A meta-analysis of alcohol consumption and the risk of 15 diseases. Prev Med. 2004;38:613–619.
45. Corrao G, Rubbiati L, Bagnardi V, et al. Alcohol and coronary heart disease: a meta-analysis. Addiction. 2000;95:1505–1523.
46. Schutze M, Boeing H, Pischon T, et al. Alcohol attributable burden of incidence of cancer in eight European countries based on results from prospective cohort study. Br Med J. 2011;342:d1584.
47. Carrao G, Bagnardi V, Zambon A. Exploring the dose-response relationship between alcohol consumption and the risk of several alcohol-related conditions: a meta-analysis. Addiction. 1999;94:1551–1573.

Chapter 14
Electronic and Other Self-Help Materials for Unhealthy Alcohol Use in Primary Care

Steven J. Ondersma and Golfo K. Tzilos

There is ample reason to think broadly about facilitating change in unhealthy alcohol use. Data from the 2009 National Survey on Drug Use and Health (NSDUH) indicate that fully 87.7 % of the estimated 19.3 million persons in the United States who need treatment for alcohol use neither received treatment in the past year, *nor wanted such treatment* [1]. At the same time, the majority of those who recover from an alcohol use disorder do not do so via formal treatment [2–4], and brief interventions (1–2 sessions, often as brief as 15 min in length) for alcohol use frequently show results that appear equivalent to those of longer interventions [5–7], sometimes even with heavier drinkers [8]. Growing evidence suggests that even pre-treatment assessment, and/or the decision to seek help and be involved in a research study, can result in significant change [9–13].

Thus, alternative approaches could be important options for those whose unhealthy drinking is not severe enough to merit formal treatment, as well as with dependent drinkers who are currently unwilling to consider formal treatment. If successfully implemented in a primary care setting, such approaches might—through their reach and accessibility—have a meaningful population impact on unhealthy alcohol use. This may be particularly true if the overall efficacy of these approaches is often similar to that of more extended interventions. The key, from the perspective of a busy primary care setting, is whether these alternative approaches can be implemented without prohibitively large investments in time or training.

Self-help approaches—broadly defined here as any non-pharmaceutical source of assistance not involving a live counselor or other professional—may meet the need for an alternative approach that is efficacious, relatively palatable to patients exhibiting unhealthy alcohol use (UAU), and minimally burdensome to medical staff.

S. J. Ondersma (✉)
Department of Psychiatry and Behavioral Neurosciences,
Merrill-Palmer Skillman Institute, Wayne State University, Detroit, MI, USA
e-mail: sondersm@med.wayne.edu

G. K. Tzilos
Center for Alcohol & Addiction Studies, Brown University, Providence, RI, USA
e-mail: Golfo_Tzilos@brown.edu

R. Saitz (ed.), *Addressing Unhealthy Alcohol Use in Primary Care,*
DOI 10.1007/978-1-4614-4779-5_14, © Springer Science+Business Media New York 2013

Notably, self-help approaches are nearly always conceptualized as being relevant for any unhealthy use of alcohol, whether or not formal criteria for abuse or dependence are met (as we will see, however, it may be a mistake to consider such approaches only with those whose drinking does not meet diagnostic criteria). In this chapter, we will review the major classes of self-help resources available and the evidence for their efficacy, with emphasis on those that are easily accessible by clinics and patients alike.

Self-help materials for UAU exist in many forms. The present chapter will organize these many forms into four broad categories based on primary method of delivery: internet-delivered approaches, interactive voice response (IVR) methods, mobile device-based approaches, and print materials (see Table 14.1 for examples of internet and print materials). Note that some have referred to 12-step programs, such as Alcoholics Anonymous, as "self-help" since they are not run by health professionals; in this text, we refer to such programs as "mutual help," since the main mechanism of efficacy comes from participation in a group. These programs are not covered in this chapter.

Within each self-help material delivery category, interventions can vary along many dimensions. For example, although most involve a single session or mailing, some interventions involve daily interaction for as long as six months. The interventions to be described here are also personalized to varying degrees. Tailored interventions provide each user with a specific set of messages that are targeted to that individual's characteristics on a number of dimensions, such as self-efficacy, motivation, or alcohol expectancies; others provide essentially the same content to all users, or tailor only in more basic ways, such as providing feedback regarding each individual's number of drinks per year, or amount spent per year (with the latter typically being referred to as personalized normative feedback interventions rather than tailored interventions). They can be targeted generally at UAU among adults, or specifically at specialized sub-groups such as heavy drinking college students. This review will focus only on interventions that have been subjected to at least minimal empirical evaluation, defined as at least one controlled trial. We will begin with the broad category of internet-based interventions for UAU.

Internet-Delivered Feedback Interventions for UAU

Internet-delivered interventions for alcohol use take many forms (see Table 14.1, for examples). They can be passively available as websites for use by individuals who seek information or assistance, or introduced proactively (for example, by staff in a primary care setting); they can be freely available to the public, or available only to those with access (purchased or otherwise); and they can be unstructured—allowing users to freely navigate to various pages within the site—or structured, walking users through an ordered set of steps. Although the approach taken by these resources is variable, the vast majority of internet-delivered interventions for alcohol

Table 14.1 Self-help resources

Internet websites	http://www.checkyourdrinking.net
	http://www.drinkerscheckup.com
	http://www.downyourdrink.org.uk
	http://www.echeckuptogo.com (for universities)
	http://college.alcoholedu.com/ (for universities)
	http://www.rethinkingdrinking.niaaa.nih.gov
Printed material	Sobell, L & Sobell, M. Healthy Lifestyles Guided Self-Change Program, Nova Southeastern University: http://www.nova.edu/gsc
	Miller WR, Munoz RF. Controlling your drinking: tools to make moderation work for you. New York: Guilford; 2005. Self-help guide, original published in 1975 by the same authors
	A 16-page booklet from the National Institute on Alcohol Abuse & Alcoholism: http://pubs.niaaa.nih.gov/publications/RethinkingDrinking/OrderPage.htm

use are web- and feedback-based, focusing on the provision of feedback such as self-reported quantity and frequency of drinking, score on a standard risk measure (such as the Alcohol Use Disorders Identification Test (AUDIT) [14], a brief, 10-item, self-report measure to detect risky levels of alcohol use), self-reported consequences of drinking, or money spent on alcohol. Internet-based feedback interventions are generally brief and single-session, and to varying degrees involve four elements: (a) an invitation to obtain feedback regarding, for example, one's drinking and how it compares with that of others, or its association with health; (b) a brief series of self-report items regarding one's alcohol use, money spent, and consequences of drinking (e.g., concern expressed by others, health problems, failing to meet expectations because of drinking); (c) feedback regarding, for example, how one's use compares to that of others, amount of money spent in a given time period on alcohol, blood–alcohol content, etc.; and (d) information on how to change one's drinking (ranging from tips for self-change to information about treatment options). Although computer-delivered interventions cannot replicate the interpersonal elements of person-delivered interventions seen as particularly crucial to approaches such as motivational interviewing (a specific, highly specified and validated form of brief counseling intervention) [15], computer-delivered approaches may seek to: (a) be consistent with those key elements by, for example, avoiding judgment or advice-giving, and eliciting reasons to change, and (b) leveraging the unique ability of computers to use multimedia in interesting and engaging ways. Content for these programs is presented as text and images on formatted web pages; videos or 'click for more' options are sometimes used.

Internet-based Feedback Interventions for College Students

Most studies have focused on websites targeting UAU within college samples. For example, the eCHECKUPTOGO program (www.eCHECKUPTOGO.com) has been evaluated repeatedly with college student samples, and is marketed to universities and other entities that wish to customize it to their specific setting by the non-profit San Diego State University Research Foundation. Their website provides an initial screening/assessment that evaluates alcohol use, spending patterns, values (e.g., activities the respondent wishes he or she engaged in more often), weight, and other information. It then provides feedback in a number of areas, including how the respondent's drinking compares to student norms at the national level as well as at the respondent's university, the student's blood alcohol level and the consequences of higher levels, and the biphasic response to alcohol (i.e., how positive effects peak at lower levels of drinking, and decline with heavier drinking). The site also provides information about the consequences of heavier drinking (in terms of accidents, sexual risk, violence, etc.) and incorporates video content for explaining some of the more complex information in the feedback report (e.g., the biphasic response). Users are invited to check potential change methods that they believe may be helpful for them, and this information is provided in the feedback report itself.

Internet-based Feedback Interventions for General Adult Samples

An example of a similar tool for general adult populations is www.checkyour-drinking.net, a commercially owned site that is freely available online (customized versions for specific uses or settings can be purchased from the website's developer). This brief (approximately 10 min, depending on the user), single-session, feedback-based intervention begins with 18 questions regarding the extent and frequency of drinking, weight, and consequences, and subsequently provides on-screen feedback in areas such as, how the respondent's use compares to national norms, number of drinks per year, the financial cost of those drinks, AUDIT score, health effects, sensible drinking guidelines, and ways to reduce risk. This report comes in the form of a single web page with tabs for the various categories of feedback (e.g., health effects). Users are able to print the report and/or email it to a health care provider.

Support for the Efficacy of Internet-Delivered Feedback Interventions: The Bottom Line

The first report of a computer-delivered intervention for alcohol use with no therapist contact appeared in the Journal of Studies on Alcohol in 2000 [16]. This field has now grown to the extent that there are currently at least ten meta-analyses, systematic reviews, or qualitative reviews that focus, either exclusively or in part, on the efficacy of computer-delivered interventions for alcohol use (see Table 14.2). These reviews are based on at least 26 available controlled studies, 19 of which focused on drinking in college samples. Taken as a whole, these reviews present encouraging evidence of the efficacy of computer-delivered interventions for alcohol use. As seen in Table 14.2, which provides a brief overview of the available reviews that provide

Table 14.2 Between-group effect sizes in meta-analyses and systematic reviews of self-help treatment for unhealthy alcohol use

Author, Year	Sample	No. of studies	Conclusions
Computer-delivered interventions (CDIs)			
Khadjesari et al. [19]	Adult	24	CDIs reduce alcohol use by 25.9 g ethanol (2 US standard drinks)/week, vs. minimally active controls
Portnoy et al. [25]	Mixed	17	CDIs effective ($d = 0.24$) in reducing substance use (included studies of alcohol and drugs) more so when delivered in greater doses
Rooke et al. [24]	Mixed	34	CDIs reduce risky alcohol use ($d = 0.22$); effects greater vs. attention placebo than active control
Carey et al. [22]	College students	43	CDIs reduced quantity/frequency of alcohol ($d = 0.15$), but were equivalent to alternative alcohol-related comparison interventions
White et al. [23]	College students	5	CDIs reduce alcohol use at post-treatment ($d = 0.42$); also peak blood alcohol content ($d = 0.66$)
Printed self-help materials			
Apodaca and Miller. [31]	Adult	22	Printed self-help materials lead to reductions in alcohol consumption, abstinence, or gamma-glutamyl transferase ($d = 0.21$) with patients identified via screening
Computer-delivered or printed			
Riper et al. [18]	Mixed	14	Single-session personalized feedback alone reduces risky alcohol use ($d = 0.22$)

a mean between-groups effect size, these reviews tend to find positive results for brief, feedback-based internet interventions, with effect sizes analogous to those found for person-delivered brief interventions [5, 6, 17]. In one review, this level of change translated into an overall number needed to treat (NNT) to achieve benefit of 8.06 [18]; another suggested that persons in intervention groups reduced their drinking by approximately 25.9 g (approximately 2 US standard drinks) per week more than those in control groups [19]. This latter distinction is important given the already-noted tendency of persons in control conditions to also show significant pre-post reductions in drinking. In terms of results in applied settings, real reductions of over 7 standard drinks per week have been reported [20]. It is for this reason (and because of similar effects seen with in-person brief intervention after screening) that screening and brief intervention for UAU is currently recommended by the US Preventive Services Task Force [21].

Support for the Efficacy of Internet-Delivered Feedback Interventions: Other Considerations

The above "bottom-line" global summary is accurate, but those interested in delving deeper should be aware of a number of relevant caveats. First, the effects of these interventions—as with person-delivered brief interventions—are generally small in size. As seen in Table 14.2, mean effect size estimates for interventions of this type range from a low of 0.15 [22] to a high of 0.39 [23] for brief, single-session web-based feedback interventions, with three separate reviews finding a mean effect size of $d = 0.22$–0.24 [18, 24, 25]. As noted by many reviews and meta-analyses in this area, even small effects can have large public health consequences, particularly when the cost and simplicity of a given intervention are low enough to give it substantial reach [18].

Second, the effects noted in these reviews are variable. At least part of this variability is likely to be a result of poor understanding of factors that moderate their efficacy. Although reviews overall report remarkable consistency of effects across a number of potential study, design, or treatment characteristics, the possible role of a number of potential moderators must be considered. For example, there is relatively consistent evidence that studies using active and/or relevant control groups tend to find no effects [19, 22, 24]. For example, Carey et al. [22] found a significant difference in drinking-quantity effect sizes between studies using active, alcohol-relevant control groups ($d = 0.02$) and studies using minimally active controls ($d = 0.20$). In addition, interventions involving a higher dose of brief intervention (more total minutes, or multiple sessions rather than just one) have also been associated with stronger effects [23, 25], although one meta-analysis failed to find a dose effect [24]. Finally, although not evaluated directly by any reviews, at least one individual study has noted that a computer-delivered brief intervention was more efficacious with persons whose UAU was more severe [26], a finding that echoes results from one study of a therapist-delivered brief intervention for injured emergency department patients (though in primary care settings, the bulk of evidence for efficacy is for brief intervention for those without dependence) [8].

Third, a great deal is still not known about the association between efficacy and the interaction of intervention characteristics, setting, context, and individual characteristics. The failure of many intervention characteristics to clearly moderate drinking outcomes, and the apparent efficacy of control groups with even modest alcohol relevance, together suggest that parsimony may be in order; specifically that, perhaps most forms of sustained attention to one's drinking may be therapeutic, and that complex efforts to improve upon computer-delivered interventions may be in vain. At the same time, this area of research is quite new, and the replicability and modularity of computer-delivered approaches render them conducive to rigorous research that evaluates the importance of individual factors. In addition, web-based approaches could allow for extremely large sample sizes that would facilitate detection of intervention characteristics—whether globally or in interaction with individual factors and context—that can result in improvements in efficacy[1]. These two factors may in fact represent the best opportunity yet seen for behavioral science to make truly cumulative gains in intervention efficacy.

Interactive Voice Response (IVR) Interventions for UAU

IVR self-help interventions also use computers to collect data from users and to present information or feedback that is at least partially targeted based on each user's responses. Rather than using a computer screen for presenting information and accepting input, however, these approaches make use of simple telephone technology. Users are queried by voice recordings, provide answers to multiple choice questions using the telephone's keypad or by speaking into the phone, and receive personalized information or guidance in return. Proponents of this approach, like many proponents of web-based interventions, suggest that their high potential for reach, cost-effectiveness, and ability to work without time investment from medical staff make them ideal for use in primary care.

The most recent example of such an approach is described by Helzer et al. [27], who developed technology that briefly evaluated drinking during daily, 2-min, toll-free, participant-initiated telephone calls to their IVR system. They then randomly assigned drinkers—all of whom were identified in a primary care setting, and who received a physician-delivered brief intervention—to one of four conditions: (1) no further intervention; (2) instructions to make daily calls to the IVR system; (3) daily calls plus a monthly, mailed graphical feedback summarizing that participant's use in the past month, along with a brief note from that participant's physician; and (4) IVR and mailed feedback along with monetary incentives to complete the daily phone calls. Helzer et al. found that 10 % of participants in this study never initiated any calls to the IVR system, and that the remaining 90 % of participants completed a mean of 180 calls over the 6-month treatment period (representing 68 % of scheduled calls). The authors noted that incentives did not appear to increase the frequency of completing daily calls, and that the group receiving feedback showed greater reductions in drinking than the group not receiving feedback.

Mobile Device Interventions for UAU

A third electronic approach involves the use of mobile devices. Mobile devices have been relatively heavily utilized for smoking [28], and many believe that they will soon play a large, many-faceted role in health care overall. At present, there is

---

[1] Similarly, Ondersma et al. [41] have suggested that during-session data such as ratings of state motivation or satisfaction could serve as a proxy measure of likely outcome, allowing a large number of treatment characteristics to be evaluated with greater speed, and less expense, than in a traditional clinical trial.

only one published trial of a mobile-device-based self-help intervention for alcohol use. Weitzel et al. [29] describe an intervention in which 40 college students who self-reported drinking more than once per week were randomly assigned to receive either daily requests to complete a brief drinking-related survey using their handheld wireless devices, or the daily survey requests plus brief messages tailored to them on extent of drinking, expected outcomes of drinking, and self-efficacy. Participants assigned to the tailored message condition reduced drinking more than those assigned to the survey-only condition. Although a small sample, this study found significant effects despite low power and despite using a relatively active comparator.

Printed Self-Help Materials for Alcohol Use

In 1978, well before computers became part of daily life, William R. Miller reported that participants in a clinical trial who were randomly selected to receive a post-treatment self-help manual showed less drinking, at a 3-month follow-up, than participants who did not receive the manual [30]. Miller and colleagues continued to examine this finding in subsequent studies, and others followed suit; Apodaca and Miller later published a meta-analysis of what they termed "bibliotherapy" interventions for UAU (see citation and summary of findings in Table 14.2) [31]. Although print interventions were variable in length and content, most sought to reduce drinking by helping persons with UAU track their drinking, understand moderate drinking guidelines, learn self-control techniques, find alternatives to drinking, and other strategies. This review separated studies examining the effects of printed materials on drinking among persons responding to newspaper ads, versus those with participants whose risk was proactively identified via screening in primary care. The mean weighted effect size for the former group averaged $d = 0.31$, whereas effects for the proactively identified group were $d = 0.21$.

These averages, however, collapse across level of contact with an interventionist such as a therapist, nurse, or physician; in fact, most studies included in the 2004 Apodaca & Miller review included at least some non-trivial contact (e.g., a brief motivational assessment or advice session along with the printed materials). In other words, even very brief contact is almost inevitable in the process of introducing the materials. However, those studies utilizing printed self-help materials without overtly therapeutic contact with a therapist or helper appear to show effect sizes consistent with the means noted above. For example, in Heather et al. [32], participants responding to a newspaper ad and receiving only a behavioral self-help book showed greater reductions in drinking than a control group receiving just alcohol-related information (with an effect size of 0.34 in the Apodaca and Miller meta-analysis). Similarly, a large World Health Organization (WHO) study found that a condition involving printed self-help materials plus 5 min of helper contact was as effective as a condition involving the same materials and 15 min of helper contact (both groups out-performed the control condition) [33].

In a relatively large study not included in the Apodaca & Miller review, Sobell and colleagues randomly assigned 825 self-referred persons with UAU to either personalized mailed information (providing normative feedback) or untailored information [34]. Participants in both groups significantly reduced their drinking, with no differences between groups. Similarly, in a rare example of true tailoring for alcohol use (as opposed to personalized feedback on drinking), Blow et al. report the results of a four-group trial with at-risk drinkers recruited at an emergency department [35]. Participants were assigned to one of four conditions involving either a tailored or untailored message booklet (of identical superficial appearance and length under all conditions), and either brief advice or no brief advice. Results overall suggested that drinking outcomes were better in participants who received brief advice, and that the tailored message booklet was not associated with better drinking outcomes than the untailored booklet. (This latter finding is inconsistent with evidence from a recent meta-analysis, which suggests that tailored materials show a small but significant advantage over non-tailored materials [36].)

Overall, studies of printed self-help materials suggest that this relatively simple approach has utility in reducing UAU. In addition, one study of internet-based personalized feedback with and without a printed self-help book found that the addition of the book resulted in greater reductions in drinking than seen with the internet session alone [37]. However, the Apodaca & Miller meta-analysis [31] suggests that this utility is more consistent and clear with persons who self-refer than with individuals who are proactively identified in primary care settings (who naturally may be less likely to resonate with specific suggestions regarding how to reduce one's drinking). There is as yet no clear guidance regarding whether minimal helper contact is necessary along with these materials (and if so, how much helper contact is needed). However, the above-noted findings from Heather et al. [32] and the WHO study [33] suggest that these approaches may be helpful with no or minimal helper contact.

Summary

Several conclusions can be drawn from this review. First, although much more research is needed, the weight of evidence suggests that self-help interventions—defined here as any non-pharmaceutical source of assistance not involving a live counselor or other professional—are often helpful in promoting reductions in alcohol use among persons with UAU. The effects from meta-analyses of web-based and print materials are relatively consistent (as seen in Table 14.1). Although small, the magnitude of a given intervention's effects is only meaningful when considered in the context of its cost, difficulty, replicability, and reach. Self-help interventions are relatively simple and inexpensive to implement; if done so widely, they have the potential for a relatively strong public health/population impact.

Making it Happen: Practical Recommendations

Clinicians may avoid discussions of alcohol use, in part out of a sense that they lack the ability to respond appropriately or effectively with patients who screen positive [38]. The ease with which the above materials can be accessed, combined with the evidence that they can be helpful with UAU, makes them an option that should be given strong consideration by health professionals in primary care settings. A number of specific steps could be considered.

1. *Don't miss an opportunity.* Universal screening in primary care can be accomplished in a number of ways (covered elsewhere in this book), is well-tolerated by patients [39], and its strong association with a number of health outcomes makes it well within the purview of primary care. (Although not the focus of this chapter, there are also many high-quality materials available to help health care professionals to implement screening and brief intervention procedures. For example, the NIAAA Clinician's Guide, 'Helping Clients Who Drink Too Much' can be found at http://pubs.niaaa.nih.gov/publications/practitioner/cliniciansguide2005/guide. pdf, and comes with video case examples to enhance training.)

2. *Make the internet available.* A waiting-room kiosk, an exam room with a computer, a notebook computer or two, or even one of the many new tablet or handheld devices can all be the means by which identified patients can be encouraged to access a free internet-based feedback intervention. These devices can cost as little as $ 300 for a simple "net book." As seen in Table 14.1, at least four free sites could be bookmarked on one or more computers dedicated for this purpose. Of these, three have been supported in at least one clinical trial for use with general adult samples (www.checkyourdrinking.net, www.drinkerscheckup.com, and http://www.downyourdrink.org.uk). The site hosted by the National Institute on Alcohol Abuse and Alcoholism (NIAAA) (http://rethinkingdrinking.niaaa.nih.gov), despite not yet being evaluated in a clinical trial, is extremely similar to the others in content, is more thorough than most, and is perhaps the simplest to access.

3. *Have printed materials available in waiting areas and in exam rooms.* The Miller and Munoz behavioral self-control strategy book [40] is available in paperback form for $ 15 or less from major online booksellers; the print materials from the Sobell Guided Self-Change Clinic at Nova Southeastern University are available at no cost at www.nova.edu/gsc. A 16-page booklet from the National Institute on Alcohol Abuse & Alcoholism, designed to mirror what is available at the "Rethinking your Drinking" website, can be downloaded or ordered at no cost at http://pubs.niaaa.nih.gov/publications/RethinkingDrinking/OrderPage.htm. Having such materials within easy reach can greatly increase the likelihood that they will find their way into the hands of patients with UAU.

4. *Develop a fact sheet that can be handed out to patients, either universally or on a targeted basis.* This sheet could provide simple information regarding the association between drinking and health, and could additionally provide links to the websites noted above. The NIAAA website offers several fact sheets that target special patient populations (e.g., women: http://pubs.niaaa. nih.gov/publications/womensfact/womensfact.htm).

These steps can be implemented either singly or in combination, and are likely to feel more routine and less burdensome the longer they are in place. Implementing these steps in a routine way can enable any primary care practice to have a genuine impact on UAU among its patients.

References

1. Substance Abuse and Mental Health Services Administration. Results from the 2009 National Survey on Drug Use and Health. Rockville: Office of Applied Studies, NSDUH Series H-38 A, HHS Publication No. SMA 10-4586; 2010.
2. Klingemann HK, Sobell LC. Introduction: natural recovery research across substance use. Subst. Use Misuse. 2001;36(11):1409–1416.
3. Bischof G, Rumpf HJ, Hapke U, Meyer C, John U. Types of natural recovery from alcohol dependence: a cluster analytic approach. Addiction. 2003;98(12):1737–1746.
4. Burman S. The challenge of sobriety: natural recovery without treatment and self-help groups. J Subst Abuse. 1997;9:41–61.
5. Moyer A, Finney JW, Swearingen CE, Vergun P. Brief interventions for alcohol problems: a meta-analytic review of controlled investigations in treatment-seeking and non-treatment-seeking populations. Addiction. 2002;97(3):279–292.
6. Burke BL, Arkowitz H, Menchola M. The efficacy of motivational interviewing: a meta-analysis of controlled clinical trials. J Consult Clin Psychol. 2003;71(5):843–861.
7. Kaner EF, Dickinson HO, Beyer F, et al. The effectiveness of brief alcohol interventions in primary care settings: a systematic review. Drug Alcohol Rev. 2009;28(3):301–323.
8. Field CA, Caetano R. The effectiveness of brief intervention among injured patients with alcohol dependence: who benefits from brief interventions? Drug Alcohol Depend. 2010;111(1–2):13–20.
9. Epstein EE, Drapkin ML, Yusko DA, Cook SM, McCrady BS, Jensen NK. Is alcohol assessment therapeutic? Pretreatment change in drinking among alcohol-dependent women. J Stud Alcohol. 2005;66(3):369–378.
10. Kypri K, Langley JD, Saunders JB, Cashell-Smith ML. Assessment may conceal therapeutic benefit: findings from a randomized controlled trial for hazardous drinking. Addiction. 2007;102(1):62–70.
11. Carey KB, Carey MP, Maisto SA, Henson JM. Brief motivational interventions for heavy college drinkers: a randomized controlled trial. J Consult Clin Psychol. 2006;74(5):943–954.
12. Clifford PR, Maisto SA, Davis CM. Alcohol treatment research assessment exposure subject reactivity effects: Part I. Alcohol use and related consequences. J Stud Alcohol Drugs. 2007;68(4):519–528.
13. McCambridge J, Day M. Randomized controlled trial of the effects of completing the alcohol use disorders identification test questionnaire on self-reported hazardous drinking. Addiction. 2008;103(2):241–248.
14. Saunders JB, Aasland OG, Babor TF, de la Fuente JR, Grant M. Development of the alcohol use disorders identification test (AUDIT): WHO collaborative project on early detection of persons with harmful alcohol consumption–II. Addiction. 1993;88(6):791–804.
15. Miller WR, Rollnick S. Motivational interviewing: preparing people for change. 2nd ed. New York: Guilford; 2002.
16. Cunningham JA, Humphreys K, Koski-Jannes A. Providing personalized assessment feedback for problem drinking on the Internet: a pilot project. J Stud Alcohol. 2000;61(6):794–798.
17. Kaner EF, Beyer F, Dickinson HO, et al. Effectiveness of brief alcohol interventions in primary care populations. Cochrane Database Syst Rev. 2007;2:CD004148.

18. Riper H, van Straten A, Keuken M, Smit F, Schippers G, Cuijpers P. Curbing problem drinking with personalized-feedback interventions: a meta-analysis. Am. J. Prev. Med. 2009;36(3):247–255.

19. Khadjesari Z, Murray E, Hewitt C, Hartley S, Godfrey C. Can stand-alone computer-based interventions reduce alcohol consumption? A systematic review. Addiction. 2011;106(2):267–282.

20. Riper H, Kramer J, Conijn B, Smit F, Schippers G, Cuijpers P. Translating effective web-based self-help for problem drinking into the real world. Alcohol Clin Exp Res. 2009;33(8):1401–1408.

21. U.S. Preventive Services Task Force. Screening and behavioral counseling interventions in primary care to reduce alcohol misuse: recommendation statement. Ann Intern Med. 2004;140(7):554–556.

22. Carey KB, Scott-Sheldon LA, Elliott JC, Bolles JR, Carey MP. Computer-delivered interventions to reduce college student drinking: a meta-analysis. Addiction. 2009;104(11):1807–1819.

23. White A, Kavanagh D, Stallman H, et al. Online alcohol interventions: a systematic review. J Med Int Res. 2010;12(5):e62.

24. Rooke S, Thorsteinsson E, Karpin A, Copeland J, Allsop D. Computer-delivered interventions for alcohol and tobacco use: a meta-analysis. Addiction. 2010;105(8):1381–1390.

25. Portnoy DB, Scott-Sheldon LA, Johnson BT, Carey MP. Computer-delivered interventions for health promotion and behavioral risk reduction: a meta-analysis of 75 randomized controlled trials, 1988–2007. Prev Med. 2008;47(1):3–16.

26. Doumas DM, Hannah E. Preventing high-risk drinking in youth in the workplace: a web-based normative feedback program. J Subst Abuse Treat. 2008;34(3):263–271.

27. Helzer JE, Rose GL, Badger GJ, et al. Using interactive voice response to enhance brief alcohol intervention in primary care settings. J Stud Alcohol Drugs. 2008;69(2):251–258.

28. Whittaker R, Borland R, Bullen C, Lin RB, McRobbie H, Rodgers A. Mobile phone-based interventions for smoking cessation. Cochrane Database Syst Rev. 2009;4:CD006611.

29. Weitzel JA, Bernhardt JM, Usdan S, Mays D, Glanz K. Using wireless handheld computers and tailored text messaging to reduce negative consequences of drinking alcohol. J Stud Alcohol Drugs. 2007;68(4):534–537.

30. Miller WR. Behavioral treatment of problem drinkers: a comparative outcome study of three controlled drinking therapies. J Consult Clin Psychol. 1978;46(1):74–86.

31. Apodaca TR, Miller WR. A meta-analysis of the effectiveness of bibliotherapy for alcohol problems. J Clin Psychol. 2003;59(3):289–304.

32. Heather N, Kissoon-Singh J, Fenton GW. Assisted natural recovery from alcohol problems: effects of a self-help manual with and without supplementary telephone contact. Br J Addict. 1990;85(9):1177–1185.

33. A cross-national trial of brief interventions with heavy drinkers. WHO Brief Intervention Study Group. Am J Public Health. 1996;86(7):948–955.

34. Sobell LC, Sobell MB, Leo GI, Agrawal S, Johnson-Young L, Cunningham JA. Promoting self-change with alcohol abusers: a community-level mail intervention based on natural recovery studies. Alcohol Clin Exp Res. 2002;26(6):936–948.

35. Blow FC, Barry KL, Walton MA, et al. The efficacy of two brief intervention strategies among injured, at-risk drinkers in the emergency department: impact of tailored messaging and brief advice. J Stud Alcohol. 2006;67(4):568–578.

36. Noar SM, Benac CN, Harris MS. Does tailoring matter? Meta-analytic review of tailored print health behavior change interventions. Psychol Bull. 2007;133(4):673–693.

37. Cunningham JA, Humphreys K, Koski-Jannes A, Cordingley J. Internet and paper self-help materials for problem drinking: is there an additive effect? Addict Behav. 2005;30(8):1517–1523.

38. Beich A, Gannik D, Malterud K. Screening and brief intervention for excessive alcohol use: qualitative interview study of the experiences of general practitioners. Br Med J. 19 2002;325(7369):870.

39. Kypri K, Stephenson S, Langley J. Assessment of nonresponse bias in an internet survey of alcohol use. Alcohol Clin Exp Res. 2004;28(4):630–634.
40. Miller WR, Munoz RF. Controlling your drinking: tools to make moderation work for you. New York: Guilford; 2005.
41. Ondersma S, Grekin E, Svikis D. The potential for technology in brief interventions for substance use, and during-session prediction of computer delivered brief intervention response. Subst Use Misuse. 2011;46(1):77–86.

Chapter 15
Screening and Brief Intervention Practice Systems and Implementation

John Muench

> *Rules of art derive their force from reason alone: and therefore*
> *whenever something better occurs, the rule followed hitherto*
> *should be changed. But "laws derive very great force from*
> *custom," as the Philosopher states (Polit. ii, 5): consequently*
> *they should not be quickly changed.*
> *Aquinas, Summa Theologica, Of Change in Laws*

Introduction

Alcohol screening and brief intervention (SBI) represents an innovation in primary health care despite its efficacy having been known for over 30 years. It is one of the highest ranked, yet least performed of the United States Preventive Services Task Force-recommended preventive services [1–3]. While primary care physicians (PCPs) are motivated to do the right thing for their patients [4] there are significant barriers that must be overcome for wide implementation of SBI to take place.

Addressing health behavior change in primary care is a complex and multifaceted undertaking, as is instituting systematic clinic processes to facilitate clinicians addressing health behaviors. There are special challenges when the behavior to be changed is unhealthy alcohol use. This chapter will review the issues that must be addressed for successful clinical implementation of SBI and offer a typical example of one such implementation process.

The Innovation

Implementation of a new health care innovation first requires consideration of what is being changed. Many clinicians who have not been trained in SBI processes undoubtedly feel they already do an adequate job in addressing and counseling for

J. Muench (✉)
Department of Family Medicine, Oregon Health & Science University, Portland, OR, USA
e-mail: muenchj@ohsu.edu

R. Saitz (ed.), *Addressing Unhealthy Alcohol Use in Primary Care,*
DOI 10.1007/978-1-4614-4779-5_15, © Springer Science+Business Media New York 2013

unhealthy alcohol use. While some PCPs may be adequately performing components of SBI, the message from patients in addictions treatment settings indicates that it isn't happening broadly or effectively [5–7]. Essential elements of SBI are fundamentally different from the way primary care doctors have traditionally addressed unhealthy alcohol use. The innovative, core components of SBI can be summarized as follows:

1. Regular and universal screening in a medical setting of all patients for unhealthy alcohol use.
2. The systematic use of validated screening instruments and validated or standardized assessment approaches [8].
3. Consideration of unhealthy alcohol use as a continuum as opposed to a dichotomous "dependent (or alcoholic, or alcohol abuse) versus not dependent."
4. The use of patient-centered change talk (including assessment of readiness) versus directive, prescriptive talk.
5. Ensuring seamless transitions (back and forth) between primary care and specialty addiction treatment.

Without systematized regular and universal screening systems in place, it's not likely that PCPs will know which of their patients have some level of unhealthy use and need further assessment and intervention, especially given time limitations and competing priorities. Without an understanding of the continuum of unhealthy alcohol use and the processes and tools used for risk-stratifying their patients, they won't be able to assess their patients' needs and provide appropriate medical advice. Without having been versed in the principles of motivational interviewing or brief motivational counseling approaches and "change talk", they won't be as effective in guiding their patients toward lower risk behavior or toward further help if needed. Any implementation of SBI in the primary care setting must ensure that these core components (universal screening, validated and standardized tools, recognition of the continuum, patient-centered behavior change counseling, and seamless transitions to and from specialty care) are in place, functioning effectively, and are sustainable.

Implementation

Implementation is defined as "the constellation of processes intended to get an innovation into use within an organization" [9]. Implementation of new health care innovations is a complex social process that is strongly interconnected with the context in which it takes place.

Medical and public health research has long focused on the discovery and testing of innovations that can improve health. However, there is a well-known gap between the acquisition of these innovations and their translation into clinical practice. It has long been assumed that evidence based practices, once known, would automatically diffuse into general practice. But such passive diffusion has proven quite insufficient, resulting in a "science to service gap". It is estimated that it takes an average of 17 years for rigorous medical evidence to make its way into common practice [10]. This has proven to be an under-estimation with regard to SBI.

Implementation Research

Over the past decade, there has been growing interest and research in the implementation processes that can more actively move innovations into common practice. Recent literature reviews have been conducted to create overarching theoretical constructs that can help to better explain what works with regard to implementation [9, 11, 12]. We will briefly review some constructs that might help to inform and guide SBI implementation.

Stages of Implementation

The implementation of an innovation like SBI doesn't take place all at once; it is an iterative process that occurs over an extended period of time. Fixsen et al. described six functional stages of implementation [11]. Although they seem linear, each stage can have a complex effect on all the others. They are as follows:

Exploration

In this stage, an organization evaluates the cost and benefits of implementing a new innovation. Questions that should be answered include: What is the specific problem that needs to be addressed? What is the innovation that will help address the problem? What changes will need to be made at the clinical level to allow effective use of the innovation? What changes are needed outside the organization that will facilitate it? What are the start-up costs and costs of ongoing support? Where will funding come from? What data systems will need to be in place to monitor changes?

At this early stage, an implementation team should be identified. It should have direct access to the organization's decision makers. Team members should have sufficient time carved out to conduct needed research, determine the appropriate processes to institute the innovation, and determine the costs and benefits of doing so.

Installation

This stage begins with the decision to implement the innovation and ends when that innovation is used for the first time with the first patient. This stage requires resources for planning and setting up work-flow processes. It may entail hiring new staff, purchasing new equipment, arranging training, and preparing supervision and coaching. Initial training of staff should begin. This stage is likely to take between 2 and 6 months.

Initial Implementation Stage

This is where the rubber hits the road; those involved in the process must be ready to perform their part of the innovation. Further training and support will be needed as practitioners are not likely to be proficient in their roles. This stage may require 9–24 months. Initial performance feedback should take place at this stage.

Full Implementation Stage

This stage is reached when at least 50 % of the practitioners perform their functions acceptably as measured by performance criteria that accurately reflect fidelity to the original innovation. Despite full functioning of the innovation, attention still needs to be paid to its maintenance. It's especially important to consider the likelihood of staff turnover and the need to train new personnel, as well as to continue to assure that all current personnel remain faithful to the original model. From the start of "exploration" to the point of first achieving full implementation often requires 2–4 years.

Innovation Stage

When the innovation has been fully implemented, the practitioners will more fully understand the process and its nuances. At this point, they can sometimes use this understanding to improve the innovation.

Sustainability Stage

The need for sustainability should be considered and incorporated into all the other stages and expanded at every opportunity. The work-flows, tools and performance feedback built into the implementation should help to ensure this. But medical settings are not static; they exist in constant states of change and require ongoing quality assurance systems that will help sustain the innovation.

Consolidated Framework for Implementation Research

In another review, Damschroder et al. exhaustively noted 39 constructs they found in the implementation research literature, resulting in a "Consolidated Framework for Implementation Research" (CFIR) [9]. These constructs were considered likely to influence the implementation of evidence based practices, and were further categorized under five overarching domains as follows:

1. The *intervention characteristics* include such things as the expected effect of the innovation, the strength of evidence behind it, its adaptability to the local context, and its cost.
2. The *outer setting* includes the economic, political, and social context within which an organization resides and will likely affect implementation.
3. The *inner setting* constitutes the characteristics of the organization within which the intervention will be implemented. It includes such things as the organization's

size, structure, communication networks, culture, change climate, and readiness to change.

4. The *characteristics of individuals* who will carry out the intervention include the knowledge and beliefs of the practitioners about the intervention and their self-efficacy and willingness to carry it out.
5. Finally, the *process of implementation* consists of all the planning, engaging and reflecting on the process.

Williams et al. used this CFIR to assess 8 different SBI implementation projects that have been described in the literature [13]. Each project was reviewed to determine the percentages of patients who were appropriately screened for unhealthy alcohol use and for brief interventions performed when patients screened positive. Then, each report was coded for the constructs of the CFIR that were reported. The project with the greatest percentage of patients screened reported having more characteristics in the outer setting, the inner setting and the process of implementation. The two studies that had the highest rates of brief interventions, however, did not exhibit any patterns of association with the CFIR elements or domains that distinguished them from the other projects. These three projects together seemed to especially emphasize their use of electronic health records along with performance accountability through measurement and feedback. The authors noted that changing clinical behavior seems possible, although it requires "multifaceted approaches at multiple levels".

One of these projects, "Cutting Back," implemented SBI in 10 primary care practices associated with managed care organizations in 5 states. Its own review noted that successful implementation was associated positively with the presence of an influential on-site coordinator, with a greater number of personnel trained at the site, with the site's willingness to make use of outside technical assistance, and with support from the managed care organization. Clinics were also more successful if they had stable patient membership and if they had providers who were already familiar with alcohol screening and other clinical preventive services. The most important barriers were found to be lack of time, and competing organizational priorities [14].

From Theory to Practice

A more practical framework that describes the necessary steps for implementation is the Johns Hopkins Quality and Safety Research Group's "translating evidence into practice model" [15]. There are five general principles of this model:

1. A focus on systems of care (as opposed to care of individual patients),
2. Engagement of local interdisciplinary teams to assume ownership of the project,
3. Creation of centralized support for the technical work,
4. Encouraging local adaptation of the intervention, and
5. Creation of a collaborative culture within the local unit and larger system.

The steps in this model are as follows:

1. *Summarize the evidence.* The leadership team should determine the best intervention to reach a specified outcome. The intervention is then turned into a set of specific practitioner behaviors. Workflows are defined, and the tools and resources needed to carry out the behaviors are gathered.
2. *Identify local barriers to implementation.* The innovation must be made to fit into the local practice setting. Once workflows are designed, the implementation team needs to carefully walk through these workflows to see where barriers and problems are likely to occur. It's helpful to ask all the stakeholders why it is or isn't easy for them to perform their part of the innovation.
3. *Measure performance.* Performance measures must be developed in order to evaluate whether the recommended innovation is taking place appropriately (process measures) or whether patient outcomes improve (outcome measures).
4. *Ensure all patients receive the intervention.* The general tactics for the initial and full implementation include the follow "four Es" approach:
    a. *Engage*—Share with staff the reasons this change is needed. Share real-life stories about how absence of the intervention has affected patient outcomes.
    b. *Educate*—Explain the problem and how the innovation has been shown to solve the problem if implemented correctly.
    c. *Execute*—Design an implementation "toolkit" that will facilitate the workflows designed in Step 1 and that addresses the barriers noted in Step 2. Standardize care processes, create independent checks, and learn from mistakes.
    d. *Evaluate*—Use performance measures to determine whether the innovation is working as desired. Be vigilant for unintended consequences of the implementation such as decreased attention to other processes of care.

SBI Implementation Process

Thus, there are many specific questions that must be answered when considering SBI implementation and how it can be adapted to a local context. We will consider these in terms of the CFIR domains.

Intervention Characteristics

Screening

What screening instrument will be used? To be faithful to the SBI model, the screening process needs to assess risky behavior by asking consumption questions as well as assess for alcohol-related consequences and dependent drinking. One example of such a process would be to use a short one item, or three item consumption screen such as the Alcohol Use Disorders Identification Test, consumption items (AUDIT-C) [16, 17]. For those whose score meets a specified cut-off, this would be followed by a more extensive screen such as the ten question AUDIT or other checklist of alcohol use disorder symptoms to further assess for harmful or dependent drinking [8, 18]. Another process could be to use the ASSIST (Alcohol, Smoking and Substance Involvement Screening Test) that incorporates substances other than alcohol. These choices must be researched early to decide which best meets the clinics' goals and can be made to fit with other workflow processes.

Who will perform the screening and where? It is possible to screen orally, asking consumption questions along with questions about harms experienced from drinking. It can also be done using paper forms, or using computer enhanced methods (tablet or kiosk). If done with screening instruments such as the AUDIT, how will it be scored to determine the level of the patient's risk? How will clinicians be supported regarding decisions they will make that depend on risk level? How will the result be placed in the medical record? What patient population will be targeted? What will be the age range? What will be the process with non-English speaking patients, with illiterate patients, or those with mild cognitive deficits? How often will the screening take place? There is no clear evidence for an optimal screening frequency for alcohol use. In a primary care setting, it may not be reasonable to ask patients to fill out the same screening assessment every time they come to the doctor. How will patients be flagged when a specified time has passed? Will outreach be done in order to ensure screening of a specified patient population, or will this be done only for those who come to the office?

Brief Interventions

What will be the process for performing brief interventions? How will those performing the intervention be trained? Will their training lead to effective brief interventions? How will achievement and maintenance of their skills be assured? Who will perform the intervention, and where and when will it take place? Depending on the clinical context, it might be better to allow clinicians to perform the brief interventions as part of their encounter, or it might be more effective to do a "warm hand-off" to another professional such as a nurse case manager, or a behavioral health provider [19, 20].

How will SBI be recorded? Can this process be systematized through check-lists in the record, or will the clinicians need to record the process in their progress note? Will the system put in place encourage good care or will it incentivize documentation only or gaming of the system? Will patients be billed for this service, and if so, how will this be done? How will patients be referred for specialty care? What other tools will be needed? It may be helpful to have patient education handouts or "cutting back agreements" easily available in each exam room.

How will success be measured? From the first exploration stages it will be important to have a general sense of the goals and expected outcomes. These ideas must be refined into specific measurable outcomes. Process measures should include the number of eligible patients appropriately screened, the number of eligible patients who receive a brief intervention, and the number of eligible patients referred or offered referral for specialty addictions treatment services. The denominators of these measures, "eligible patients" can be tricky to define and accurately measure. "Eligibility" should also take into account the patient's readiness to accept these processes while at the same time not encouraging practitioners to assume patients are not interested or ready. A patient drinking risky amounts who has had some consequences might turn out to be pre-contemplative about their behavior and not willing to accept a brief intervention or referral. Outcome measures are more difficult to measure and track. Short term outcome measures might include reduction in risky drinking, drinking with consequences or dependent drinking. Long-term outcome measures might include decreases in the biological, psychological, and social consequences of unhealthy alcohol use.

Implementation Process Questions

Who will make up the implementation team? Implementation research emphasizes the importance of clinical champions who are respected and have a firm belief in the importance of the innovation [21]. How will the SBI process be fit into the clinical workflow? How will any needed tools be designed and created, including electronic health record (EHR) tools, and who will do so? Who will carry out necessary training sessions, especially with regard to performance of brief interventions?

Inner Setting

How ready is this organization to implement a systematic SBI process? Does it have a firm sense of a mission, and how well does SBI fit with this? Is there sufficient stability in clinic personnel? Are there stable clinical teams and a sense of "teamness" and community? How are new work processes typically communicated? What are the resources available within the clinic that might facilitate SBI, such as a Chronic Disease Care Management model, or an integrated Behavioral Health model [22, 23]?

Outer Setting

Are there project requirements or mandates coming from outside agencies and if so, how will the current implementation meet them? This is especially likely if there is outside funding for the project or if targets set by external performance measures need to be met. Are there relationships with other organizations undergoing a similar implementation with which ideas and resources could be shared? Are there adequate relationships and communication links with specialty addictions services?

Characteristics of Individuals

Do the staff believe that unhealthy alcohol use is a medical risk factor or condition that should be addressed in the clinic? Resistance can be met when trying to introduce new workflows and duties with staff who might already feel stretched. Can in-service sessions be held that will help them better understand the clinical importance of addressing unhealthy alcohol use? Will staff feel empowered to actively take part and give feedback about the process and therefore be invested in it? What kind of training and support will be needed [24]? Are there ways to help staff gain insight into how their own personal and family issues shape their attitudes with regard to alcohol use?

An SBI Implementation Fictional Example

As part of a "primary care renewal" project, Managed Care, Inc. (a local Medicaid managed care organization) offered to provide seed money to their member clinics to provide SBI services to all their adult patients. These funds were meant to defray the administrative, training, and material costs involved with the first three years of the project in hopes that it would then be self-sustaining. They also provided information from the state health department on the local costs of alcohol abuse, and national statistics on the poor rate of addressing this problem in the primary care setting. Four of the community health centers agreed to participate, and an implementation process was begun. A joint implementation committee was formed that included one physician and the office manager from each of the clinics. They decided that the overall purpose of the project should be to decrease risky, harmful, and dependent drinking in their adult populations. This committee was given a four hour training session on SBI, including sessions on brief interventions that were given by a motivational interviewing trainer. They reviewed the literature and decided upon a core process that they could all undertake as follows: All adults presenting to their clinics would receive an annual alcohol screening using the AUDIT-C. All who screened positive would receive further assessment with the remaining seven AUDIT questions. Those who scored in the risky, harmful, or dependent zones using standard AUDIT scoring would receive at least a brief intervention, and all those in the dependent zones would be advised referral to specialty addictions treatment center. It was agreed that one year after initiating the project, 75 % of all eligible adults who presented to the clinics would receive an annual screen, 85 % of those who screened positive would receive a full AUDIT, and 75 % of those in the risky, harmful or dependent zones would receive a brief intervention. Having set those standards, the implementation team representatives were allowed to determine how to adapt the intervention to their own setting, workflows, and office processes.

Clinic A was a small rural health center. Its patient population of 13,000 (just over 11,000 adults) was cared for by 5 primary care physicians and 2 nurse practitioners. The physician who had been on the central implementation team, Dr. Jim W., agreed to take on the role of "physician champion for the project." He asked for volunteers and identified Demo S. from the front desk, and two medical assistants, Carol S. and Tami H. who agreed to be part of the clinic SBIRT implementation team.

This team met once weekly over lunch for the next six weeks to set up the work-flows and processes that would work best for their office. They began by assessing the clinic resources that would be needed. They felt hampered by the lack of pro-fessional counseling services within the clinic, but felt their clinicians would be up to the task of performing brief interventions. They did, however, worry that their office clinicians would run even later than normal, and they agreed it would be best to otherwise minimize the clinicians' role in the process. They also decided that they would like to integrate the screening process as much as possible into the electronic health record (EHR) they had implemented two years previously. They decided to begin the implementation using only English materials because this was the primary language for over 95 % of their rural population.

The process they devised was as follows. A half sheet AUDIT-C screening form was designed to be handed out on a small "privacy clipboard" at the front desk. The front desk staff would be alerted to the need to give out the clipboard annually by way of a tickler built into the EHR registration module. When the medical assistant brought the patient back to the exam room, they would note the brightly colored "privacy clipboard," quickly review and score the AUDIT-C as part of the vital sign process, determine whether or not the patient qualified for a further assessment, and if so, ask the patient to fill out the remaining AUDIT questions while waiting for their primary care clinician. The PCP would review the full AUDIT results with the patient during the encounter and perform any needed intervention or referral. Upon completion of the visit, the medical assistant would enter the results of the AUDIT-C and/or AUDIT into a flow-sheet in the EHR for tracking purposes. After their third weekly meeting, the group was ready to present this process during an "all-clinic" lunch meeting. They received general agreement from the rest of the staff to proceed as planned, although there were some concerns raised about making patients feel uncomfortable.

Several jobs needed to be done prior to implementation. First, the forms had to be designed and printed, and sufficient quantities stored in designated places for easy access; a standard file pocket in each exam room was created so that medical assistants could easily find and deliver AUDIT forms to patients. Twenty special privacy clipboards were ordered. A meeting was held with their EHR vendor to create a tickler process for the front desk, as well as a place for the medical assistant to record the result of the screening in the electronic record. They also discussed building an automated report that would measure their main performance outcomes.

The planning group realized that special training would be needed so that all mem-bers of the team would be able to perform their roles. The front desk personnel were given a demonstration of the EHR tickler system as well as a brief non-judgmental script that they could use to feel more comfortable handing patients an alcohol screen as part of the check-in process. Similarly, the medical assistants gathered for a brief training session to demonstrate the scoring of the AUDIT-C and the cut-off scores for which they would hand patients the remaining AUDIT questions. Scripted text was demonstrated using role plays to demonstrate how to perform this task non-judgmentally and how to handle resistance from patients. Finally, the clinician staff needed to be able to use the AUDIT to help risk-stratify patients into severity of unhealthy alcohol use and to provide appropriate interventions depending upon patient needs and readiness to change. Jim arranged a two hour in-service with the other six clinicians. He demonstrated the use of the AUDIT form to help determine severity. The motivational interviewing expert from Managed Care, Inc. used most of this session teaching how to perform brief interventions. The clinicians voiced some reservations about having the time to do this during their typical 15-min office visits. They were receptive to learning and practicing the brief intervention process, especially as they quickly realized these were skills that could be efficiently used for many other patient behaviors such as tobacco use and physical inactivity. By the end of the session, the clinicians were able to demonstrate the ability to perform brief interventions and expressed that they felt comfortable doing so.

Jim realized that to fully implement SBIRT they would need better links with referral resources to assist patients who had more severe alcohol related problems. He and the office manager took time to visit the closest county addictions treatment center to ensure that they could efficiently refer and advise their patients on access to inpatient and outpatient services, and especially detoxification. Demo was given the task of researching online listings of local AA meetings. Carol and Tami designed an exam room "toolkit" that consisted of a small poster clearly stipulating the definitions of "standard drink", risky drinking limits, and consequences of overdrinking. A pocket card was created to help the clinicians remember the steps of the brief intervention. A patient education handout was written for patients who drank too much. This included information on access to local treatment facilities as well as a "drinking diary" and a "drinking goals form" that could be signed by the patient to firmly define the plan that might come about as a result of the brief intervention. Jim piloted these materials with his own patients during development to ensure they all worked appropriately. The team relied greatly on the NIAAA publication "Helping Patients Who Drink Too Much: A Clinician's Guide" [25]. Finally, the team felt that everything was ready to begin their implementation. They presented their completed materials and processes during the next "all-clinic lunch", and set a Monday morning start date. On the Saturday afternoon before their start, the implementation team gathered one last time to step through the process, making sure all the materials were ready and in place, and ensuring all the bugs were worked out.

At 8:00 am on Monday morning, the first 20 adult patients were handed the privacy clip-board during check-in, and asked to fill out the form with a brief explanation that this was a new screening process for all of the clinic's patients. The implementation team had forgotten to consider that during the first few weeks nearly every patient would receive the annual screening and hadn't planned how to quickly return empty clipboards to the front desk. Waiting for their return, an unacceptably long line formed at the check-in desk. An ad hoc decision was made that for the first week, only new patients and patients scheduled for "check-ups" or "complete physicals" would receive the screening to allow for a slower ramp-up of the process. More clipboards were purchased. The remainder of that week, the process continued without major problems, and the next week, they were ready to move forward with screening all adults (except the few follow-up patients who had already been screened).

One month after start-up, the implementation team again met with the entire clinic for their first SBI assessment report. They presented the EHR generated report showing that they had had 1,823 adult visits in that time period, accounting for 1,760 unique patient visits. Of those, 1,020 patients, or 58 % of those eligible actually received the "annual screen" at the front desk. This number was likely diluted by the unexpected slow-down during the first week in which not everyone could be given an AUDIT-C. The front desk personnel felt they were now on track giving the clipboard to most patients, but did admit to missing a few when they had several patients waiting in line to check in.

From those 1,020 who received and filled out the AUDIT-C, 183 (18 %) scored in a way that warranted further assessment but only 64 %, or 117 patients had appropriately received the full AUDIT in the exam room. The medical assistants felt they would have trouble meeting their 85 % goal. They had several tasks to do during the rooming process, and at times their partner clinician would be left waiting and impatient to start their part of the encounter. They noted that they sometimes missed the small clipboard if it was hidden under patients' purses and coats.

Of the 117 patients who received the full AUDIT screening, 18 scored in the non-risky zone, 37 in the risky zone, 44 in the harmful zone, and 6 in the dependent zone. Twelve patients declined to fill out the full AUDIT. Thus, 87 patients were eligible for at least a brief intervention in this first month, or around 12 per clinician. However, the tracking and chart review process showed that only 52 patients actually received any form of a brief intervention from their doctor. The clinician staff offered several reasons for this. Some felt that their 15-min schedule made it very difficult to address alcohol given that patients often came in with several other problems to be addressed. Some of the clinicians also admitted that it still felt awkward to do brief interventions, especially with patients they had known for many years and wondered if they might benefit from a quick review session with the motivational interviewing specialist. The clinicians discussed how to overcome some of these barriers.

Discussion of the Barriers and Facilitators for Implementing SBI in Primary Care

As can be inferred from the above, implementation of SBI is associated with several barriers. Many of these are similar to those associated with implementation of other preventive health and behavior counseling procedures. But there are some unique barriers associated with SBI that must be considered [26–28].

The National Center on Addiction and Substance Abuse conducted a survey of a nationally representative sample of primary care physicians as well as patients in addictions treatment facilities [7]. Three out of four of the patients said that their primary care physician was not involved in their decision to seek treatment, and 16.7 % said that their physician was only involved "a little". From the other direction, only 32 % of the physicians reported carefully screening for substance abuse. When asked what prevented their doing so, they responded as follows:

- 57.7 % believed that their patients would lie about their substance use
- 35.1 % reported that time constraints prevented such discussions
- 29.5 % did not want to "question their patient's integrity"
- 25 % were afraid of frightening/angering their patients
- 15.7 % were uncertain about treatments
- 12.6 % were personally uncomfortable with the subject
- 11 % were afraid doing so would cause their patient to switch to another doctor
- 10.6 % were concerned that insurance didn't reimburse for a physician's time for this service.

These barriers can be grouped under three general headings:

1. Psychosocial issues
2. Knowledge gap
3. Time and money.

Psychosocial Issues

Many of the barriers affecting SBI implementation are due to a cultural mindset in which mental health and physical health are considered separate, split into two different arenas with their own clinics and payment systems. This can negatively affect the treatment of problems such as unhealthy alcohol use in which there are components of both mental and physical health. While there is much ongoing work to resolve this problem, it continues to interfere with physicians trying to effectively address unhealthy alcohol use. Another barrier comes from the sometimes ingrained belief that alcohol use disorders are a moral problem, not a health problem, and therefore not a legitimate part of medical care [28, 29]. Even when physicians believe that addressing unhealthy substance use is an important part of primary care, such ingrained beliefs can affect their emotional response to discussing alcohol with their patients (even through subconscious body language). If these responses are detected by patients, they might affect the doctor–patient relationship. Doctors sometimes perceive these issues as patient resistance—worried that patients lie about their substance use, that patients become irritated and upset when asked about it [7, 30], and that treatment is ineffective, despite strong evidence to the contrary [31]. Additionally, alcohol drinking is a behavior shared by most physicians and this can result in another level of emotional response. Some will avoid discussions with patients that would require having to consider their own unhealthy alcohol use. Some have been shown to use their own consumption as the benchmark of appropriate use by their patients [32].

SBI implementation projects must take these issues into consideration. It's necessary to minimize the impact on the doctor-patient relationship through processes and attitudes that normalize addressing unhealthy alcohol use in medical clinics as a health problem and not a stigmatized moral problem (in fact, the term used consistently in this text, unhealthy alcohol use, may help do just that). Physicians sometimes need to step back and examine their own attitudes and perceptions and how they might be influencing their practice. Being able to discuss these issues with colleagues in support groups or Balint groups can be extremely helpful and gratifying [33].

Knowledge Gap

Some of the discomfort experienced by physicians when addressing unhealthy substance use occurs because of uncertainty in how to proceed. There is uncertainty in their ability to assess unhealthy alcohol use [34, 35], lack of confidence in ability to perform brief interventions [36], and confusion over how to refer patients who need a higher level of service than they can provide, especially given the current fragmentation in addictions resources in most states, and the fact that many patients are not ready to take such a step [37]. There has traditionally been inadequate training in medical schools and post-graduate residency education concerning unhealthy substance use, especially concerning SBI [7, 38]. Any implementation of SBI needs to consider how best to assure that those performing the various components are well-versed in the use of screening tools, performance of brief interventions, and referral to local treatment settings.

Time/Money

Implementation of preventive services and behavioral health counseling requires start-up and maintenance resources [21]. Unfortunately, the current US healthcare payment system is based on providing procedural or management services for medical diagnoses, with little attention to screening or preventive behavioral interventions. Lack of time and inadequate/misaligned reimbursement are major barriers to wide dissemination of SBI [26, 39].

Primary care visits encompass some combination of acute, chronic, and preventive care. Patients sometimes present primarily for preventive services offered within the context of the "complete physical exam," but much more often, patients present sporadically for acute care problems or chronic disease management whereby it's harder to offer preventive health measures [40]. Additionally, there are multiple preventive health services to be considered, sometimes creating competition even among themselves [21, 41].

Systematizing screening processes using EHR tools and logic models might facilitate the provision of these services to the right patients at the right time. Several preventive health implementation projects have shown the value of using team-based approaches [42–44]. Some have made good use of ancillary staff to efficiently carry out SBIs at less cost than using clinicians [19]. Clinics already operating with integrated behavioral health models will be able to do so more easily [22].

Remuneration for SBI is being instituted in some states, but is currently complex and less rewarding than for most other services in primary care [45]. Under the right circumstances, it is possible to submit bills to insurance companies for alcohol behavioral counseling, but the complexity of doing so, and the questionable and low level of reimbursement make it unlikely physicians will do so. Preventive delivery economic analyses show that small rewards don't motivate physicians to change their routines [27]. It's not known what level of remuneration will be sufficient to encourage physicians to perform brief interventions. It is also clear that remuneration isn't the sole barrier preventing clinicians from performing SBI for unhealthy alcohol use. Clinicians much more commonly screen for hypertension, cancer, and even tobacco despite the fact that these aren't billed as separate procedures. The cultural and knowledge barriers discussed above likely play a more significant role.

As of July 2010, 28 state Medicaid authorities had instituted Current Procedural Technology (CPT) and Healthcare Common Procedure Coding System (HCPCS) billing codes for SBI provision but of these only 19 had actually assigned monies to the use of the codes. CPT code 99408 requires 15–30 min of time (potentially cumulative from an office team), and 99409 for over 30 min. Screening takes less than 15 min and could be billed using a health assessment code or could be remunerated in part by performance improvement incentive programs (details associated with such options are beyond the scope of this chapter in part because they may change and differ by locale and insurer). Of the 19 states who had assigned monies, reimbursement rates for 99408 ranged from $20 in Iowa to $116 in Alaska [45].

These time and money disincentives are being recognized more and more with regards to SBI and other preventive health services [39, 46]. New models of care have been proposed and are being implemented and tested, including such concepts as patient centered medical homes, chronic disease care management and integrated behavioral medicine. These models offer renewed hope that changes will take place to facilitate SBI implementation, especially changes in the primary care reimbursement rules that discourage performance of evidence-based preventive and behavioral counseling services. Until there is change in the health care payment system, these will be difficult barriers to overcome [47].

Conclusion

Alcohol SBI is clearly an effective public health innovation, but widely translating this innovation into day to day clinical settings has proven difficult. While there are core elements of SBI that should be part of any implementation process, there is insufficient evidence to argue for any one office workflow or any one implementation process. It is important to adapt the core SBI process to fit local clinical contexts. Current experience with SBI implementations, as with other preventive and behavioral counseling innovations shows the importance of using local clinician champions, performance feedback processes, and team based approaches to both the SBI workflow and its implementation. We have narrated an example of one possible process that could work within a "patient centered medical home" model. SBI implementation will become generally self-sustaining once reimbursement improves or payment models shift from "encounter-centric" fee for service models, to models that emphasize population health and pay-for-performance [46, 48]. Until that time, SBI dissemination will likely be limited to clinical arenas that receive outside support to help seed and sustain it. The ongoing evaluation of current federally funded SBI projects [49] is likely to provide more evidence on the best practices for its implementation in the future.

References

1. Coffield AB, Maciosek MV, McGinnis JM, et al. Priorities among recommended clinical preventive services. Am J Prev Med. 2001;21:1–9.
2. Kuehn BM. Despite benefit, physicians slow to offer brief advice on harmful alcohol use. JAMA. 2008;299:751–753.
3. Solberg LI, Maciosek MV, Edwards NM. Primary care intervention to reduce alcohol misuse ranking its health impact and cost effectiveness. Am J Prev Med. 2008;34:143–152.
4. Cohen DJ, Tallia AF, Crabtree BF, Young DM. Implementing health behavior change in primary care: lessons from prescription for health. Ann Fam Med 2005;3 Suppl 2:S12–19.
5. Cheeta S, Drummond C, Oyefeso A, et al. Low identification of alcohol use disorders in general practice in England. Addiction. 2008;103:766–773.
6. D'Amico EJ, Paddock SM, Burnam A, Kung FY. Identification of and guidance for problem drinking by general medical providers: results from a national survey. Med Care. 2005;43:229–236.
7. National Center on Addiction and Substance Abuse. Missed Opportunity: CASA National Survey of Primary Care Physicians and Patients on substance abuse. New York: Columbia University, CASA; 2000.
8. Fiellin DA, Reid MC, O'Connor PG. Screening for alcohol problems in primary care: a systematic review. Arch Intern Med. 2000;160:1977–1989.
9. Damschroder LJ, Aron DC, Keith RE, Kirsh SR, Alexander JA, Lowery JC. Fostering implementation of health services research findings into practice: a consolidated framework for advancing implementation science. Implement Sci. 2009;4:50.
10. Balas EA, Boren SA. Managing clinical knowledge for health care improvement. In: Bemmel J, McCray AT, editors. Yearbook of Medical Informatics 2000: patient-centered systems. Stuttgart: Schattauer Verlagsgesellschaft mbH; 2000. pp. 65–70.
11. Fixsen DL, Naoom SF, Blasé KA, Friedman RM, Wallace F. Implementation Research: A Synthesis of the Literature. Tampa, FL: University of South Florida, Louis de la Parte Florida Mental Health Institute, The National Implementation Research Network (FMHI Publication 231, 2005. Accessed 10 May 2011, at http://cfs.cbcs.usf.edu/_docs/publications/NIRN_Monograph_Full.pdf.
12. Greenhalgh T, Robert G, Macfarlane F, Bate P, Kyriakidou O. Diffusion of innovations in service organizations: systematic review and recommendations. Milbank Q. 2004;82:581–629.
13. Williams EC, Johnson ML, Lapham GT, et al. Strategies to implement alcohol screening and brief intervention in primary care settings: a structured literature review. Psychol Addict Behav. 2011.
14. Babor TE, Higgins-Biddle J, Dauser D, Higgins P, Burleson JA. Alcohol screening and brief intervention in primary care settings: implementation models and predictors. J Stud Alcohol. 2005;66:361–368.
15. Pronovost PJ, Berenholtz SM, Needham DM. Translating evidence into practice: a model for large scale knowledge translation. Br Med J. 2008;337:a1714.

16. Hawkins EJ, Kivlahan DR, Williams EC, Wright SM, Craig T, Bradley KA. Examining quality issues in alcohol misuse screening. Subst Abuse. 2007;28:53–65.

17. Vinson DC, Kruse RL, Seale JP. Simplifying alcohol assessment: two questions to identify alcohol use disorders. Alcohol Clin Exp Res. 2007;31:1392–1398.

18. Maisto SA, Saitz R. Alcohol use disorders: screening and diagnosis. Am J Addict. 2003;12 Suppl 1:S12–25.

19. Babor TF, Higgins-Biddle JC, Dauser D, Burleson JA, Zarkin GA, Bray J. Brief interventions for at-risk drinking: patient outcomes and cost-effectiveness in managed care organizations. Alcohol Alcohol. 2006;41:624–631.

20. Spandorfer JM, Israel Y, Turner BJ. Primary care physicians' views on screening and management of alcohol abuse: inconsistencies with national guidelines. J Fam Pract. 1999;48:899–902.

21. Crabtree BF, Miller WL, Tallia AF, et al. Delivery of clinical preventive services in family medicine offices. Ann Fam Med. 2005;3:430–435.

22. Hunter CL, Goodie JL. Operational and clinical components for integrated-collaborative behavioral healthcare in the patient-centered medical home. Fam Syst Health. 2009;28:308–321.

23. Saitz R, Larson MJ, Labelle C, Richardson J, Samet JH. The case for chronic disease management for addiction. J Addict Med. 2008;2:55–65.

24. Kaner EF, Lock CA, McAvoy BR, Heather N, Gilvarry E. A RCT of three training and support strategies to encourage implementation of screening and brief alcohol intervention by general practitioners. Br J Gen Pract. 1999;49:699–703.

25. NIAAA: helping patients who drink too much. http://www.niaaa.nih.gov/Publications/EducationTrainingMaterials/Pages/guide.aspx. Accessed 10 May 2011.

26. Johnson M, Jackson R, Guillaume L, Meier P, Goyder E. Barriers and facilitators to implementing screening and brief intervention for alcohol misuse: a systematic review of qualitative evidence. J Public Health (Oxf). 2010.

27. Nilsen P. Brief alcohol intervention—where to from here? Challenges remain for research and practice. Addiction. 2010;105:954–959.

28. Roche AM, Hotham ED, Richmond RL. The general practitioner's role in AOD issues: overcoming individual, professional and systemic barriers. Drug Alcohol Rev. 2002;21:223–230.

29. Beich A, Gannik D, Malterud K. Screening and brief intervention for excessive alcohol use: qualitative interview study of the experiences of general practitioners. Br Med J. 2002;325:870.

30. McCormick KA, Cochran NE, Back AL, Merrill JO, Williams EC, Bradley KA. How primary care providers talk to patients about alcohol: a qualitative study. J Gen Intern Med. 2006;21:966–972.

31. Whitlock EP, Polen MR, Green CA, Orleans T, Klein J. Behavioral counseling interventions in primary care to reduce risky/harmful alcohol use by adults: a summary of the evidence for the U.S. Preventive Services Task Force. Ann Intern Med. 2004;140:557–568.

32. Kaner E, Rapley T, May C. Seeing through the glass darkly? A qualitative exploration of GPs' drinking and their alcohol intervention practices. Fam Pract. 2006;23:481–487.

33. Kjeldmand D, Holmstrom I, Rosenqvist U. Balint training makes GPs thrive better in their job. Patient Educ Couns. 2004;55:230–235.

34. Kaner EF, Heather N, Brodie J, Lock CA, McAvoy BR. Patient and practitioner characteristics predict brief alcohol intervention in primary care. Br J Gen Pract. 2001;51:822–827.

35. Rush B, Ellis K, Crowe T, Powell L. How general practitioners view alcohol use. Clearing up the confusion. Can Fam Physician. 1994;40:1570–1579.

36. Roche AM, Guray C, Saunders JB. General practitioners' experiences of patients with drug and alcohol problems. Br J Addict. 1991;86:263–275.

37. Town M, Naimi TS, Mokdad AH, Brewer RD. Health care access among U.S. adults who drink alcohol excessively: missed opportunities for prevention. Prev Chronic Dis. 2006;3:A53.

38. Miller NS, Sheppard LM, Colenda CC, Magen J. Why physicians are unprepared to treat patients who have alcohol- and drug-related disorders. Acad Med. 2001;76:410–418.

39. Nutting PA, Gallagher K, Riley K, et al. Care management for depression in primary care practice: findings from the RESPECT-Depression trial. Ann Fam Med. 2008;6:30–37.

40. Buckley DI, Calvert JF, Lapidus JA, Morris CD. Chronic opioid therapy and preventive services in rural primary care: an Oregon rural practice-based research network study. Ann Fam Med. 2010;8:237–244.
41. Yarnall KS, Pollak KI, Ostbye T, Krause KM, Michener JL. Primary care: is there enough time for prevention? Am J Public Health. 2003;93:635–641.
42. Ferrer RL, Mody-Bailey P, Jaen CR, Gott S, Araujo S. A medical assistant-based program to promote healthy behaviors in primary care. Ann Fam Med. 2009;7:504–512.
43. Grumbach K, Bodenheimer T. Can health care teams improve primary care practice? JAMA. 2004;291:1246–1251.
44. Hung DY, Rundall TG, Crabtree BF, Tallia AF, Cohen DJ, Halpin HA. Influence of primary care practice and provider attributes on preventive service delivery. Am J Prev Med. 2006;30: 413–422.
45. Fussell HE, Rieckmann TR, Quick MB. Medicaid reimbursement for screening and brief intervention for substance misuse. Psychiatr Serv. 2011;62:306–309.
46. Goroll AH. The future of primary care: reforming physician payment. N Engl J Med. 2008;359:2087, 2090.
47. Bodenheimer T, Grumbach K, Berenson RA. A lifeline for primary care. N Engl J Med 2009;360:2693–2696.
48. Martin JC, Avant RF, Bowman MA, et al. The future of family medicine: a collaborative project of the family medicine community. Ann Fam Med. 2004;2 Suppl 1:S3–32.
49. See SAMHSA Grantee website at http://www.samhsa.gov/prevention/sbirt/grantees/index.aspx.

Chapter 16
Confidentiality

Richard Saitz

Introduction

Confidentiality is an important issue for any health condition but it is particularly important for conditions that are associated with stigma. If not kept private, knowledge that a patient has such a condition could harm their reputation, place them at risk for criminal or civil liability, or damage their financial standing, employability or insurability. These consequences are potentially true for patients with a chronic medical condition, for example, heart disease, diabetes, asthma or cancer, but they are even more likely when the condition is alcohol dependence or drug addiction. Conditions associated with unhealthy alcohol and other drug use likely also place patients at risk of such consequences, such as depression, HIV and other sexually transmitted diseases and hepatitis C.

General Approach

In general, patients should be able to have a reasonable expectation of privacy and confidentiality of their healthcare visit. The primary care setting has a major advantage in this regard over specialty addiction treatment programs in that simply being present in the waiting room does not indicate any particular diagnosis, or even any diagnosis at all since the visit might be for preventive care. Collection of information by survey, interview or examination should be conducted in private space outside the earshot (or sight, if written documents) of others. Those documents should be

R. Saitz (✉)
Clinical Addiction Research and Education (CARE) Unit,
Section of General Internal Medicine, Department of Medicine,
Boston Medical Center and Boston University School of Medicine, Boston, MA, USA
e-mail: rsaitz@bu.edu

Department of Epidemiology, Boston University School of Public Health, Boston, MA, USA

Office of Clinical Research and Clinical Translational Science Institute, Boston University
Medical Campus, Boston, MA, USA

R. Saitz (ed.), *Addressing Unhealthy Alcohol Use in Primary Care,*
DOI 10.1007/978-1-4614-4779-5_16, © Springer Science+Business Media New York 2013

secured (locked cabinets, electronically) and accessible to people taking care of the patient and to the patient on request.

But for good patient care, when assessed, information about unhealthy alcohol and other drug use should be recorded in the medical record. Such information should be recorded, and recorded accurately for the protection of the clinician and the patient. For example, if a patient requests that alcohol and drug information not be recorded, and the clinician accedes to the request, this would be a failure of standards of medical practice, and in addition to professional consequences and legal consequences, could end up harming the patient if another clinician relies on inaccurate records and prescribes an inappropriate treatment. Similarly, just as with other medical conditions, alcohol and drug conditions should be documented with the most accurate description known. "Drinker," "social alcohol," "alcohol," "drug addict," are not informative and are likely inaccurate. Appropriate terms could include, for example, "unhealthy alcohol use," "risky consumption of alcohol," "drug use," "alcohol abuse," "drug dependence," and "substance use with consequences."

Of note, proper documentation is not only medically appropriate but it can affect the implications of a breach of confidentiality (or appropriate release of records) and even stigma associated with it. For example, documentation of use of risky amounts of alcohol should not be interpreted as alcohol or drug dependence, and therefore should not be associated with the same consequences (unless the reader of the record is ignorant regarding terminology and proper assessment and diagnosis).

The Privacy Rule (HIPAA [1])

Once the information is in a medical record, it can be useful for patient care by any clinician with access to it. Medical records are protected by the Privacy Rule. In December, 2000, the Department of Health and Human Services (HHS) issued the "Standards for Privacy of Individually Identifiable Health Information" final rule (known as the "Privacy Rule"), pursuant to the Administrative Simplification provisions of the Health Insurance Portability and Accountability Act of 1996 (HIPAA). HIPAA spells out what uses of the medical record are permitted, and they include access to take care of the patient. The patient can authorize release of that information to specific entities or people with an expiration date.

But the contents of medical records will be seen by anyone the patient authorizes, and by anyone involved in the transaction (including, for payment). Therefore, the health insurer may become aware of a diagnosis, as might the owner of an insurance plan who might be the patient's family member. The patient may authorize release of their records to life or disability insurance companies, and subpoenas could lead to release of records for legal purposes. These are all examples of legal and authorized releases of records that could lead to adverse consequences for patients. For example, the Uniform Individual Accident and Sickness Policy Provision model law (UPPL) written in 1947 is in effect in many states in the United States [2]. It states that the insurer shall not be liable for any loss sustained or contracted in consequence of the insured's being intoxicated or under the influence of any narcotic, unless administered on the advice of a physician. As a result, an insurer might not pay for treatment of a condition related to alcohol intoxication if the physician documents intoxication. The insurer generally has access to these records without patient authorization since HIPAA permits it for payment purposes.

Special Confidentiality Protection (CFR 42 Part II)

However, some records of alcohol and drug condition-related care have additional protection. In 1972, the Code of Federal Regulations (CFR) 42 Part II was enacted because of stigma and the fear people had about entering treatment since disclosure of their condition could have serious consequences [3]. The purpose was to encourage help-seeking and decrease the risk of discrimination. The law has provided special protection for patients with alcohol and drug use disorders, but questions have been raised regarding whether the law has interfered with high quality of care because of perceived and real barriers the law imposes on sharing information between clinicians and health care entities. Furthermore, despite the existence of the law, stigma and discrimination continue. In fact, the separation of addiction-related records and other medical records, and separate privacy rules, do not facilitate integration of care and may even contribute to continued stigma. Problems of stigma and discrimination and even poor care and treatment of people who suffer from addictions in general health setting are real and of great concern, but special confidentiality protections do not appear to have helped the situation. In addition, because they only apply in certain circumstances some have recognized the protections to be inadequate.

What Does CFR 42 Part II Require and When Does It Apply?

The details are important because in general, it does not apply in primary care, though there may be exceptions. It is about here that I must remind readers that I am a physician who has read the regulations but not a lawyer; I may be wrong, and this chapter does not constitute legal advice. But this is my understanding based on reading and practice that is shared by a number of primary care addiction experts. It is also important to note that state or local regulations can supersede Federal regulations if they are stricter, so the information herein may not be applicable (and the laws of course do not apply outside the United States, though other countries may have similar protections and similar considerations apply).

CFR 42 Part II applies to health care entities when they receive Federal assistance (e.g., Medicare, Veterans Affairs payments, have Controlled Substances Act registration to prescribe controlled substances to treat addiction (e.g., benzodiazepines for withdrawal, buprenorphine for opioid dependence [though, not naltrexone for alcohol dependence]), or have tax exempt status from the Internal Revenue Service). The regulations apply when a treatment program or identified unit within a general medical facility *holds itself out* as a provider and provides *alcohol or drug diagnosis, treatment or referral for treatment.* They also apply to staff whose *primary function* is as a provider who provides alcohol or drug diagnosis, treatment or referral for treatment [4–6]. So, a clinic with a sign that says "Alcohol and drug treatment clinic" or a clinician who spends most of his time diagnosing, treating, or referring patients for alcohol and drug conditions would keep records that need to be compliant with CFR 42 Part II. Exceptions to CFR 42 Part II applicability are the Department of Veterans Affairs, within the Armed Forces, a medical emergency (defined as an immediate threat and need for immediate treatment), and a general medical facility unless it holds itself out or has a primary function as described above.

When CFR 42 Part II applies, it requires written authorization from the patient to disclose (*and to re-disclose*) the information to other health providers. The authorization must be more detailed than that required under HIPAA. It must be to a named provider for a specific purpose and with an expiration date (or event). Although the law has no discrimination prohibitions or protections, it does include fines for release of records not consistent with the regulation of $500 and up to $5,000.

In the primary care management of unhealthy alcohol use, what might come under CFR 42 Part II? Screening, brief intervention, assessment, pharmacotherapy, and referral to 12-step groups and specialized treatments, if done by a clinician who does not provide these services as their primary function and does not provide the service in an entity that holds itself out as providing the service, does not likely come under the regulations. Although controversial, the same provision of care in the same setting might come under CFR 42 Part II if it is provided by a health promotion advocate or health educator whose primary role in the practice is to provide those services. Although not the focus of this book, some patients with unhealthy alcohol use will also have opioid dependence and be treated with buprenorphine for that condition in primary care. There has been some difference of opinion regarding whether CFR 42 Part II applies in that case. If the physician has many other patients and this is a small part of their practice and they do not advertise as a program, the practice may not fall under the regulation. However, if it is a large part of their practice and they define themselves to the public as a program, CFR 42 Part II may apply.

Conclusions

Confidentiality is a serious consideration in the identification and management of patients with unhealthy alcohol use in primary care. Clinicians need to be aware of Federal and other regulations that are relevant. They should also be aware of the risk of stigma and discrimination their patients face. Nonetheless, clinicians caring for such patients should document encounters accurately and use common sense in collecting sensitive information and in sharing it with other clinicians, within the bounds of applicable regulations. Some regulations may not be crystal clear, and as with many practices in medicine, protection and use of information will need to be based on sound judgment.

References

1. Summary of the HIPAA privacy rule. http://www.hhs.gov/ocr/privacy/hipaa/understanding/summary/index.html. Accessed 17 March 2012.
2. Chezem L. Legal barriers to alcohol screening in emergency departments and trauma centers. Alcohol Res Health. 2004/2005;28(2):73–77.
3. Code of Federal Regulations (CFR) 42 Part 2. http://www.gpo.gov/fdsys/pkg/CFR-2002-title42-vol1/pdf/CFR-2002-title42-vol1.pdf. Accessed 17 March 2012.
4. Substance Abuse and Mental Health Services Administration U.S. Department of Health and Human Services. Applying the Substance Abuse Confidentiality Regulations 42 CFR Part 2 (revised). http://www.samhsa.gov/about/laws/SAMHSA_42CFRPART2FAQII_Revised.doc. Accessed 17 March 2012.
5. Frequently asked questions. Applying the substance abuse confidentiality regulations to Health Information Exchange. http://www.samhsa.gov/HealthPrivacy/docs/EHR-FAQs.pdf. Accessed 17 March 2012.
6. Applying the Substance Abuse Confidentiality Regulations 42 CFR Part 2 (REVISED). Substance Abuse and Mental Health Services Administration. U.S. Department of Health and Human Services. http://www.samhsa.gov/about/laws/SAMHSA_42CFRPART2FAQII_Revised.pdf

Chapter 17
Choices for Patients and Clinicians: Ethics and Legal Issues

Michael Weaver

Introduction

Physicians deal with legal issues regarding patient safety and confidentiality on a regular basis, and these can be challenging when patients have problems related to alcohol. Ethical issues arise when there are conflicts between principles of patient autonomy, physician beneficence, and justice that may relate to both public safety and individual health. Legal concerns often relate to privacy and confidentiality and vary from state to state. This chapter addresses some common legal and ethical issues that may be encountered in primary care when addressing issues related to alcohol use or its consequences.

Physician Duties

To Document Unhealthy Alcohol Use or Not?

Disclosure of unhealthy alcohol use, particularly when it involves health and social effects and alcohol dependence, can have consequences for patients. Disclosure could affect insurance payments or coverage, employability or driving privileges. Patients may ask physicians not to document alcohol or other substance use issues out of fear of consequences. Confidentiality is critical for patients to be able to reveal information that is essential to identifying unhealthy alcohol use and for the diagnosis and treatment of alcohol use disorders (AUD). However, an office bill generated to an insurance company for a blood alcohol level or other testing may prompt an insurance company inquiry. Similarly, a diagnostic code for alcohol abuse or dependence or for an alcohol-related condition may also prompt scrutiny. The Uniform Accident and Sickness Policy Provision Law (UPPL) is a model law that

M. Weaver (✉)
Virginia Commonwealth University School of Medicine, Richmond, VA 23298-0109, USA
e-mail: mweaver@mcvh-vcu.edu

R. Saitz (ed.), *Addressing Unhealthy Alcohol Use in Primary Care,*
DOI 10.1007/978-1-4614-4779-5_17, © Springer Science+Business Media New York 2013

allows insurance carriers to exclude coverage for alcohol and drug-related injuries [1]. Thirty-eight states have provisions consistent with this law in their insurance codes. Confidentiality regulations don't provide protection from disclosure because patients sign consent forms authorizing release of this information to the insurance carrier for payment.

Despite these consequences the physician has a duty to document the patient's health issues in the medical record, for good care and for protection of the physician (ability to document diagnosis and treatment that could stand up to any review, legal or otherwise). Clinicians can do other forms of screening for AUD besides biological testing that may generate fewer specific bills. In fact other methods are generally preferred for screening, such as interview, and written or computer-based questionnaires. When unhealthy use without dependence is identified, no diagnostic code exists (e.g., for risky drinking) and thus the record will appropriately list a risk factor but will not reflect an alcohol use disorder diagnosis. Keeping records related to AUD in a separate file in an office setting may help preserve confidentiality, even with an electronic medical record, although this may be complicated to set up, and more importantly has two major drawbacks—(1) separate records risk poor quality care when all necessary information to care for a patient is not easily available when it is needed and (2) it perpetuates the separate and thus less well coordinated care for unhealthy alcohol use that is the norm in most health systems.

Is There Mandated Reporting?

Driving

Physicians are required to report patient health conditions that impact public safety in many states, such as reporting tuberculosis and certain sexually transmitted diseases to public health agencies. Some states require reporting to the department of motor vehicles for diagnoses of diabetes or epilepsy, including alcohol withdrawal seizures. A survey revealed that physicians agree that patients treated for injuries due to driving while intoxicated by alcohol should be reported to the police, but only a minority of physicians would actually report those patients themselves [2]. This discrepancy is due to concern about physician-patient confidentiality or threat of civil action by the patient against the physician. The state has the primary responsibility for traffic safety, not the physician [3]. A public policy statement by the American Society of Addiction Medicine (ASAM) emphasizes that physicians should not be required to report patients who might at some future time cause harm because of the nature of their illness, such as, required reporting to a state motor vehicle licensing agency or other state or federal agencies [4]. The National Highway Traffic Safety Administration recommends that physicians document history and physical findings consistent with unhealthy alcohol use and provide brief intervention to patients, as well as consider reporting unhealthy alcohol use with consequences in accordance with state laws [2]. Physicians should be familiar with mandatory reporting laws in their state for drivers with specific chronic conditions, including seizures resulting from an AUD.

Professional Drivers and Pilots

Professional drivers (long-distance truck drivers and train engineers) are required to undergo random testing for alcohol and drugs according to federal regulations from the U.S. Department of Transportation (DOT). This extends to compensated or voluntary drivers of school buses and church buses, even if drivers do not cross state lines. The rules state that a driver who fails an alcohol test must be removed immediately from his or her driving responsibilities. The driver may not return to these responsibilities until he or she has been evaluated by an addiction professional and has complied with any recommended rehabilitation. Pilots must comply with the regulations of the Federal Aviation Administration (FAA) requiring random testing for alcohol and drugs. There is a very low prevalence of alcohol violations in aviation employees [5] and the number of aviation accidents attributable to alcohol is correspondingly small [6]. Having an AUD is not a disqualifying medical condition for a pilot. However, pilots must report any charges of driving under the influence of alcohol or drugs (DUI) or related charges to the FAA within 60 days. Convictions for DUI have been shown to be associated with reported past aviation accidents in all pilot groups [7].

The onus of reporting in a timely fashion is on the professional driver or pilot, and DOT/FAA regulations are strict about this, including having professional drivers and pilots give consent for release of medical information about alcohol testing or impairment. Physicians should encourage patients who are professional drivers or pilots to report alcohol-related problems to the DOT or FAA, as required. This benefits the individual patient as well as the public, since impairment by a public transportation worker is both a personal and a public safety issue. Professional drivers and pilots have workplace employee assistance programs that address AUD and provide addiction treatment specific to those occupations. There are strict requirements for follow-up testing as well as returning to work. Alcoholics Anonymous groups specific to pilots are available and are known as "Birds of a Feather."

Pregnancy and Parenting

Patient history or physician examination may lead a physician to request laboratory screening for substances in a pregnant woman and/or newborn child, in the interest of both the woman's and the child's health. Testing should not be done without the patient's (woman's) knowledge. A request for bodily fluid testing must be accompanied by informed consent, because testing without this violates the constitutional rights of the mother and child [8] and the patient's autonomy. The physician must balance the maternal right to privacy with the imperative to protect the fetus [9]. Most physicians favor mandatory screening for unhealthy alcohol use, although there is concern that fear of prosecution and potential loss of custody of the child or her other children would cause women to avoid prenatal care [10]. Some states have laws that present terrible dilemmas to clinicians because they equate positive drug testing with child abuse or criminal offenses, which can interfere with successful treatment of substance dependence [11, 12]. However, in many cases across the nation, legislators and the courts have ruled that addiction in pregnancy is not a criminal matter [8] and there is no evidence that punitive approaches work [10].

Clinicians should be familiar with legislation in their community regarding the legal duty to report positive results to Child Protective Services (CPS). The CPS worker is then responsible for further investigation of risk to the child and a determination is made about the mother's and family's suitability to retain custody of the newborn infant and any other children in the household [13]. Legal coercion may help the mother to enter addiction treatment and improve outcomes, especially when allowed to retain custody of her infant [14].

Unlike in the case of the pregnant woman, alcohol use, nondependent unhealthy alcohol use and even alcohol dependence by a parent are not de facto evidence of child harm, although they may raise concerns regarding child safety. Thus, although unhealthy alcohol use should not automatically be reported to CPS, suspicion of child harm (e.g., neglect, endangerment) must be reported by mandated reporters.

Addressing Documentation and Reporting Issues with Patients

Federal regulations for transportation workers are clear and place the burden of reporting on the patient, not the physician. Requirements for reporting a patient with an identified AUD or specific alcohol-related consequences to various agencies vary from state to state. Familiarity with state reporting requirements regarding the potential for impaired driving or fetal exposure to alcohol is important for physicians. Furthermore, consistent with good medical practice, physicians must document the clinical encounter; it is not appropriate to fail to document even at a patient's request. Instead, patients should be aware that their health issues (including alcohol-related ones) will be documented in their medical record. Patients can then be informed about limits to confidentiality. Address reporting issues with the patient in a compassionate, nonjudgmental manner. Consequences related to employment or custody issues may help patients recognize the severity of problems related to alcohol or the existence of an AUD. This recognition can be an opportunity to discuss concerns about drinking and its consequences, and provide additional motivation for the patient to contemplate changes in drinking or entering treatment. External pressure from employers or legal authorities can increase the likelihood that the patient will enter treatment and remain adherent with treatment for alcohol dependence.

How do you Handle an Intoxicated Patient in the Office?

A patient may be recognized to be intoxicated during an office visit. The patient should be isolated from others in the waiting area when noticed to be intoxicated, especially if the patient is disruptive. The decision about degree of impairment should be based on clinical observation at the time, not just a diagnosis of an AUD or a blood alcohol level (because a patient with tolerance may not be impaired despite a "high" level). The impaired patient should not be allowed to drive. Alternate transportation should be secured. This may involve having a family member or friend come to pick up the patient from the physician's office, or calling a taxicab or arranging for suitable public transportation to convey the patient back home safely.

An intoxicated patient should be reported to the authorities only in unusual situations in which the patient is considered by the physician to be an immediate threat to public safety [4]. The office should contact the police or CPS (if the impaired patient is accompanied by a minor) only if a discussion with the patient fails to result in a safe and satisfactory solution. The patient may require transport to the emergency department for evaluation. Voluntary emergency department evaluation affords protection (for public safety, as well as liability by the physician) without breach of confidentiality.

Seek advice from competent legal counsel to have an appropriate office policy for the practice setting and state. Outlining standard office procedure for this type of incident helps prevent the appearance of discrimination. It also helps office staff recognize and respond to a potentially difficult situation consistently. Of note, an intoxicated patient in the office by definition has unhealthy alcohol use, which should be addressed clinically.

What About Underage Drinking?

Consumption of alcohol before age 21 years is underage drinking. Underage drinking is culturally and statistically normative in the United States though purchase is illegal, as is supplying alcohol to minors in certain circumstances. Alcohol use among college students is often tolerated although not sanctioned. Initiation of drinking in early adolescence increases the risk for development of an AUD [15, 16]. The hazards of underage drinking are well documented. Parents are often unaware of their teen's drinking and related problems [17]. Assurances of confidentiality from physicians have been shown to increase adolescents' willingness to discuss topics such as alcohol and substance use, and increase willingness to return for future visits [18].

A physician may be a credible source of information to an adolescent about adverse health effects of alcohol. Adolescents engaging in underage drinking may be referred to age-appropriate websites for more information. The National Institute on Alcohol Abuse and Alcoholism of the National Institutes of Health has a website for young teens about alcohol and resisting peer pressure called "The Cool Spot" (www.thecoolspot.gov).

It is rarely appropriate to perform a urine drug screen (UDS) or test breath or blood for alcohol in an adolescent without permission even at the request of a parent. The physician should obtain information from the parent about their concerns, then discuss these with the adolescent without the parent's presence. The adolescent often agrees to the UDS after discussion. The physician can then address plans by the patient and parent for responding to positive or negative results.

When an adolescent is identified with an AUD, formal addiction treatment may be necessary. Adolescents have widely varying levels of competence at any age, but many adolescents are competent to make health care decisions at age 12 years. All states require parental consent for medical care to minors and all states have laws that permit adolescents to consent to specific services, including addiction treatment, but there is significant variability between states, including age of consent, age at and condition/treatment for which an adolescent may make decisions without parental involvement (so-called mature minor), and parental notification requirements. Federally funded programs prohibit parental notification without the consent of the minor [19]. Parental involvement is positive and to be encouraged. If an adolescent is not competent to make a health care decision based on the determination by the physician, document this rationale in the medical record. Then inform the adolescent that confidentiality will be broken and involve the adolescent in the process of informing the parents.

Advice to Patients

Should Physicians Give Advice to Abstain?

When an AUD is identified by a physician, it is often accompanied by medical or mental health problems as well as social consequences. Addressing drinking behavior in an office practice setting can prevent additional consequences for the patient. A nonjudgmental attitude is essential, and increases the likelihood that the patient will answer honestly and consider recommendations. The physician should give clear advice to abstain when that is the best medical course (e.g., for dependence). A strong and clear recommendation to change drinking behavior is essential. A sample statement of this is, "Based on the information you have provided, you are at high risk of having or developing an alcohol use disorder. It is medically in your best interest to stop drinking." This can be followed up by specific medical reasons to quit drinking before problems (or more problems) develop. To fulfill the ethical responsibility to the patient, the physician should not only raise the patient's drinking as an issue, but also provide appropriate information and engage the patient in discussion [20]. This may include discussion of various treatment options available to the patient. If the patient is resistant to changing drinking behavior, the physician should follow up at future visits and continue to offer clear advice to abstain. Such clear and strong advice, however, is best done using an empathic, nonjudgmental approach that respects patient autonomy.

Is Coerced Treatment Ethical?

Coercion by Significant Others

Family and friends can be an effective source of social pressure for patients with AUD to enter addiction treatment [21, 22]. Family members or an employer may give the patient an ultimatum to force the patient into addiction treatment. This form of social pressure is a type of coercion. The patient may not like the consequences (losing the spouse or job), but retains autonomy to make a decision to enter treatment or refuse. Coercion raises retention rates in addiction treatment, which helps improve the odds of a positive outcome.

Drug Courts

In the criminal justice system, incarceration alone is insufficient in addressing AUD or recidivism to criminal behavior [23]. Drug courts address this problem with judicially supervised treatment-driven programs for nonviolent addicted criminal offenders. These courts are a collaboration between judges, prosecutors, defense attorneys, probation officers, and addiction treatment providers. Participation by offenders is voluntary, and by choosing to participate in drug court, criminal defendants avoid serving a substantial period of incarceration, as well as gain sobriety and a crime-free lifestyle. This form of legal coercion is ethical because the offender retains the autonomy to make a choice about whether to go to addiction treatment, although the alternative is incarceration and is less desirable. The coercive powers of the court system can contribute to recovery from AUD. Program participation requires abstinence from alcohol, attending addiction treatment for 12–18 months, court dates, 12-step meetings, and urine drug screens. A person coerced to enter addiction treatment by the criminal justice system is as likely to do well as a person who goes to addiction treatment voluntarily [24, 25]. Drug courts are an efficacious and cost-effective way to rehabilitate alcohol- and drug-related offenders [26].

Treatment Against a Patient's Will?

A family member may ask a physician to admit a patient into an addiction treatment program against the patient's will. Having a diagnosis of an AUD alone—even with the denial commonly seen in AUD patients—is insufficient to deem a patient incompetent to make health care decisions [27]. Therefore, the patient with an AUD retains the autonomy to choose or refuse to enter treatment for an AUD.

Informed consent is a legal and ethical duty in medical treatment. Patients entering addiction treatment may have limited awareness of alcohol problems and are not prepared for full discussion of consequences or the need for addiction treatment. The consent process itself may help the patient move into a new stage of change.

Practitioners may seek consent incrementally. Most of the risks from participating in addiction treatment that are discussed as part of the informed consent process involve confidentiality.

The physician (and family) must respect the right of the patient to choose a less effective addiction treatment or refuse treatment. The patient's refusal should not be met with a punitive response by the physician. However, social pressure by family or an employer can have a beneficial impact on treatment entry and retention.

What About Medical Marijuana?

Some states have enacted medical marijuana laws by voter initiative, which reduce or eliminate state criminal penalties for possessing marijuana for medical use. However, the U.S. federal government continues to enforce the Controlled Substances Act, which lists marijuana as Schedule I, so recommending or prescribing marijuana is not supported by the Drug Enforcement Administration, the Department of Justice, or the Department of Health and Human Services. A patient may request documentation by a physician regarding medical marijuana, so physicians must be aware of state statutes.

A survey of providers revealed that only 36 % of physicians believe prescribed marijuana should be legal and 26 % were neutral [28]. Safety concerns about medical marijuana include harms due to smoking as a delivery system, psychological dependence, and risks of injury due to acute intoxication [29].

Physicians can use this request for documentation by a patient as an opportunity to discuss alcohol as well as drug use. Patients obtaining marijuana ostensibly for medical purposes may also engage in use of alcohol, and the combination of these substances can be discussed in the context of increasing risks for impairment. Combining medical marijuana with alcohol for recreational purposes can be dangerous. Physicians may be able to make a better determination about medical versus recreational use of marijuana by a patient after appropriately gathering more information about use of alcohol and other illicit substances. This is essential if a physician is in a community where state statutes allow medical marijuana with physician approval.

What is Harm Reduction and is it Ethical?

Some patients may not be ready to stop or decrease drinking despite discussion with the physician. The physician should acknowledge the patient's autonomy, but address the issue at subsequent visits with an expression of concern regarding risks from use, and inquiry about interest in changing drinking behavior. "Harm reduction" is a set of practical strategies to reduce negative consequences of alcohol use (without necessarily eliminating the risk), which incorporates a range of strategies from safer use to managed use to less use to abstinence. It also may involve avoiding heavy drinking in hazardous situations (e.g., when unwanted sexual encounters may occur, while operating heavy machinery, or even avoidance of hangovers on work days). These strategies meet drinkers "where they're at" and address the conditions of drinking along with the drinking itself. If the patient continues to drink despite clear advice to abstain, the physician can provide additional information about harm reduction strategies to help improve the patient's safety. The ethical nature of the discussion is supported in two realms—(1) the patient retains autonomy and (2) the physician fulfills a duty to inform the patient regarding the ideal treatment goal along with alternatives that can also reduce risks to health.

Patients should be cautioned against drinking and driving. Physicians can discuss planning ahead to avoid having to drive after drinking by using a designated driver, drinking in a location where the patient will not have to leave (the home of the patient or a trusted friend), or giving the car keys to a nondrinking individual. These harm reduction strategies can help establish the physician's concern for the patient's safety while respecting the patient's autonomy to choose to continue to drink.

Caution adolescents against underage drinking and refer to an age-appropriate website. Once an AUD has been identified, the physician should advise abstinence and recommend appropriate treatment. However, this may not be welcomed by the adolescent with an AUD. Initial goals may be to reduce use and obtain further help.

Caution patients against combining alcohol and prescription medications to avoid interactions. Effects of antihypertensive medications may be acutely intensified, causing dizziness or weakness from hypotension, and chronic heavy alcohol consumption will negate the beneficial effects of these medications. Regular and/or heavy drinking may put a patient into a category that is too high-risk for specific medications, especially anticoagulants, due to potential for falls with bleeding. Heavy drinking may make tighter control of diabetes too risky (due to hypoglycemia). Combining alcohol with controlled substance prescriptions such as sedatives or opioid analgesics may result in significant harm due to synergistic effects, including unintentional overdose with respiratory depression.

Frank discussions of harm reduction may help the patient to consider a change in drinking while showing respect for the patient's autonomy. The issue can be raised at subsequent visits to evaluate continuance of risky behaviors. Awareness of the risks and of the physician's concern may enhance the patient's motivation for changing drinking behavior.

Conclusion

Legal and ethical issues can pose challenges for physicians, and planning ahead is helpful. Awareness of applicable state regulations regarding reporting requirements and consent for treatment is essential. Having office policies in place, for difficult situations and patients, helps prevent confusion at the time of an incident such as an impaired patient. A nonjudgmental attitude is important when addressing sensitive issues with patients, especially those involving problem drinking. Patients should be informed about limits of confidentiality under specific circumstances, but this can be an opportunity to discuss consequences of drinking as well as readiness for changing this behavior. Physicians have an ethical duty to offer clear advice to abstain from drinking if an AUD is identified, but physicians should also respect the patient's autonomy to choose to continue to drink. Harm reduction strategies can be offered and these issues can be revisited at subsequent office visits.

References

1. National Association of Insurance Commissioners (NAIC). Model laws regulations and guidelines. NAIC: Model regulation service. Kansas City: Uniform Individual Accident and Sickness Policy Provisions Law. 2004; Vol. II, p. 180–181.
2. Mello MJ, Nirenberg TD, Lindquist D, et al. Physicians' attitudes regarding reporting alcohol-impaired drivers. Subst. Abuse. 2003;24:233–242.
3. Krumholz A, Fisher RS, Lesser RP, Hauser WA. Driving and epilepsy: a review and reappraisal. JAMA. 1991;265:622–626.
4. American Society of Addiction Medicine (ASAM). Public policy statement of reporting of patient information related to fitness for driving or other potentially dangerous activities. J Addictive Dis. 2000;19:125–127.
5. Guohua L, Brady JE, DiMaggio C, et al. Validity of suspected alcohol and drug violations in aviation employees. Addiction. 2010;105:1771–1775.
6. Cook CCH. Alcohol and aviation. Addiction. 1997;92:539–555.
7. Platenius PH, Wilde GJS. Personal characteristics related to accident histories of Canadian pilots. Aviation Space and Environmental Medicine. 1989;60:42–45.
8. Harris LH, Paltrow L. The status of pregnant women and fetuses in U.S. criminal law. JAMA. 2003;289:1697–1699.
9. Lambert B, Scheiner M, Campbell D. Ethical issues and addiction. J Addictive Diseases. 2010;29:164–174.
10. Abel EL, Kruger M. Physician attitudes concerning legal coercion of pregnant alcohol and drug abusers. Am J Obstet Gynecol. 2002;186:768–772.
11. Ferguson v. City of Charleston: US Court of Appeals, Fourth Circuit. Wests Fed Rep. 1999;186:469–489.
12. Kimbel AS. Pregnant drug abusers are treated like criminals or not treated at all: a third option proposed. J Contemp Health Law Policy. 2004;21:36–66.
13. Wunsch MJ, Weaver MF. Alcohol and other drug use during pregnancy: management of the affected mother and child. In: Ries R, Fiellin D, Miller S, Saitz R, editors. Principles of addiction medicine. 4th ed. Chevy Chase: American Society of Addiction Medicine; 2009. p. 1111–1124.
14. Nace EP, Birkmayer F, Sullivan MA, et al. Socially sanctioned coercion mechanisms for addiction treatment. Am J Addict. 2007;16:15–23.
15. Clark DB. The natural history of adolescent alcohol use disorders. Addiction. 2004;99 Suppl 1:5–22.
16. Hingson RW, Heeren T, Winter MR. Age at drinking onset and alcohol dependence: age at onset, duration, and severity. Arch Pediatr Adolesc Med. 2006;160:739–746.
17. Young TL, Zimmerman R. Clueless: parent knowledge of risk behaviors of middle school students. Arch Pediatr Adolesc Med. 1998;152:1137–1139.
18. Ford CA, Millstein SG, Alpern-Felsher BL, Irwin CE. Influence of physician confidentiality assurances on adolescents' willingness to disclose information and seek future health care. JAMA. 1997;278:1029–1034.
19. Gittler J, Quigley-Rick M, Saks MJ. Adolescent health care decision making: the law and public policy. Washington, DC: Carnegie Council on Adolescent Development; 1990.

20. Clark HW, Bizzell AC. Ethical issues in addiction practice. In: Ries R, Fiellin D, Miller S, Saitz S, editors. Principles of addiction medicine. 4th ed. Chevy Chase: American Society of Addiction Medicine; 2009. p. 1485–1490.
21. Wild TC, Newton-Taylor B, Alleto R. Perceived coercion among clients entering substance abuse treatment: structural and psychological determinants. Addictive Behav. 1998;23:81–95.
22. Hasin DS. Treatment/self-help for alcohol-related problems. Relationship to social pressure and alcohol dependence. J Stud Alcohol. 1994;55:660–666.
23. Hora PF, Schma WG. Drug courts and the treatment of incarcerated populations. In: Ries R, Fiellin D, Miller S, Saitz R, editors. Principles of addiction medicine. 4th ed. Chevy Chase: American Society of Addiction Medicine; 2009. p. 1513–1518.
24. Cooper CS. Drug courts—just the beginning: getting other areas of public policy in sync. Subst Use Misuse. 2007;42:243–256.
25. McMurran M. What works in substance misuse treatments for offenders. Crim Behav Ment Health. 2007;17:225–233.
26. Klag S, O'Callaghan F, Creed P. The use of legal coercion in the treatment of substance abusers? An overview and critical analysis of thirty years of research. Subst Use Misuse. 2005;40:1777–1795.
27. Spike J. A paradox about capacity, alcoholism, and noncompliance. J Clin Ethics. 1997;8:303–306.
28. Charuvastra A, Friedmann PD, Stein MD. Physician attitudes regarding the prescription of medical marijuana. J Addict Dis. 2005;24:87–93.
29. Joy JE, Watson SJ, Benson JA. Marijuana and medicine: assessing the science base. Washington, DC: National Academy Press; 1999.

Chapter 18
Hospital Management

Richard D. Blondell and Mohammadreza Azadfard

Introduction

Compared to the general population, the prevalence of unhealthy alcohol use is higher among hospitalized patients [1]. A process that is known as screening and brief intervention has been implemented at some institutions and observational studies suggest benefit [2] though the results of randomized trials have been decidedly mixed (in hospital settings). Patients with alcohol dependence and recent alcohol use in these settings may require management to prevent or treat the alcohol withdrawal syndrome (AWS).

Prevalence and Epidemiology

Estimates of the prevalence of alcohol use disorders among patients in hospital settings vary with the patient population that is selected and the study methodology that is used. For example, one study of 2,040 admissions to non-federal short-stay general hospitals in the 48 contiguous US states determined the overall prevalence of alcohol use disorders was 7.4 % (95 % confidence interval, 5.6–9.1 %) for all admissions and 24.0 % (95 % confidence interval 18.7–29.4 %) among those who were current drinkers [3]. However, in one large multi-hospital study of 59,760 patients in the Houston area, systematic screening by physicians, nurses and medical technician generalists identified 15,241 (26 %) as appropriate candidates for additional services [2]. In another study conducted in Dutch emergency departments, data on alcohol use by patient self-report and staff judgment combined resulted in prevalence rate estimates of 4.9–18.2 % [4]. Drinking problems appear to be more common among medical than surgical inpatients [5]. Rates of intoxication among victims of traumatic injuries approach 50 %, with the highest rates among men aged 21–33 years

R. D. Blondell (✉) · M. Azadfard
Department of Family Medicine, University at Buffalo, Buffalo, NY 14215, USA
e-mail: blondell@buffalo.edu

R. Saitz (ed.), *Addressing Unhealthy Alcohol Use in Primary Care,*
DOI 10.1007/978-1-4614-4779-5_18, © Springer Science+Business Media New York 2013

Table 18.1 Risk stratification and action to be taken

Level of use	Characteristics	Suggested action
No use	Abstinent from alcohol, no prior alcohol use disorder	Inform abstinence can be a healthy choice
Prior disorder	Currently abstinent with a past alcohol use disorder	Support that abstinence likely the safest choice
		Caution when using controlled substances, and explore risk for relapse
Low risk use	Consumption of alcohol does not exceed low-risk limits, no evidence of alcohol-related consequences	Support low risk drinking as a reasonably healthy choice
At-risk use	Consumption of alcohol exceeds low-risk limits, no evidence of alcohol-related consequences	Brief intervention with advice to cut-down or to quit drinking
"Problem" use and Abuse	Consumption of alcohol exceeds low-risk limits, with evidence of alcohol-related consequences that do not meet criteria for dependence or that meet criteria for abuse (recurrent consequences)	Brief intervention with advice to cut-down or to quit drinking
Dependent use	Meets criteria for dependence, with or without risk factors for alcohol withdrawal	Brief intervention with goal of abstinence and referral to treatment if the patient agrees
		Treatment to prevent or manage withdrawal

old [6]. Comorbid psychiatric problems (e.g., organic brain syndromes, depressive disorders, phobias) are common among inpatients with alcohol problems who have been admitted to general hospitals. A lifetime diagnosis of alcoholism was associated with a 41.3 % prevalence of lifetime psychiatric comorbidity, and current alcoholism was associated with a 44.4 % prevalence of current psychiatric comorbidity [7].

Case Finding, Screening and Assessment

Case finding identifies those with symptoms related to consumption of alcohol, whereas screening is used to identify patients who have risky alcohol consumption or those with disorders without regard to symptoms. Individuals who are identified as potentially having a drinking problem by case finding or screening may need further assessment to determine their level of risk, which would serve to guide the clinician in taking the appropriate therapeutic action (See Table 18.1).

Case Finding

When a patient presents to a hospital, it may be clinically obvious that drinking with health consequences exists due to the nature of the primary diagnosis (e.g., pancreatitis), the past medical history (e.g., prior treatment for alcoholism), the physical examination (e.g., intoxication) or the results of toxicology. Other patients may freely admit using alcohol excessively. In instances such as these, no additional screening is indicated (assessment for severity would be the next step).

At other times the clinician may suspect the presence of unhealthy alcohol use among some patients based on the presenting complaint (e.g., hematemesis), past domestic problems (e.g., divorce, domestic violence), financial difficulty (e.g., lost jobs) or criminal activity (e.g., arrests for driving while intoxicated, public intoxication or drug-related crimes). The physical examination may also yield clues to an underlying alcohol use disorder (e.g., parotid hypertrophy, hepatomegaly). The results of routine laboratory tests (e.g., macrocytosis, elevated liver enzymes) that were obtained as part of the admission process may be the result of an alcohol use disorder.

Screening

Screening patients (regardless of symptoms or signs) for the presence of an alcohol use disorder during their hospital stay may become the standard-of-care in many hospitals. This screening is coupled with an appropriate "brief intervention" that is designed to reduce drinking or encourage linkage with treatment for alcohol dependence, which hopefully would improve clinical outcomes, and reduce overall health care costs. Whether health care cost savings and improved clinical outcomes can actually be achieved among a population screened universally, remains to be determined [8].

Screening for unhealthy alcohol use is typically done with questionnaires. Items that relate to the "quantity and frequency" of alcohol use are the most straightforward to use, but some patients may under-report the amount they consume. To address this problem, questionnaires that focus on the "patterns and consequences" of alcohol consumption can be used during the clinical interview. One example is the so-called CAGE questionnaire, which has been used for decades [9]. The CAGE acronym is based on the questions that relate to *cutting* down, *annoyed* by the criticism of others, *guilt* associated with drinking, and drinking first thing in the morning (i.e., an "eye-opener"). The main limitation of this questionnaire is that it identifies disorders (like dependence) and not the entire spectrum of unhealthy use. Another common screening questionnaire that does identify the spectrum and has been used for years is the Alcohol Use Disorders Identification Test (AUDIT) [10].

There is no consensus on which questions are best to use in emergency departments or on inpatient wards. The effectiveness (yield and validity) of screening questions seems to vary by gender, ethnicity, and presenting problem (e.g., medical disorder, traumatic injury, pregnancy) [11, 12]. Some experts recommend using a few "quantity and frequency" questions based on the AUDIT questionnaire that are followed by a few "patterns and consequences" questions based on the CAGE questions as a good strategy for routine screening [13]. Estimates of the daily consumption of alcohol are useful in determining who may be at risk for the development of the alcohol withdrawal syndrome.

A number of biological markers or clinical laboratory tests have been used to identify patients who have excessive alcohol consumption [14]. Because the liver is adversely affected by alcohol, liver enzyme serum levels are frequently used as a marker of problem drinking. The most common are gamma-glutamyltransferase (GGT) and aspartate aminotransferase (AST). Injuries to the liver and chronic hepatitis C are common among hospitalized patients which limits the value of liver enzymes as a screening test. Another item used as a marker for heavy alcohol use is the serum carbohydrate deficient transferrin (CDT) level, which has a sensitivity of about 70 % for very heavy regular drinking [15]. Alcohol interferes with the maturation of red blood cells, which leads to macrocytosis and an elevated erythrocyte mean cell volume (MCV) in some patients with extensive alcohol use. Because there is no single biological marker that appears to be effective for screening patients for alcohol use disorders, investigators have evaluated a combination of markers [16, 17]. Using the combination of CDT and GGT increases sensitivity to about 90 % above either marker alone for very heavy regular alcohol use, without compromising specificity [18]. Toxicology (alcohol and other drugs) can identify those who are intoxicated or who have abused illicit drugs. Since alcohol and drug problems are common among victims of traumatic injuries, routine toxicology testing is recommended for trauma services [19]. Whether a single test or a combination of other tests is of practical value for routine screening of all hospitalized patients remains to be determined. For withdrawal risk we recommend asking about daily heavy (e.g. , >4 or 5 standard drinks) drinking or signs of dependence (e.g., CAGE questions, or dependence items from the AUDIT or dependence criteria).

Assessment

Patients who have been identified as having hazardous drinking may need a clinical assessment to determine the extent of their problems so as to guide the clinician in taking appropriate action. Among hospitalized patients, it is especially important to assess for risk factors associated with AWS (See Table 18.2). Treatment may be required to prevent AWS or to manage the complications of AWS (e.g., Wernicke's encephalopathy, seizures, and delirium) (See Table 18.3).

Family members may provide useful information suggestive of an alcohol use disorder, but not always. Sometimes family members simply do not know the extent of the patient's use of alcohol. At other times, family members may not give accurate information because they also drink heavily, or are trying to protect the patient from legal action (e.g., an arrest related to driving under the influence of alcohol).

One third or more of the patients who drink excessively also use other drugs [28, 29]. It is important to evaluate patients with unhealthy alcohol use for concurrent illicit drug use, because a concurrent drug withdrawal syndrome complicates the management of AWS [30].

Table 18.2 Risk factors for more severe alcohol withdrawal or delirium tremens. (Based on Refs. [20–24])

Characteristic	Comment
Recent drinking	Drinking >60–100 g/day (e.g., >1 pint of liquor, >5–8 standard alcohol content 12 ounce beers)
Current withdrawal	Symptoms when not drinking, drinking to prevent symptoms
Prior withdrawal	Past severe alcohol withdrawal with seizures or delirium
Past heavy drinking	At-risk daily drinking >8–10 years
Any acute illness	Medical, surgical, or psychiatric
Cirrhosis	Especially if elevated bilirubin
Renal disease	Elevated Blood Urea Nitrogen (BUN) or serum creatinine
Neurological disease	Seizures, brain injury, and cerebral vascular events
Macrocytosis	Elevated mean corpuscular volume (MCV)
Intoxication	Any random blood alcohol concentration (BAC) > 150 mg/dL
Sedative use	The concurrent abuse of sedatives may increase withdrawal risk and severity

Table 18.3 Medications used to prevent and manage alcohol withdrawal. (Information based on FDA approved package inserts and references [25–27])

Medication	Comments
Thiamine	Used to prevent Wernicke-Korsakoff syndrome
	Must be given before glucose containing fluids
	Initial parenteral doses are recommended
Long-acting benzodiazepines	Recommended as the drugs-of-choice for monotherapy
	Symptom-triggered, front loading, and fixed schedule dosing
Short-acting benzodiazepines	An alternative to long-acting benzodiazepines for elderly, those with hepatic synthetic dysfunction or risk for respiratory failure
	Can prevent second seizure in emergency department
	Should not be stopped abruptly without tapering
Sympatholytics	Beta-blockers and clonidine have been used
	Given to control severe hypertension and tachycardia
	Used after adequate sedation with benzodiazepines
Neuroleptics	May be used for severe agitation or hallucinations
	May lower seizure threshold
	Used after adequate sedation with benzodiazepines
Magnesium	Use is controversial as a specific treatment for alcohol withdrawal symptoms per se
	Causes little harm in routine use to treat deficiency which is common and difficult to diagnose, as long as renal insufficiency is excluded
	Used to manage hypomagnesemia and hypokalemia

Management of the Alcohol Withdrawal Syndrome (AWS)

Alcohol withdrawal is a common problem in hospital practice and is a complex management issue that involves anticipating and preventing withdrawal symptoms, monitoring withdrawal signs and symptoms with objective rating scales, and treating complications (e.g., fluid and electrolyte abnormalities, liver failure). The specific goals of AWS management are to prevent the Wernicke–Korsakoff syndrome (that may occur with or without withdrawal symptoms), severe withdrawal symptoms, withdrawal seizures, delirium tremens, and death.

The Progression of AWS

The symptoms and signs of AWS tend to progress over time. Those with early mild symptoms can be managed on general medical or surgical wards, whereas others with more severe signs may need to be transferred to a critical care setting [31]. Patients with delirium tremens who require the use of restraints or who develop hyperthermia are at increased risk of death [32].

Symptoms and signs of AWS can begin within five to eight hours after the last drink, but these may be subtle as patients are usually coherent, with only mild cognitive impairment, anxiety, restlessness or a poor appetite. Tremor is most common. Later, patients may develop agitation, nausea with a decreased appetite; sleep disturbances, facial sweating, fluctuating tachycardia and mild hypertension. As AWS progresses, marked restlessness, agitation and tremulousness, with constant eye movement may develop. Sometimes the patient may appear mildly disoriented and confused, but re-orientation is often possible. There may also be pronounced tachycardia and systolic hypertension. Diaphoresis, moderate nausea, vomiting, anorexia, and diarrhea are common.

"Alcoholic hallucinosis," which consists of auditory, tactile or visual hallucinations, may be present and often is not accompanied by other symptoms of withdrawal.

Similarly, seizures, which are typically grand mal, may occur but are not always preceded by other symptoms of withdrawal. Seizures usually are single and last less than five minutes, but some patients have seizures in salvos of two or three, or even status epilepticus though status should prompt evaluation for another etiology besides alcohol withdrawal [33].

Delirium tremens, can occur from 72 to 96 h after the last drink. They are always preceded by other symptoms (autonomic) of withdrawal. Patients appear severely ill with unstable vital signs. This is associated with fever, severe hypertension (though neither are cardinal features) and tachycardia, delirium, drenching sweats, and marked tremulousness. Delirium (acute transient confusional state) is the sine qua non, and re-orientation is difficult or impossible. Causes of death during this stage include head trauma, cardiovascular complications, infections, aspiration pneumonia, and fluid and electrolyte abnormalities. Long-term mortality is increased in patients who have a history of severe AWS [34].

Nonpharmacological Interventions

Nonpharmacologic interventions are important in the management of AWS and include frequent reassurance, reality orientation, and nursing care [35]. Patients seem to do best when they are kept in an evenly lit, quiet room; and dark shadows, bright lights, loud noises, and other excessive stimuli are avoided. Since volume depletion is a potential complication of AWS, the liberal intake of caffeine-free fluids is important and judicious use of intravenous fluids may be required [36]. The vital signs, fluid intake and output, and serum electrolytes should be monitored, especially with cases of moderate-to-severe AWS.

The clinical course of the AWS should also be monitored with an objective rating scale such as the Clinical Institute Withdrawal Assessment-Alcohol, revised (CIWA-Ar) [37]. The CIWA-Ar can be used by the nursing staff to monitor patient progress and by physicians as a guide for pharmacotherapy. Higher scores indicate greater severity and risk for the development of more severe withdrawal. One caution, particularly in patients hospitalized for reasons other than alcohol withdrawal, is that the assessment is nonspecific—many medical and psychiatric conditions can produce high CIWA-Ar scores even if the patient doesn't have alcohol dependence or withdrawal. Each item must be scored based on the clinician's expert opinion that the symptom or sign is related to alcohol withdrawal, based on a complete clinical evaluation. Another related caution is to only use the CIWA-Ar and treat alcohol withdrawal when the diagnosis is in fact present. Numerous examples exist of patients being treated for withdrawal, based on the CIWA-Ar scale, when they have not had recent regular heavy drinking that could put them at risk for withdrawal, or when they do not have the ability to be assessed by this scale because of cognitive impairments (the scale can only be used with cognitively intact patients).

Thiamine

Thiamine (vitamin B_1) deficiency is frequent among patients with alcohol dependence and can lead to a serious complication, the Wernicke–Korsakoff syndrome. Thiamine (100 mg) must be given before glucose-containing fluids are given, and the initial dose should be given parenterally [38]. Oral thiamine supplementation is widely used, despite the absence of comparative trials; high doses must be used to compensate for poor absorption [39, 40]. Intravenous or intramuscular administration is best if patients have a poor nutritional status, if there is any question regarding malabsorption, or severe complications such as Wernicke encephalopathy (a medical emergency), even though rare anaphylactic reactions have been reported after thiamine injection [41].

Benzodiazepines

Benzodiazepines are considered to be the drugs of choice as monotherapy for the prevention and treatment of AWS [42]. Current evidence suggests that long-acting benzodiazepines (i.e., chlordiazepoxide, diazepam) are superior to short-acting

Table 18.4 Benzodiazepine regimens for alcohol withdrawal. (Information based on FDA-approved package inserts or from other references [25, 44, 45] when "off-label" use is noted)

Regimen	Agents
Symptom triggered	Chlordiazepoxide: FDA approved dosage: 50–100 mg PO for symptoms with a max of 300 mg/day. Off-label dosage: 25–100 mg PO every hour for CIWA > 8 until agitation resolves as evidenced by randomized trials Diazepam: FDA approved dosage: 10 mg-QID X 24 h PRN, then 5–10 mg PRN TID-QID. Off-label dosage: 20 mg every 1–2 h at first sign of withdrawal until symptoms are improved (referred to as "front loading") as demonstrated in randomized trials
Fixed schedule	Chlordiazepoxide can be used off-label as demonstrated in randomized trials: 50 mg every 6 h for four doses, then 25 mg every 6 h for eight doses, with additional doses given as needed based on symptoms. Hold for sedation
Short-acting benzodiazepines	Oxazepam: FDA approved dosage: 15–30 mg PO TID-QID. Off-label dosage: substitute for chlordiazepoxide or diazepam in the above regimens as was done in randomized trials, but with a taper over several days if more than a day of dosing is administered Lorazepam: Not FDA-approved for alcohol withdrawal. FDA approved dosage: none. Off-label dosage: 1–4 mg Q3–4 h as needed, then taper off over 3–5 days in a symptom-triggered or fixed schedule regimen, e.g., 2 mg 4 times on day 1, 2 mg 3 times on day 2, 1 mg 3 times on day 3, and 1 mg 2 times on day 4

benzodiazepines (i.e., lorazepam, oxazepam), owing to the gradual decrease in serum benzodiazepine levels of the long half-life drugs that leads to a "self-tapering" effect [25]. Compared with other drugs, the benzodiazepines appear to be superior for symptom control, seizure and delirium management, and for the prevention of life-threatening events [43]. As summarized in Table 18.4, benzodiazepines may be administered as needed on a "symptom triggered" basis or on a "fixed schedule."

Fixed dose schedules are used in settings when nursing expertise in monitoring or availability to adequately monitor AWS is limited, when the likelihood of AWS is increased (e.g., a patient with past severe AWS, particularly AWS complications that occur without prior warning or symptoms or when the patient has a high risk for withdrawal such as acute medical, psychiatric or surgical illness, or is having withdrawal symptoms at a high (>100–150 mg/dL blood alcohol level)—cases in which at least one dose should be given regardless of symptoms) or when outpatient detoxification is indicated [36, 46]. A typical dosing schedule would be chlordiazepoxide 50 mg every 6 h for four doses then 25 mg every 6 h for eight doses. "As-needed" dosing should always be available even if the patient is on a fixed dose schedule.

With symptom-triggered protocols, patients are monitored with an objective rating scale such as the CIWA-Ar and are administered medications when the symptoms or signs of AWS are noted [47]. A typical dosing regimen would be 25–100 mg of chlordiazepoxide every 1–4 h as needed. Once medication is no longer required for symptoms for 24 h, symptoms are very unlikely to re-emerge. With this regimen assuming long-acting medications are used, no taper is required nor is there any need to gradually decrease the dose. In addition, it is not possible to specify a maximum dose since patients' requirements are based on symptoms. However, clinicians may wish to re-evaluate the clinical circumstances when daily doses of 300 mg or more of chlordiazepoxide are reached to minimize inappropriate over-sedation. But these doses are easily reached appropriately in many patients with substantial symptoms. A variation of this symptom-triggered approach is a protocol known as "front-loading" treatment [36]. In this regimen, 20 mg of diazepam is given at the first sign of AWS and repeated every 1 to 2 h until symptoms resolve. Generally, patients can be treated with lower total doses of benzodiazepines using symptom-triggered protocols than with fixed dose schedules. Symptom-triggered and front-loading arose from two different types of studies but the approaches are essentially the same with the exception that in the latter approach an initial dose is given regardless of symptoms (it was studied in people with substantial symptoms whereas symptom-triggered therapy studies have included patients with minimal symptoms initially).

Short-acting benzodiazepines (e.g., oxazepam, lorazepam) can be used for patients with an impaired ability to metabolize long-acting benzodiazepines (e.g., compromised liver function as evidenced by low serum albumin or high bilirubin or international normalized ratio (INR)) or when over-sedation must be avoided (e.g., patients with respiratory impairments that risk respiratory failure). Patients who present to emergency departments with alcohol withdrawal seizures can be treated with 2 mg of intravenous lorazepam to present a second seizure, but other causes of seizures need to be excluded if the clinical picture is inconsistent with an alcohol withdrawal seizure (e.g., the history and time course are not what would be expected, the neurological examination finds focal signs, there is fever) or it is the first ever seizure for the patient [48]. Symptom-driven lorazepam has also been used successfully in the intensive care unit [49]. However, the doses of short-acting benzodiazepines must be gradually reduced over several days as the abrupt discontinuation of these medications can lead to a re-emergence of the withdrawal syndrome, including seizures.

Physicians who are not familiar with the management of AWS tend to prescribe inadequate doses of benzodiazepines and are often surprised at the large doses can be tolerated by some patients. Nevertheless, patients who receive large doses require extremely close monitoring since respiratory depression and death can occur. Some patients with severe AWS may require continuous infusions of benzodiazepines, barbiturates or propofol to adequately control AWS; intensive care unit monitoring and mechanical ventilation are usually required in such cases. Special care may be needed for the elderly or those with liver disease, as the metabolism of long-acting benzodiazepines may be compromised in these patients. Shorter acting benzodiazepines are preferred in the elderly and renally metabolized benzodiazepines (e.g., lorazepam) are preferred for those with liver disease.

Other Medications

Other medications can be used in the management of AWS as long as benzodiazepines are already being given (the only medications proven to prevent the mortal complications of withdrawal, seizures and DTs) [25]. Beta-adrenergic antagonists (i.e., "beta-blockers") and clonidine have been used to manage hypertension and tachycardia associated with AWS following the administration of adequate doses of benzodiazepines; however, these medications may increase the risk of hallucinations and sleep disturbances, and can also interfere with clinicians' ability to determine the severity of withdrawal (by lowering the heart rate and other autonomic symptoms). Neuroleptics are commonly used to manage delirium and severe agitation; however, since they increase the risk of seizures, they should only be given after adequate sedation with benzodiazepines has been achieved. Furthermore, it is not clear that neuroleptics add any benefit to benzodiazepine treatment alone. Nonetheless it does appear that some patients continue to have severe symptoms despite adequate and high doses of benzodiazepines. This may be because other receptor pathways are involved in the pathophysiology of withdrawal beyond those affected by benzodiazepines. As a result, clinicians may need to try other medications. There are no convincing data to support the routine use of magnesium sulfate for the management of AWS, but it may be indicated in case of magnesium deficiency (and the serum level often does not reflect the deficiency—as a result, provided renal function is normal, it is reasonable to assume deficiency and treat it; deficiency should be assumed if hypokalemia is present). Although useful for patients who are attempting to maintain abstinence from alcohol, acamprosate, naltrexone, and disulfiram are not beneficial in alcohol withdrawal per se though acamprosate may help with symptoms of protracted withdrawal.

Brief Interventions

The hospitalization of a patient with an unhealthy alcohol use may provide a unique opportunity for brief interventions and referral to treatment designed to improve clinical outcomes and reduce health care costs. The practice has been tested in hospital settings with mixed results [50–55]. In general, there is very little evidence that dependent drinking (the most common pattern in hospitalized adults with unhealthy use) is reduced or completion of a referral (or any beneficial impact of referral or its completion) is accomplished by brief intervention in this circumstance. But some authorities believe there is enough evidence for clinical and policy action, while others view this (particularly, universal screening with the expectation that individual patients so identified will decrease their drinking or enter treatment and become abstinent) as premature [56]. Nevertheless, patients with unhealthy alcohol use who are identified during hospitalization should have this problem addressed along with their other problems as part of the routine discharge planning process. And patients willing to discuss their use and healthy changes should be encouraged to address their drinking. Furthermore, alcohol use should be identified in all hospitalized patients for proper diagnosis of symptoms and treatment just like all nonprescription medications taken are identified.

Prevention

Those without unhealthy alcohol use may benefit from routine health advice regarding the use of alcohol: Continue abstinence or low-risk levels of drinking, don't drink and drive, or avoid drinking while taking certain medications (e.g., sedatives, opioids). Controlled substances should be used with great caution in patients with a current or past alcohol use disorder.

Summary

Unhealthy alcohol use is common among hospitalized patients, and those with dependence need to be assessed for withdrawal risk. Thiamine should always be given to these patients; they should be monitored with a structured withdrawal rating scale (e.g., CIWA) and treated with benzodiazepines as the drug-of-choice for monotherapy of alcohol withdrawal. Referral to alcohol counseling rehabilitation services should be part of discharge planning when appropriate.

References

1. Roson B, Monte R, Gamallo R, et al. Prevalence and routine assessment of unhealthy alcohol use in hospitalized patients. Eur J Intern Med. 2010;21:458–464.
2. SBIRT outcomes in Houston: final report on InSight, a hospital district-based program for patients at risk for alcohol or drug use problems. Alcohol Clin Exp Res. 2009;33:1374–1381.
3. Smothers BA, Yahr HT, Sinclair MD. Prevalence of current DSM-IV alcohol use disorders in short-stay, general hospital admissions, United States, 1994. Arch Intern Med. 2003;163:713–719.
4. Vitale SG, Van De Mheen D, Van De Wiel A, Garretsen HF. Alcohol and illicit drug use among emergency room patients in the Netherlands. Alcohol Alcohol. 2006;41:553–559.
5. Sri EV, Raguram R, Srivastava M. Alcohol problems in a general hospital—a prevalence study. J Indian Med Assoc. 1997;95:505–506.
6. Blake RB, Brinker MR, Ursic CM, Clark JM, Cox DD. Alcohol and drug use in adult patients with musculoskeletal injuries. Am J Orthop (Belle Mead NJ). 1997;26:704–709; discussion 709–710.
7. Arolt V, Driessen M. Alcoholism and psychiatric comorbidity in general hospital inpatients. Gen Hosp Psychiatry. 1996;18:271–277.
8. Bray JW, Cowell AJ, Hinde JM. A systematic review and meta-analysis of health care utilization outcomes in alcohol screening and brief intervention trials. Med Care. 2011;49:287–294.
9. Ewing JA. Detecting alcoholism. The CAGE questionnaire. JAMA. 1984;252:1905–1907.
10. Bohn MJ, Babor TF, Kranzler HR. The Alcohol Use Disorders Identification Test (AUDIT): validation of a screening instrument for use in medical settings. J Stud Alcohol. 1995;56:423–432.
11. Cherpitel CJ. Screening for alcohol problems in the emergency department. Ann Emerg Med. 1995;26:158–166.
12. Cherpitel CJ. Screening for alcohol problems in the U.S. general population: a comparison of the CAGE and TWEAK by gender, ethnicity, and services utilization. J Stud Alcohol. 1999;60:705–711.

13. National Institute on Alcohol Abuse and Alcoholism. Helping patients who drink too much: a clinician's guide. NIH Publication No. 07-3769; 2007.
14. Conigrave KM, Saunders JB, Whitfield JB. Diagnostic tests for alcohol consumption. Alcohol Alcohol. 1995;30:13–26.
15. Spies CD, Emadi A, Neumann T, et al. Relevance of carbohydrate-deficient transferrin as a predictor of alcoholism in intensive care patients following trauma. J Trauma. 1995;39:742–748.
16. Nilssen O, Ries R, Rivara FP, Gurney JG, Jurkovich GJ. The WAM score: sensitivity and specificity of a user friendly biological screening test for alcohol problems in trauma patients. Addiction. 1996;91:255–262.
17. Hoeksema HL, de Bock GH. The value of laboratory tests for the screening and recognition of alcohol abuse in primary care patients. J Fam Pract. 1993;37:268–276.
18. Hietala J, Koivisto H, Anttila P, Niemela O. Comparison of the combined marker GGT-CDT and the conventional laboratory markers of alcohol abuse in heavy drinkers, moderate drinkers and abstainers. Alcohol Alcohol. 2006;41:528–533.
19. Parran TV Jr, Weber E, Tasse J, Anderson B, Adelman C. Mandatory toxicology testing and chemical dependence consultation follow-up in a level-one trauma center. J Trauma. 1995;38:278–280.
20. Glickman L, Herbsman H. Delirium tremens in surgical patients. Surgery. 1968;64:882–890.
21. Ferguson JA, Suelzer CJ, Eckert GJ, Zhou XH, Dittus RS. Risk factors for delirium tremens development. J Gen Intern Med. 1996;11:410–414.
22. Wojnar M, Bizon Z, Wasilewski D. The role of somatic disorders and physical injury in the development and course of alcohol withdrawal delirium. Alcohol Clin Exp Res. 1999;23:209–213.
23. Blondell RD, Looney SW, Hottman LM, Boaz PW. Characteristics of intoxicated trauma patients. J Addict Dis. 2002;21:1–12.
24. Lukan JK, Reed DN Jr, Looney SW, Spain DA, Blondell RD. Risk factors for delirium tremens in trauma patients. J Trauma. 2002;53:901–906.
25. Mayo-Smith MF. Pharmacological management of alcohol withdrawal. A meta-analysis and evidence-based practice guideline. American Society of Addiction Medicine Working Group on Pharmacological Management of Alcohol Withdrawal. JAMA. 1997;278:144–151.
26. Sellers EM, Naranjo CA, Harrison M, Devenyi P, Roach C, Sykora K. Diazepam loading: simplified treatment of alcohol withdrawal. Clin Pharmacol Ther. 1983;34:822–826.
27. Saitz R, Mayo-Smith MF, Roberts MS, Redmond HA, Bernard DR, Calkins DR. Individualized treatment for alcohol withdrawal. A randomized double-blind controlled trial. JAMA. 1994;272:519–523.
28. Kouimtsidis C, Reynolds M, Hunt M, et al. Substance use in the general hospital. Addict Behav. 2003;28:483–499.
29. Busto U, Simpkins J, Sellers EM, Sisson B, Segal R. Objective determination of benzodiazepine use and abuse in alcoholics. Br J Addict. 1983;78:429–435.
30. Busto UE, Sellers EM. Anxiolytics and sedative/hypnotics dependence. Br J Addict. 1991;86:1647–1652.
31. McKeon A, Frye MA, Delanty N. The alcohol withdrawal syndrome. J Neurol Neurosurg Psychiatry. 2008;79:854–862.
32. Khan A, Levy P, DeHorn S, Miller W, Compton S. Predictors of mortality in patients with delirium tremens. Acad Emerg Med. 2008;15:788–790.
33. McMicken D, Liss JL. Alcohol-related seizures. Emerg Med Clin North Am. 2011;29:117–124.
34. Campos J, Roca L, Gude F, Gonzalez-Quintela A. Long-term mortality of patients admitted to the hospital with alcohol withdrawal syndrome. Alcohol Clin Exp Res. 2011;35:1180–1186.
35. Naranjo CA, Sellers EM, Chater K, Iversen P, Roach C, Sykora K. Nonpharmacologic intervention in acute alcohol withdrawal. Clin Pharmacol Ther. 1983;34:214–219.
36. Blondell RD. Ambulatory detoxification of patients with alcohol dependence. Am Fam Physician. 2005;71:495–502.

37. Sullivan JT, Sykora K, Schneiderman J, Naranjo CA, Sellers EM. Assessment of alcohol withdrawal: the revised clinical institute withdrawal assessment for alcohol scale (CIWA-Ar). Br J Addict. 1989;84:1353–1357.
38. Ploner M, Schnitzler A. Wernicke's encephalopathy. Lancet. 2003;361:1000.
39. Meier S, Daeppen JB. Prevalence, prophylaxis and treatment of Wernicke encephalopathy. Thiamine, how much and how do we give it?. Rev Med Suisse. 2005;1:1740–1744.
40. Paparrigopoulos T, Tzavellas E, Karaiskos D, Kouzoupis A, Liappas I. Complete recovery from undertreated Wernicke-Korsakoff syndrome following aggressive thiamine treatment. In Vivo. 2010;24:231–233.
41. Thorarinsson BL, Olafsson E, Kjartansson O, Blondal H. Wernicke's encephalopathy in chronic alcoholics. Laeknabladid. 2011;97:21–29.
42. Holbrook AM, Crowther R, Lotter A, Cheng C, King D. Meta-analysis of benzodiazepine use in the treatment of acute alcohol withdrawal. CMAJ. 1999;160:649–655.
43. Amato L, Minozzi S, Vecchi S, Davoli M. Benzodiazepines for alcohol withdrawal. Cochrane Database Syst Rev. 2010. doi:10.1002/14651858.CD005063.pub3.
44. Prater CD, Miller KE, Zylstra RG. Outpatient detoxification of the addicted or alcoholic patient. Am Fam Physician. 1999;60:1175-1183.
45. Solomon J, Rouck LA, Koepke HH. Double-blind comparison of lorazepam and chlordiazepoxide in the treatment of the acute alcohol abstinence syndrome. Clin Ther. 1983;6:52–58.
46. Hayashida M, Alterman AI, McLellan AT, et al. Comparative effectiveness and costs of inpatient and outpatient detoxification of patients with mild-to-moderate alcohol withdrawal syndrome. N Engl J Med. 1989;320:358–365.
47. Wartenberg AA, Nirenberg TD, Liepman MR, Silvia LY, Begin AM, Monti PM. Detoxification of alcoholics: improving care by symptom-triggered sedation. Alcohol Clin Exp Res. 1990;14:71–75.
48. D'Onofrio G, Rathlev NK, Ulrich AS, Fish SS, Freedland ES. Lorazepam for the prevention of recurrent seizures related to alcohol. N Engl J Med. 1999;340:915–919.
49. DeCarolis DD, Rice KL, Ho L, Willenbring ML, Cassaro S. Symptom-driven lorazepam protocol for treatment of severe alcohol withdrawal delirium in the intensive care unit. Pharmacotherapy. 2007;27:510–518.
50. Saitz R, Palfai TP, Cheng DM, et al. Brief intervention for medical inpatients with unhealthy alcohol use: a randomized, controlled trial. Ann Intern Med. 2007;146:167–176.
51. Freyer-Adam J, Coder B, Baumeister SE, et al. Brief alcohol intervention for general hospital inpatients: a randomized controlled trial. Drug Alcohol Depend. 2008;93:233–243.
52. Gentilello LM, Rivara FP, Donovan DM, et al. Alcohol interventions in a trauma center as a means of reducing the risk of injury recurrence. Ann Surg. 1999;230:473–480; discussion 480–473.
53. Chick J, Lloyd G, Crombie E. Counselling problem drinkers in medical wards: a controlled study. Br Med J (Clin Res Ed). 1985;290:965–967.
54. Bien TH, Miller WR, Tonigan JS. Brief interventions for alcohol problems: a review. Addiction. 1993;88:315–335.
55. Anderson P, Scott E. The effect of general practitioners' advice to heavy drinking men. Br J Addict. 1992;87:891–900.
56. Cowell AJ, Bray JW, Mills MJ, Hinde JM. Conducting economic evaluations of screening and brief intervention for hazardous drinking: methods and evidence to date for informing policy. Drug Alcohol Rev. 2010;29:623–630.

Chapter 19
Perioperative Management

Daniel P. Alford

Surgery may be required for complications of alcohol use such as the management of traumatic injuries and cancers. Patients with unhealthy alcohol use will also be among those who are planning to undergo surgery for conditions that are unrelated to alcohol use. Alcohol use disorders (AUDs), alcohol-associated chronic medical conditions, and even heavy drinking without an AUD can increase the risk of postoperative complications. Hospitalization for surgery may be the first time that an alcohol-dependent patient does not have access to alcohol, putting them at risk for withdrawal. Acute withdrawal syndromes may complicate surgery and the postoperative course with tachycardia, hypertension, anxiety, delirium, pain, and seizures. Therefore, providers of perioperative care must identify unhealthy alcohol use and be comfortable with the management of withdrawal syndromes. Careful evaluation may detect clinical signs of chronic diseases secondary to alcohol use that increase surgical risk, such as diseases affecting the cardiovascular system, liver, bone marrow, nervous system, and pancreas. In addition, the physiological stress associated with surgery may bring out sub-clinical co-morbidities not obvious during routine preoperative evaluation. This chapter focuses on relevant perioperative issues in the patient with unhealthy alcohol use.

Perioperative Care for Unhealthy Alcohol Use

AUD are common especially in patients seeking medical and surgical care [1]. The prevalence of alcohol use disorders is as high as 40 % in emergency department and various surgical inpatient settings and up to 50 % in patients with trauma [2]. Many chronic medical conditions that can complicate or necessitate surgery including dilated cardiomyopathy, cirrhosis, pancreatitis, and oral and esophageal cancers are attributable to alcohol. Unhealthy alcohol use is associated with in-hospital mortality

D. P. Alford (✉)
Section of General Internal Medicine, Clinical Addiction Research and Education (CARE) Unit, Boston Medical Center, Boston University School of Medicine, Boston, MA, USA
e-mail: dan.alford@bmc.org

R. Saitz (ed.), *Addressing Unhealthy Alcohol Use in Primary Care,*
DOI 10.1007/978-1-4614-4779-5_19, © Springer Science+Business Media New York 2013

in surgical patients [3]. The incidence of symptomatic alcohol withdrawal in hospitalized patients is as high as 8 % and is 2–5 times higher in hospitalized trauma and surgical patients [4–6]. Chronic alcohol use can increase the risk of postoperative complications through immune suppression, reduced cardiac function, dysregulated homeostasis including alterations in platelet production and aggregation, changes in fibrinogen levels, and poor wound healing [4, 7–9]. Postoperative complications appear to show a dose-response relationship with alcohol consumption, that is, the more alcohol consumed the higher risk for postoperative complications [10]. Therefore preoperative screening for unhealthy alcohol use and withdrawal risk is important.

Preoperative Evaluation

In addition to a complete history and physical examination, the preoperative evaluation should assess for the risk of acute alcohol withdrawal and the presence of diseases associated with chronic alcohol use. Physicians often fail to identify alcohol use disorders in medical patients [11]. In one study, only 16 % of people with AUD were identified in the perioperative setting [4]. The amount of alcohol consumed is a risk factor for hospital admission [12] and postoperative complications [7]. When screening, it is important to remember that patients with unhealthy alcohol use are often asymptomatic and often minimize consumption. Quantity and frequency questions are essential but are generally not sensitive or specific, with the exception of specific items that have been validated for this purpose. Laboratory tests such as blood alcohol levels, liver function tests are not sensitive or specific. Adults undergoing preoperative evaluation should be screened using validated questionnaires such as the alcohol use disorder identification test (AUDIT), the AUDIT-C, or a single-item screening question (see Chap. 2). Asking patient's family members about alcohol consumption during the preoperative assessment can also be helpful [9]. Other historical findings suggestive of unhealthy alcohol use include a history of traumatic injuries, marital, social and legal problems, homelessness, and a history of withdrawal and blackout episodes [13]. Screening preoperatively in the surgical setting differs from screening in other settings. In the surgical setting, screening for risk of withdrawal and medical co-morbidities are the priorities. Identifying likely dependence with the CAGE questions or a dependence checklist can be helpful but to further identify withdrawal risk, consider including one or more of the following questions in the preoperative evaluation:

a. Have you ever gone through alcohol withdrawal such as having the shakes?
b. Have you ever had problems, or gotten sick when you stopped drinking?
c. Have you ever had a seizure or DTs, been confused, after cutting down or stopping drinking?

The spectrum of withdrawal ranges from mild tremor or hallucinosis, to seizures and delirium tremens. In the postoperative period withdrawal can mimic many postoperative complications including delirium, acute pain and sepsis. Risk factors associated with severe and prolonged alcohol withdrawal include amount and duration of alcohol use, prior withdrawal episodes, recurrent detoxifications, older age, and comorbid diseases [14]. It is also important to note that sedatives (e.g., benzodiazepines) and analgesics (e.g., opioids) given during surgery and the postoperative period may delay, partially treat, or obscure some symptoms of alcohol withdrawal. It is important to assess for other drug use as well, as many patients with unhealthy alcohol use, use other substances such as benzodiazepines and cocaine. Physical examination should evaluate for evidence of liver, pancreatic, nervous system, and cardiac disease. The spectrum of alcoholic liver disease ranges from fatty liver with normal or mild elevations in liver enzymes, to acute hepatitis, and cirrhosis. Clinical evidence of cirrhosis including jaundice, palmar erythema, gynecomastia, testicular atrophy, spider telangiectasias, as well as findings consistent with portal vein hypertension namely splenomegaly, ascites, hemorrhoids, and caput medusa (dilatation of the periumbilical veins on the abdominal wall) should be sought. Pancreatitis can present as acute and chronic abdominal pain as well as exocrine (i.e., malabsorption) and endocrine dysfunction (i.e., glucose intolerance to diabetes mellitus). Pancreatitic calcifications seen on abdominal imaging studies are another clue to chronic pancreatitis. Alcohol associated dementia occurs in approximately 9 % of people with alcohol dependence [15]. Korsakoff's syndrome, hepatic and Wernicke encephalopathy, myelopathies, and polyneuropathies are other nervous system disorders associated with chronic alcohol use disorders. These neurological conditions can worsen during the perioperative period and may be confused with other postoperative neurological complications. Therefore, preoperative baseline mental status and cognition should be assessed and documented. Preoperative evaluation for congestive heart failure should be considered as up to one third of patients with long standing alcohol use disorders have a decreased cardiac ejection fraction [16]. Because of the association between unhealthy alcohol use and nicotine dependence, smoking related co-morbidities such as coronary heart disease and chronic obstructive pulmonary disease (COPD) should also be evaluated for. Up to 20 % of alcohol dependent patients were found to suffer from COPD in one series [17]. Preoperative laboratory studies should include electrolytes, liver enzyme and synthetic tests, coagulation studies, and a complete blood count. Anemia is common in patients with alcohol dependence as well as decreased platelet count from alcohol-associated bone marrow suppression and splenic sequestration. Preexisting anemia may need to be treated preoperatively as these patients are at increased risk of perioperative bleeding secondary to coagulopathies and thrombocytopenia [18]. It is also important to identify patients who are in recovery preoperatively as they may have concerns and questions about perioperative exposure to sedative hypnotics and opioid analgesics.

Management of Alcohol Withdrawal

One of the most common complications in hospitalized alcohol dependent patients is withdrawal, with up to 15 % at risk for developing seizures and/or delirium tremens

[19]. The spectrum of alcohol withdrawal ranges from minor symptoms of autonomic hyperactivity including diaphoresis, tachycardia, systolic hypertension, tremor, and insomnia, to hallucinations, nausea, vomiting, psychomotor agitation, anxiety, grand mal seizures, and life-threatening delirium tremens. In one study, 20 % of the alcohol dependent patients admitted to a surgical service developed delirium tremens after admission [20]. Withdrawal symptoms may appear within hours of decreased intake, however, during the perioperative period the administration of anesthetics, sedatives, and analgesics may delay the onset of withdrawal for up to 14 days [21]. Recognizing withdrawal risk and treating early withdrawal can often prevent the complications of severe withdrawal. Because alcohol withdrawal is especially dangerous during the postoperative period, asymptomatic but at-risk patients should receive prophylactic treatment to prevent withdrawal. Although many medications have been used to treat alcohol withdrawal, benzodiazepines are the medications of choice for both the prevention and management of alcohol withdrawal [22, 23]. Preferably benzodiazepines with a long half-life such as diazepam or chlordiazepoxide should be chosen. However patients with severe liver disease should receive a shorter acting agent such as lorazepam to avoid excessive and prolonged sedation. Treatment of withdrawal should be based on the severity of symptoms and signs. The Clinical Institute Withdrawal Assessment Scale for Alcohol, revised (CIWA-Ar) is a validated tool that can be used to rate the severity for alcohol withdrawal [24]. This 10-item scale can be completed rapidly and easily at the bedside. It may be impossible to use the CIWA-Ar in the postoperative period if patients are unable to communicate, and the scale may be less reliable in patients with acute medical or surgical illnesses that can affect the scores. Goals for management of alcohol withdrawal include: treatment of withdrawal symptoms, prevention of initial and recurrent seizures, and prevention and treatment of delirium tremens [19].

Alcohol Use and Surgical Risk

In addition to alcohol withdrawal, numerous observational studies have demonstrated that heavy alcohol use, even in the absence of clinical liver disease or the absence of alcohol dependence per se, is an independent risk factor for postoperative complications. Higher rates of postoperative complications were seen after transurethral prostatectomy, colonic surgery, and hysterectomy [25–27]. There is a dose–response effect, with increased alcohol consumption being associated with both increased postoperative complications and prolonged hospital stay. The most dramatic differences were in groups who drank greater than 60 g of alcohol (> 4 drinks) per day [18]. The postoperative complications reported were an increased rate of infection, bleeding, and delayed wound healing. In a prospective study of patients having colorectal surgery, Tonnesen and colleagues found an increase in postoperative arrhythmias [28]. Patients with alcohol dependence also have longer intensive care unit stays, more postoperative septicemia and pneumonia requiring mechanical ventilation as well as increased overall mortality [29]. Five possible pathological mechanisms have been identified to account for the increased rate of postoperative complications including immune incompetence, subclinical cardiac insufficiency, hemostatic imbalances, abnormal stress response, and wound healing dysfunction [4, 7]. Chronic alcohol use suppresses T-cell-dependent activity and decreases macrophage, monocyte and neutrophil mobilization, and phagocytosis. This immune dysfunction is reversible after abstinence [18]. The decreased cardiac function associated with unhealthy alcohol use is thought to be secondary to direct alteration in the electromechanical coupling and contractility of cardiac myocytes. This alcohol-associated cardiac dysfunction may be reversible, with 50 % of patients showing improvement after 6 months of abstinence [30]. The hemostatic dysfunction associated with unhealthy alcohol use is due to a modification in coagulation and fibrinolysis pathways as well as a decrease in the number and function of platelets [18]. Wound healing problems seem related to poor accumulation of collagen [18]. Abstinence before surgery decreases postoperative morbidity. Tonnesen and colleagues preoperatively randomized adults who drank at least 5 drinks per day and who were scheduled for elective colorectal surgery to abstinence for 1 month before surgery versus a usual care group [31]. They observed fewer complications in the abstinent group compared to the usual care group, however, there was no difference in length of stay or mortality. This is the first study to demonstrate that preoperative abstinence can lead to improved postoperative outcomes. It suggests that when possible, treatment of alcohol dependence should occur preoperatively, with treatments proven to decrease alcohol use or achieve abstinence (e.g., pharmacotherapies like disulfiram, and proven psychosocial approaches).

Alcoholic Liver Disease

The spectrum of liver disease associated with the spectrum of unhealthy alcohol use includes asymptomatic fatty liver, to acute hepatitis, and finally chronic cirrhosis. Each form of liver disease carries some degree of surgical risk and requires special preoperative considerations.

Alcoholic Fatty Liver Alcoholic fatty liver (hepatic steatosis) occurs in 90 % of heavy drinkers and is often asymptomatic and reversible. It can occur after "binge" (heavy drinking episode) or "social" drinking (that is excessive but without other recognized consequences). Signs and symptoms, when present, include nausea, vomiting and right upper quadrant pain and tenderness. Laboratory tests often demonstrate a mild elevation in liver transaminases but with preserved liver (synthetic) function with normal bilirubin, albumin and coagulation studies. These signs and symptoms usually resolve within two weeks of abstinence. Patients with fatty liver seem to tolerate surgery well [32], however there are no known studies evaluating perioperative risk in these patients. It is prudent to delay elective surgery until resolution of clinical signs and symptoms and if possible, abstinence is achieved.

Alcoholic Hepatitis Alcoholic hepatitis is a serious inflammatory disease of the liver, which occurs in up to 40 % of heavy drinkers. The pathological mechanisms include hepatocyte swelling, liver infiltration with polymorphonuclear cells, and hepatocyte necrosis. These patients often present extremely ill with nausea, vomiting, anorexia, abdominal pain, fever, and jaundice. Elevated transaminases and prolonged coagulation studies are common. Surgical risk is very high in this group with 100 % mortality rates reported in older series [33]. Therefore, alcoholic hepatitis should be considered a contraindication to elective surgery. It is recommended that elective surgery be delayed until clinical and laboratory parameters normalize, sometimes taking up to 12 weeks.

Alcoholic Cirrhosis Cirrhosis occurs in 15–20 % of long-term heavy drinkers and refers to the irreversible necrosis, nodular regeneration and fibrosis of the liver, accompanied by synthetic dysfunction. Cirrhosis is associated with abnormal hepatic circulation, resulting in portal vein hypertension. Clinically, patients may present with ascites, peripheral edema, poor nutritional status, muscle wasting, coagulopathies, gastrointestinal bleeding from esophageal varices, encephalopathy, and renal insufficiency as well as hypoxia secondary to hepatopulmonary syndrome and pulmonary hypertension. The need for surgery is common in patients with cirrhosis, with up to 10 % requiring a surgical procedure during the last 2 years of life [34]. Depending on the stage of cirrhotic disease, surgery can be extremely risky. The most common causes of perioperative mortality in cirrhotic patients are sepsis, hemorrhage, and hepatorenal syndrome [35]. Although currently used anesthetic agents are not hepatotoxic, surgical stress in itself causes hemodynamic changes in the liver resulting in postoperative elevations in liver function tests in patients with no underlying liver disease [36]. Patients with underlying liver dysfunction are at increased risk for hepatic decompensation during surgical stress as anesthetic agents decrease hepatic blood flow by as much as 50 % and therefore decrease hepatic oxygen uptake [37]. Intraoperative traction on abdominal viscera may also decrease hepatic blood flow.

Effect of Cirrhosis on Surgical Risk Surgery in patients with cirrhosis is high risk. A study of patients undergoing total knee arthroplasty found that both local and systemic complications were as high as 44 % in patients with cirrhosis versus 6 % in a control group [38]. The preoperative factors associated with increased surgical morbidity and mortality include: emergent surgery, upper abdominal surgery, poor hepatic synthetic function, anemia, ascites, malnutrition, and encephalopathy [39]. These patients are at increased risk for uncontrolled bleeding, infections and delirium. Coagulopathies and thrombocytopenia result in difficult perioperative hemostasis. Ascites increases the risk of intraabdominal infections, abdominal wound dehiscence, and abdominal wall herniation. Nutritional deficiencies result in poor wound healing and an increased risk of skin breakdown, and encephalopathy decreases the patient's ability to effectively participate in postoperative rehabilitation. The action of anesthetic agents may be prolonged and increases the risk of delirium. Cholecystectomy is a particularly risky surgery in patients with cirrhosis and portal

Table 19.1 Pugh classification. (Modified Child and Turcotte classification) [44]

	Points		
	1	2	3
Encephalopathy (grade)	None	1–2	3–4
Ascites	Absent	Slight	Moderate
Bilirubin (mg/dl)	1–2	2–3	> 3
Albumin (g/dl)	> 3.5	2.8–3.5	< 2.8
Prothombin time			
(seconds prolonged)	1–3	4–6	> 6
Internal normalized ratio (INR)	< 1.7	1.7–2.3	> 2.3
Class A 5–6 points			
Class B 7–9 points			
Class C 10–15 points			

hypertension because of intra-abdominal collateral circulation. This collateral circulation increases the vascularity of the gallbladder bed and places the patient at greater risk for severe perioperative hemorrhage. In a group of patients with cirrhosis undergoing cholecystectomy, those considered decompensated preoperatively by presence of ascites and prolonged coagulation studies had an 83 % mortality rate compared to 10 % in compensated patients [40]. In trying to risk stratify patients preoperatively it is important to look for clinical signs of cirrhosis and portal hypertension. There are two scoring systems in use to predict whether patients with advance liver disease will survive surgery [41]. Using a multivariate clinical assessment, the Child and Turcotte classification made it possible to risk stratify patients with cirrhosis preoperatively. In 1964, the Child and Turcotte classification stratified cirrhotic patients into three classes based on "hepatic reserve" and therefore surgical risk prior to portocaval shunt surgery [42]. Class "A" was the most compensated while class "C" was the most decompensated group. Variables included laboratory values of bilirubin and albumin, as well as clinical ascites, encephalopathy, and nutritional status. Garrison found good correlation between Child and Turcotte class and abdominal surgical mortality with classes A, B, and C mortality rates of 10, 31, and 76 %, respectively [43]. Some of the limitations of the Child and Turcotte classification scheme included the subjective nature and interobserver variation in the assessment of nutritional status, encephalopathy, and ascites. In addition, there was variability in the assigning of patients to classes A, B, and C and no accounting for the nature and urgency of the surgical procedure. In an attempt to decrease the subjective nature of the classification scheme, Pugh and colleagues modified the Child and Turcotte classification (see Table 19.1) [44]. The Pugh modification separates hepatic encephalopathy into five grades depending on various signs and symptoms (see Table 19.2). The subjective evaluation of nutritional status is changed to objective measured prolongation in prothrombin time and the assignment of class based on a total point score. Using pooled surgical data, the Pugh Classification scheme has proven to be a good preoperative risk stratifier (see Table 19.3).

A second scoring system is the model for end-stage liver disease (MELD) which was designed to predict survival after transjugular intrahepatic portosystemic shunt

Table 19.2 Encephalopathy grade [45]

Grade 0	Normal
Grade I	Consists of personality changes with altered sleep patterns (e.g., sleep-night reversal) and inappropriate behavior, constructional apraxia
Grade II	Consists of mental confusion, disorientation to time and place, drowsiness, asterixis, and fetor hepaticus
Grade III	Consists of severe mental confusion, stuperous but arousable, incoherent, asterixis, fetor hepaticus, rigidity, and hyperreflexia
Grade IV	Consists of deep coma, unresponsive to stimuli, not arousable, decerebrate and decorticate posturing, fetor hepaticus, decreased muscle tone, and decrease reflexes

Table 19.3 Pugh class, operative risk, and operability [46]

Child-Pugh A:—2–10 % mortality risk	No limitation
	Normal response to all operations
	Normal ability of liver to regenerate
Child-Pugh B:—6–31 % mortality risk	Some limitation in liver function
	Altered response to all operations but good tolerance with preparation
Child-Pugh C:—20–76 % mortality risk	Severe limitation of liver function
	Poor response to all operations regardless of preparation

(TIPS) treatment of bleeding esophageal varices [47]. The MELD score is used to prioritize patients for liver transplantation and more recently as a predictor of survival after non-transplant surgery [48]. The MELD score is calculated using the patient's international normalized ratio (INR), and serum creatinine and bilirubin. Since the MELD formula is complex, scores can be calculated by using an online MELD score calculator at http://optn.transplant.hrsa.gov/resources/MeldPeldCalculator.asp.

Preoperative Considerations in Patients with Cirrhosis Preoperative abstinence should be the goal before all elective procedures. Since coagulopathies may develop as a result of vitamin K deficiency due to malnutrition or intestinal bile salt deficiency, attempts at correction should start with the administration of vitamin K. If there is no effect in 12 h, it is most likely secondary to decreased hepatic production of coagulation factors, and perioperative use of fresh frozen plasma (FFP) should be considered. Thrombocytopenia secondary to bone-marrow suppression, hypersplenism, and splenic sequestration should be treated with prophylactic platelet transfusions when counts fall below 20,000/mm^3 [34]. In addition, units of packed red blood cells should be on hold in the blood bank. Ascites secondary to portal hypertension and hypoalbumenemia can impede abdominal wall healing, increase the risk of abdominal wall dehiscence and herniation, and restrict effective mechanical ventilation. Therefore, ascites should be optimally managed preoperatively with sodium restriction and appropriate diuretic therapy. In patients with peripheral edema, a more aggressive approach including large volume paracentesis (≥ 5 L) should be considered. Electrolytes should be monitored closely. Perioperative hemodynamic monitoring is often needed as these patients may have large fluid shifts especially during abdominal surgeries. Preoperative broad spectrum antibiotics (e.g., norfloxacin or ciprofloxacin) should be considered as prophylaxis against secondary and spontaneous bacterial peritonitis. Renal function should be monitored closely. Perioperative changes in volume status and hemodynamics may adversely affect renal function. These patients are at risk for renal insufficiency secondary to prerenal azotemia as well as hepatorenal syndrome. Any potential nephrotoxic agent (e.g., aminoglycoside antibiotics) should be used with extreme caution. Non-steroidal antiinflammatory drugs and acetaminophen should be used sparingly. Many perioperative conditions can exacerbate hepatic encephalopathy such as gastrointestinal bleeding, constipation, azotemia, hypoxia, and the use of sedatives [39]. Aggressive preoperative treatment of hepatic encephalopathy using lactulose and dietary protein restriction is recommended. Patients with known gastroesophageal varices should be monitored closely for gastrointestinal bleeding and should be considered for beta-blocker prophylaxis preoperatively. The nutritional status of these patients is usually poor and often deficient in thiamine, folate, vitamin C, and B vitamins. Nutritional status should be optimized with multivitamins, thiamine, folate, and nutritional supplementation preoperatively. From a pulmonary standpoint, decompensated cirrhotics may desaturate due to the development of pulmonary shunts in hepatopulmonary syndrome, therefore continuous monitoring of oxygen saturation should be part of postoperative care. General class-specific guidelines are shown in Table 19.3. There is increasing evidence that laparoscopic procedures in cirrhotic patients may be safer than open procedures, regardless of Child's classification [32]. Patients with cirrhosis undergoing surgery may benefit from a multidisciplinary approach including a hepatologist (and nephrologist if the patient has renal insufficiency).

Liver Transplantation in Patients with Alcohol Dependence

Alcoholic liver disease is one of the most common causes of end stage liver disease requiring liver transplantation in the United States. In the past, patients with a history of an addictive disorder have been kept off of transplantation lists because of fears of post-transplant noncompliance, with subsequent loss of graft, but also because of moralistic arguments that the patients had "self inflicted" diseases. In fact, some studies have demonstrated post-transplant relapse rates as high as 49 %, with lower overall survival rates in patients who failed to complete addiction treatment [49]. Other studies found no difference in one-year survival rate between alcoholic patients who maintained sobriety and patients who had no history of alcohol dependence [50]. In fact, at least among people with alcohol dependence selected for liver transplant, most (71 %) abstain or nearly completely abstain, and only 7 % return to heavy drinking. Furthermore, outcomes (mortality) after liver transplant may be even better among people with alcohol dependence than among those with other causes of liver failure because those who abstain have no ongoing cause for recurrence whereas those with hepatitis C infection, for example, often have recurrence. Patients with alcohol dependence who undergo liver transplant are more likely to eventually die from cancer and recurrent infectious hepatitis than they are from recurrent heavy alcohol use complications [51]. A recent study identified preoperative risk factors that were predictive of relapse after transplantation which included shorter length of abstinence before transplantation, greater than one episode of alcohol withdrawal before transplantation, younger age at time of transplantation, and alcohol abuse in first-degree relatives [52]. A survey of U.S. liver transplantation programs found that most accept applicants with histories of heavy alcohol use [53]. It is clear that patients with addiction disorders need to be assessed for risk of relapse, and regarding social support systems before being accepted for transplantation. As organ transplantation in patients with addiction is unusually complex, some medical centers have added addiction specialists to the transplant team [49].

Conclusions

Patients with unhealthy alcohol use have high rates of hospitalization and surgery. The underlying history of addiction may not be apparent initially, but thorough history-taking and the use of effective screening tools can elicit information about past or current unhealthy alcohol use. Because of the high prevalence of alcohol and other drug use, patients who acknowledge an addiction to one substance should be asked about all other substances of abuse. Careful evaluation can also detect clinical signs of chronic diseases of the cardiovascular system, lungs, and liver related to alcohol use. The importance of identifying alcohol use disorders preoperatively cannot be overstated. Perioperative morbidity associated with acute abstinence syndromes can be prevented with proper preoperative treatment. If possible, elective surgery should be postponed to allow time for a period of abstinence. Sedative-hypnotics and opioid analgesics should be used as indicated during the perioperative period. Management of patients with alcohol use disorders going for surgery often requires consultation with addiction specialists. All patients with active addiction should be encouraged to engage in addiction treatment preoperatively if possible, and certainly, postoperatively.

References

1. Saitz R. Unhealthy alcohol use. N Engl J Med. 2005;352(6):596–607.
2. D'Onofrio G, Bernstein E, Bernstein J, et al. Patients with alcohol problems in the emergency department, Part 1: Improving detection. Acad Emerg Med. 1998;5(12):1200–1209.
3. Delgado-Rodriguez M, Gomez-Ortega A, Mariscal-Ortiz M, Palma-Perez S, Sillero-Arenas M. Alcohol drinking as a predictor of intensive care and hospital mortality in general surgery: a prospective study. Addiction. 2003;98(5):611–616.
4. Spies C, Tonnesen H, Andreasson S, Helander A, Conigrave K. Perioperative morbidity and mortality in chronic alcoholic patients. Alcohol Clin Exp Res. 2001;25(5 Suppl ISBRA):164S–170S.

5. Foy A, Kay J. The incidence of alcohol-related problems and the risk of alcohol withdrawal in a general hospital population. Drug Alcohol Rev. 1995;14(1):49–54.
6. Gordon AJ, Olstein J, Conigliaro J. Identification and treatment of alcohol use disorders in the perioperative period. Postgrad Med. 2006;119(2):46–55.
7. Tonnesen H. Influence of alcohol on several physiological functions and its reversibility: a surgical view. Acta Psychiatr Scand Suppl. 1992;369:67–71.
8. Zhang P, Bagby GJ, Happel KI, Raasch CE, Nelson S. Alcohol abuse, immunosuppression, and pulmonary infection. Curr Drug Abuse Rev. 2008;1(1):56–67.
9. de Wit M, Jones DG, Sessler CN, Zilberberg MD, Weaver MF. Alcohol-use disorders in the critically Ill patient. Chest. 2010;138(4):994–1003.
10. Tonnesen H, Nielsen PR, Lauritzen JB, Moller AM. Smoking and alcohol intervention before surgery: evidence for best practice. Br J Anaesth. 2009;102(3):297–306.
11. Kitchens JM. Does this patient have an alcohol problem? JAMA. 1994;272(22):1782–1787.
12. Andreasson S, Allebeck P, Romelsjo A. Hospital admissions for somatic care among young men: the role of alcohol. Br J Addict. 1990;85(7):935–941.
13. Chiang PP. Perioperative management of the alcohol-dependent patient. Am Fam Physician. 1995;52(8):2267–2273.
14. Saitz R. Recognition and management of occult alcohol withdrawal. Hosp Pract (Minneap). 1995;30(6):49–58.
15. Eklund J. Alcohol abuse and postoperative complications. Do we ask the right questions? Acta Anaesthesiol Scand. 1996;40(6):647–648.
16. Regan TJ. Alcohol and the cardiovascular system. JAMA. 1990;264(3):377–381.
17. Frost EA, Siedel MR. Preanesthetic assessment of the drug abuse patient. Anesthesiol Clin North Am. 1990;8:829–841.
18. Tonnesen H, Kehlet H. Preoperative alcoholism and postoperative morbidity. Br J Surg. 1999;86(7):869–874.
19. Saitz R, O'Malley SS. Pharmacotherapies for alcohol abuse. Withdrawal and treatment. Med Clin North Am. 1997;81(4):881–907.
20. Glickman L, Herbsman H. Delirium tremens in surgical patients. Surgery. 1968;64(5):882–890.
21. Spandorfer J. The patient with substance abuse going to surgery. In: Merli GJ, Weitz HH, editors. Medical management of the surgical patient. 2nd ed. Philadelphia: WB Saunders Company; 1998. p. 255–262.
22. Mayo-Smith MF. Pharmacological management of alcohol withdrawal. A meta-analysis and evidence-based practice guideline. American Society of Addiction Medicine Working Group on Pharmacological Management of Alcohol Withdrawal. JAMA. 1997;278(2):144–151.
23. Mayo-Smith MF, Beecher LH, Fischer TL, et al. Management of alcohol withdrawal delirium: an evidence-based practice guideline. Arch Intern Med. 2004;164(13):1405–1412.
24. Sullivan JT, Sykora K, Schneiderman J, Naranjo CA, Sellers EM. Assessment of alcohol withdrawal: the revised clinical institute withdrawal assessment for alcohol scale (CIWA-Ar). Br J Addict. 1989;84(11):1353–1357.
25. Tonnesen H, Schutten BT, Jorgensen BB. Influence of alcohol on morbidity after colonic surgery. Dis Colon Rectum. 1987;30(7):549–551.
26. Tonnesen H, Schutten BT, Tollund L, Hasselqvist P, Klintorp S. Influence of alcoholism on morbidity after transurethral prostatectomy. Scand J Urol Nephrol. 1988;22(3):175–177.
27. Felding C, Jensen LM, Tonnesen H. Influence of alcohol intake on postoperative morbidity after hysterectomy. Am J Obstet Gynecol. 1992;166(2):667–670.
28. Tonnesen H, Petersen KR, Hojgaard L, et al. Postoperative morbidity among symptom-free alcohol misusers. Lancet. 1992;340(8815):334–337.
29. Jensen NH, Dragsted L, Christensen JK, Jorgensen JC, Qvist J. Severity of illness and outcome of treatment in alcoholic patients in the intensive care unit. Intensive Care Med. 1988;15(1):19–22.
30. La Vecchia LL, Bedogni F, Bozzola L, Bevilacqua P, Ometto R, Vincenzi M. Prediction of recovery after abstinence in alcoholic cardiomyopathy: role of hemodynamic and morphometric parameters. Clin Cardiol. 1996;19(1):45–50.

31. Tonnesen H, Rosenberg J, Nielsen HJ, et al. Effect of preoperative abstinence on poor postoperative outcome in alcohol misusers: randomised controlled trial. Br Med J. 1999;318(7194):1311–1316.

32. Rizvon MK, Chou CL. Surgery in the patient with liver disease. Med Clin North Am. 2003;87(1):211–227.

33. Greenwood SM, Leffler CT, Minkowitz S. The increased mortality rate of open liver biopsy in alcoholic hepatitis. Surg Gynecol Obstet. 1972;134(4):600–604.

34. Patel T. Surgery in the patient with liver disease. Mayo Clin Proc. 1999;74(6):593–599.

35. Wong R, Rappaport W, Witte C, et al. Risk of nonshunt abdominal operation in the patient with cirrhosis. J Am Coll Surg. 1994;179(4):412–416.

36. Friedman LS, Maddrey WC. Surgery in the patient with liver disease. Med Clin North Am. 1987;71(3):453–476.

37. Cowan RE, Jackson BT, Grainger SL, Thompson RP. Effects of anesthetic agents and abdominal surgery on liver blood flow. Hepatology. 1991;14(6):1161–1166.

38. Shih LY, Cheng CY, Chang CH, Hsu KY, Hsu RW, Shih HN. Total knee arthroplasty in patients with liver cirrhosis. J Bone Joint Surg Am. 2004;86-A(2):335–341.

39. Grimm IS, Almounajed G, Friedman LS. Management of the surgical patient with liver disease. In: Merli GJ, Weitz HH, editors. Medical management of the surgical patient. 2nd ed. Philadelphia: WB Saunders Company; 1998. p. 193–213.

40. Aranha GV, Sontag SJ, Greenlee HB. Cholecystectomy in cirrhotic patients: a formidable operation. Am J Surg. 1982;143(1):55–60.

41. Suman A, Carey WD. Assessing the risk of surgery in patients with liver disease. Cleve Clin J Med. 2006;73(4):398–404.

42. Child CG, Turcotte JG. Surgery and portal hypertension. Major Probl Clin Surg. 1964;1:1–85.

43. Garrison RN, Cryer HM, Howard DA, Polk HC, Jr. Clarification of risk factors for abdominal operations in patients with hepatic cirrhosis. Ann Surg. 1984;199(6):648–655.

44. Pugh RN, Murray-Lyon IM, Dawson JL, Pietroni MC, Williams R. Transection of the oesophagus for bleeding oesophageal varices. Br J Surg. 1973;60(8):646–649.

45. Trey C, Burns DG, Saunders SJ. Treatment of hepatic coma by exchange blood transfusion. N Engl J Med. 1966;274(9):473–481.

46. Stone HH. Preoperative and postoperative care. Surg Clin North Am. 1977;57(2):409–419.

47. Malinchoc M, Kamath PS, Gordon FD, Peine CJ, Rank J, ter Borg PC. A model to predict poor survival in patients undergoing transjugular intrahepatic portosystemic shunts. Hepatology. 2000;31(4):864–871. doi:10.1053/he.2000.5852.

48. Suman A, Barnes DS, Zein NN, Levinthal GN, Connor JT, Carey WD. Predicting outcome after cardiac surgery in patients with cirrhosis: a comparison of Child–Pugh and MELD scores. Clin Gastroenterol Hepatol. 2004;2(8):719–723.

49. Stowe J, Kotz M. Addiction medicine in organ tansplantation. Prog Transplant. 2001;11(1):50–57.

50. Starzl TE, Van Thiel D, Tzakis AG, et al. Orthotopic liver transplantation for alcoholic cirrhosis. JAMA. 1988;260(17):2542–2544.

51. Dimartini A. Natural history of alcohol use disorders in liver transplant patients. Liver Transpl. 2007;13(11 Suppl 2):S76–78.

52. Perney P, Bismuth M, Sigaud H, et al. Are preoperative patterns of alcohol consumption predictive of relapse after liver transplantation for alcoholic liver disease? Transpl Int. 2005;18(11):1292–1297.

53. Koch M, Banys P. Liver transplantation and opioid dependence. JAMA. 2001;285(8):1056–1058.

Chapter 20
Physicians with Unhealthy Alcohol Use

Luis T. Sanchez

Introduction

As physicians, we devote our professional lives to providing competent care to the patients we treat. That is what we learned in medical school and how we were trained in our residencies. But what is often left out of our training and medical lives, is that we are susceptible to all the illnesses and disorders that our patients can get. After all, to be good doctors, we need to be good patients [1]. A common physician failing is that we tend not to recognize signs and symptoms in ourselves and then not get ourselves diagnosed and treated if an illness is present. The stress of medical practice, time constraints, and patient demands can foster our own denial and resistance to seek help. Even having our own primary care physician who we trust, can be honest with, and meet with on a yearly or regular basis, is a difficult accomplishment for many doctors.

Similar concerns involve the use of alcohol and other addictive drugs. Physicians have a similar occurrence of lifetime alcohol and drug use disorders of 12–14 % as does the general population [2]. In that regard, we again are no different than our patients, no less susceptible. After all, whether we are going to develop unhealthy alcohol use does not depend on which medical school we attended or the quality of our residency, but is more reflective of our family history and the genetics of our parents and families. As with our patients, if a parent or relative had an alcohol use disorder, then we are more susceptible to developing a problem. One would hope that this is where the depth of our medical training would assist us in developing caution with our own alcohol use and even abstinence if particularly concerned. But because medical practice can be stressful, and because physicians can have risk factors for alcohol use disorders just like anyone else, physicians need to be fully aware of the triggers and traps that they can fall into, that have the potential to seriously affect their medical careers.

L. Sanchez (✉)
Physician Health Services, Inc., A subsidiary of the Massachusetts
Medical Society, Waltham, MA, USA
e-mail: lsanchez@mms.org

R. Saitz (ed.), *Addressing Unhealthy Alcohol Use in Primary Care*,   233
DOI 10.1007/978-1-4614-4779-5_20, © Springer Science+Business Media New York 2013

"Moderate" Drinking

"Moderate" drinking is use of quantities generally associated with a lower risk of health consequences. If we choose to drink and can do so safely, we should restrict ourselves to amounts that do not increase health risks. Recommendations for the general population regarding numbers of drinks per day or week should be carefully considered by physicians, given patient care responsibilities. Occasional heavy episodic use or "binge" drinking can be problematic. Beyond quantity, the timing of alcohol use may be important. A nightly cocktail or occasional several drinks in the evening can affect our medical performance the next day [3]. Primary care practice, similar to other specialties, requires attentiveness, intact executive functioning and no evidence of drinking, for example, alcohol on breath. Less than competent care can lead to suspiciousness from nurses, colleagues, assistants and patients. We need to remember that once we have been granted our medical license following medical school graduation, we are doctors 24 h/day, 7 days a week no matter if we are practicing or not, on vacation, relaxing in the weekend or on call. The expectation of our patients, the public and the licensing authority, is that we will conduct ourselves with professionalism. Our attendance at social functions, weddings and parties are events where we are being watched and expected to conform to the standards of a doctor's behavior, even if not well defined. Improper conduct in social settings is noticed and can contribute to professional problems if drinking behavior is excessive, associated with consequences, and continues or escalates.

Recognizing our Own Problem

Unhealthy alcohol use is easier to see in others than it is in ourselves. However, as physicians, the earlier we can recognize it, the better for our own health, our family, and our career. It is often said that the last important part of our life that we lose, as drinking problems escalate, is our medical profession. We are so well trained and accomplished in our clinical roles that our lives can be crashing down around us and we hold on to being a doctor, despite the tragedies unfolding. So in order to preserve our career and maintain a medical license, it is crucially important that we recognize our vulnerabilities and early signs of drinking with consequences.

Similar to taking a patient's history, if there is a family history of alcohol use disorders, our own risk increases. An inventory of drinking patterns needs to be recalled and acknowledged including the first drink, high school, college, and medical school drinking amounts, patterns and consequences. Current quantities and frequency of drinking should be compared to nationally recommended limits. Alcohol tolerance, frequency of drinking, and alcohol preferences need to be reviewed. Are there episodes of forgetfulness, mood changes, behavioral instability, 'gray-outs' or blackouts? Answer the CAGE screening questions. And be attentive to concerns by our loved ones, colleagues and friends as to our well being and the effects of alcohol. Despite this, physicians can be difficult to reach, with our attentiveness first to patient care, our professionalism, and denial. In addition, our obsessive nature coupled with our training and intolerance of mistakes, can lead to an avoidance of feeling shamed and embarrassed, which only fortifies our avoidance and failure to recognize problematic drinking.

Recognizing a Drinking Problem in Colleagues

It is far easier to recognize aberrant behavior in a colleague that is alcohol-related than ourselves. However, it is also easy to ignore, deny, and avoid uncomfortable situations involving colleagues who are also friends and business partners, or the senior member of the practice, a mentor, teacher or supervisor. But we cannot forget that alcohol does not spare important people or friends. There are so many examples of doctors with an alcohol problem with the familiar refrain, "I would never think that he had a problem," "but she's such a competent doctor," or "who would ever think . . . ?"

Signs include changes in behavior over time, deteriorating dress, lateness, inattentiveness, patient complaints, poor treatment of staff and trainees, disruptive outbursts at work, absences from work, isolation from others, and eventually the noticing of alcohol on breath and drunkenness. Excessive drinking at social functions, medical practice or hospital parties, nurse and assistant concerns, are important indicators of trouble. The physician who is arrested for a DUI and appears in the newspapers for that or similar reasons is obviously of concern.

Responsibilities as a Physician

Our professionalism and our state licensing authorities require that we be responsible physicians not only to ourselves but that we be watchful of our physician colleagues. Every state has its own statutes, regulations and policies in this regard, but there are similarities. Physicians are expected to conduct themselves in a clinically competent and a professional manner [4]. Included in the regulation's listing of unacceptable behaviors are, the misuse, abuse, or dependence on alcohol and other addictive drugs, in part because they can affect our practice of medicine.

In this regard, it is important to understand the difference between illness and impairment which are often confused. Illnesses, such as alcohol dependence, can be diagnosed and treated prior to becoming impairing. Impairment implies the inability to practice medicine at a reasonable and expected standard due to an illness, injury, or physical disability. A physician who is diagnosed with alcohol dependence but treated prior to any patient harm or other significant consequence and is abstinent and in recovery, is not impaired. The understanding of this important difference allows us not to use the often misused term "the impaired physician" as it can unfairly label a physician who is sober, in good recovery, and not only not impaired but often never was impaired, despite having been diagnosed with the illness of alcohol dependence or another drug use disorder.

A physician is also responsible for being fully aware of the state's medical licensing regulations, including whether there is a mandating reporting obligation, which is common in many states. Such obligations require physicians and/or other health care professionals to report to the licensing authority any physician who is in violation of the regulations , including unhealthy alcohol or other drug use [5]. Each state has specific wording in this regard which the physician needs to be aware of or consult with legal advisors if there are questions or concerns on how to proceed if a physician is being identified with an alcohol or drug use-related problem.

Most state statutes or regulations include a particularly important provision that supports the ability to divert or refer a physician with alcohol or drug-related problems, to a recognized assessment or treatment program in lieu of a report to the licensing authority as long as specific provisions are met . These provisions exist because licensing boards have recognized that alcohol and drug use disorders are illnesses and it is far better to offer an incentive to doctors to seek help early before there are patient or practice problems and in lieu of board discipline. Such provisions help address one of the main barriers to connecting physicians who have alcohol use disorders with appropriate care instead of punishment.

Treating a Doctor who is a Patient

First, just like any other patients, physicians should be screened for unhealthy alcohol use, assessed if screening is positive, and provided with feedback and advice as appropriate. In addition, however, the treating physician needs to have or develop a level of confidence and competence in treating a physician patient. A thorough history, respectful discussion, and directness in confronting if need be, and supporting the physician are crucial to the patient doctor relationship. Primary care physicians need to be aware of the responsibilities and requirements of the state if a physician who is a patient has a drinking problem and importantly is exhibiting symptoms of being impaired with current drinking and treating patients. Consultation with a colleague, or the designated hospital individual or committee [6], or consulting with the state physician health program (PHP) can be very useful in determining the best referral options for the physician and also how to fulfill any treatment and reporting obligations.

Seeking Help

As much as we can encourage or expect that people with illness symptoms will seek medical attention, physicians in general are reluctant to seek help. This is an arena where the existing culture of medicine needs to change. It needs to become an expectation for medical students, residents and practicing doctors to not only have their own primary care physician (PCP), but to choose a doctor without conflicts (not a partner nor friend that could bias the physician-patient's honesty or willingness to share medical concerns), and to meet with the PCP as regularly as needed. Additionally, the PCP needs to be provided an accurate alcohol and other drug use history, and to have comfort in seeking assistance if needed. That unfortunately is not the norm today, so that the PCP, if there is one, is often the last to know that his or her physician-patient has a problem.

Physicians need to develop sufficient self awareness and comfort in seeking help and to avoid the well-known tendency to self diagnosis and self treatment. The adage that we all know is remarkably true. We can too easily end up with a fool for a doctor.

Physician Health Programs (PHPs)

It is essential that physicians are aware of their state PHP. Information can be found on the website of the Federation of State Physician Health Programs (FSPHP) www.fsphp.org [7]. These confidential programs in 46 member states are available to physicians with health-related problems, including alcohol and other drug use disorders, and mental health, behavioral, and physical problems. Doctors (and their doctors) can easily access their state PHP to confidentially discuss health issues including alcohol concerns. Assessments, referrals for treatment, support groups, and monitoring are available and have been demonstrated to be very effective.

Monitoring

Each state PHP has the availability of monitoring contracts for physicians with an alcohol or other drug use disorder and can benefit from an abstinence-based structured aftercare program including random toxicology testing, therapy, support groups, workplace monitoring, and documentation of compliance. Because of their comprehensive nature and structure, these programs support continuation of or return to practice, and help avoid the end of a career due to an alcohol use disorder. The length of the monitoring is usually 3–5 years [8]. The monitoring can be confidential and not disclosed to the state licensing authority if allowed by state regulations . If there is contract noncompliance, usually the licensing board is notified for its review and the monitoring continues with board awareness and a possible disciplinary sanction. Although many evidence-based counseling techniques (such as those discussed elsewhere in this book) do not involve coercion (e.g., brief motivational interventions), in the context of treatment for alcohol use disorders in practicing physicians, the threat of disciplinary action and loss of license are effective. These contractual arrangements have been shown to be very helpful to physicians in their recovery with high success rates over time (higher, in fact, than treatment for alcohol use disorders among non-physicians) [2, 9].

Relapses

As with our patients with addictions, physicians in recovery can relapse. Or doctors, who have recognized that their drinking is a problem, will attempt to stop or make pledges to themselves and loved ones, to not drink for a period of time or never, then relapse, return to drinking, and view themselves as a failure. If this occurs, it becomes a more urgent reason for the physician to seek help from addiction professionals and/or contact the state PHP for a confidential assessment and referral to treatment if indicated. As with other patients, the PCP can encourage the physician patient who experiences a relapse of a chronic condition (as can be the case with alcohol dependence), with a reminder of past success with regard to drinking, and a discussion of the value of career and family as motivation to seek help and recovery once again.

"Binge" Drinking

"Binge" drinking is heavy (>3 standard drinks on an occasion for women, >4 for men) episodic drinking. Physicians need to be careful of situations that can lead to excessive or binge drinking such as hospital or practice holiday parties, family gatherings, weddings, or other occasions where there can be a tendency to drink too much. Residents can be particularly vulnerable when feeling stressed, sleep deprived and with limited times when not on call to socialize with colleagues or friends in a party setting.

Educating Others

Inherent in being a physician is being a leader and teacher. As primary care physicians, there are opportunities to provide guidance and awareness of alcohol problems to not only our patients, but to our colleagues, medical staff, medical students, and our families, friends and society. As we know, alcohol issues are omnipresent. A recovering physician is important to the medical community as a role model, mentor and teacher if the physician is comfortable in those roles.

Driving While Intoxicated (DWI)

Driving soon after any drinking has the potential of unsafe driving and a crash with or without bodily injury to the driver or others. Driving after drinking can also result in an arrest. Although the unsafe driving and arrest is a problem for all drinking drivers, it can be a larger problem for physicians with a possibility of loss of standing in the community and respect as a physician, and licensing board involvement and a potential impact on the physician's medical license. Prevention is crucial—avoid driving after drinking. In the event of a crash or arrest, the physician should consider contacting the state PHP for advice and an assessment. Attorneys are not always aware of the flow of possible consequences when a physician is arrested, including the requirement in many states to inform the licensing board of the arrest either at the time of license renewal or sooner. Regardless, the physician should seek advice. Medical students who have been arrested or cited for DWI also need to be made aware of the importance of seeking advice, often best from the state PHP which can provide a confidential consultation and can help avoid damaging professional consequences.

Alcohol, Other Drugs, and Mental Disorders

In addition to alcohol, physicians are susceptible to the abuse of other drugs including prescription medications , which can be easily accessible in the practice or hospital, or have been prescribed to the physician, patients or to family members. The abuse of opioids, benzodiazepines, stimulants, and others alone or in combination with alcohol are particularly troublesome and can lead to impairment. Physicians also need to avoid the use and abuse of any illicit substances, including marijuana, cocaine, heroin, and stimulants. Mental health disorders are common among people with alcohol and other drug use disorders. Physicians with alcohol use disorders therefore may also have treated or untreated depression, bipolar disorder, anxiety, attention, and other mental health diagnoses, all of which their PCP needs to be aware of and to facilitate appropriate care [10].

Wellness, Sobriety, and Recovery

The physician practice of health and wellness should be an essential part of our work/life balance . Exercise, good nutrition, not smoking, and no or "moderate"use of alcohol are important to good medical practice and the health of our patients. Healthy doctors lead to healthy patients [1]. Paying attention to our physician and other colleagues in this regard is also good practice.

Practical Advice for PCPs

All physicians should consider the following for their personal and professional wellbeing.

1. Protect the privilege of "moderate" drinking by drinking lower risk amounts responsibly and safely.
2. Do not drink during the work day.

3. Do not drink if on call.
4. Be careful of evening or weekend drinking which could affect the next day's work performance.
5. Be cautious of drinking if prescribed other medications, especially controlled substances.
6. Do not drive after drinking.
7. Contact the state PHP for confidential advice, consultation, assessment or referral to treatment if concerned about your or a colleague's use of alcohol and its consequences.
8. Be aware of state reporting obligations if you know of a physician with possible impairment from alcohol and the relevant exceptions to reporting.
9. If medical or legal issues arise as a result of alcohol use, consult with an attorney with expertise in medical and physician matters.

Conclusion

Physicians need to be responsible in their use of alcohol and be willing to seek help and support if unhealthy use, including abuse or dependence, develops. Self awareness is often the first step to taking the next healthy step. Confidential referrals, assessments and treatment are available to physicians and treatment can be very successful—both career- and life-saving. Being willing and able to assist our colleagues is also a physician's responsibility.

References

1. Frank E. Physician health and patient care. JAMA. 2004, 291: 637.
2. DuPont RL, McClellan T, Carr G, Gendel M, Skipper GE. How are addicted physicians treated? A national survey of physicians health programs. J Subst Abuse Treat. 2009;37:1–7.
3. Gallagher A, Boyle E, Toner P, et al. Persistent next day effects of excessive alcohol consumption on laparoscopic surgical performance. JAMA. 2011;146: 419–426.
4. Model Medical Staff Code of Conduct. American Medical Association. http://www.ama. assn.org/ama1/pub/upload/mm/21/ama-medical-staff-code-of-conduct.pdf. Accessed 4 March 2011.
5. Desroches C, Rao S, Fromson J, et al. Physicians' perceptions, preparedness for reporting, and experiences related to impaired and incompetent colleagues. JAMA. 2010;304:187–193.
6. Hospital accreditation standards 2011. The Joint Commission. MS.11.01.01;41–42.
7. Federation of state physician health programs. www.fsphp.org. Accessed 30 April 2011.
8. Federation of state physician health programs. Physician health program guidelines. 2005. www.fsphp.org/2005FSPHP_Guidelines.pdf. Accessed 30 April 2011.
9. Knight J, Sanchez L, Sherrit L, Bresnahan L, Fromson J. Outcomes of a monitoring program for physicians with mental and behavioral health problems. J Psych Prac. 2007; 13: 25–32.
10. Domino KB, Hornbein TF, Polissar NL et al. Risk factors for relapse in health care professionals with substance use disorders. JAMA. 2005;293:1453–1460.
11. Council on Mental Health. American Medical Association. The sick physician: impairment by psychiatric disorders, including alcoholism and drug dependence. JAMA. 1973; 223:684–687.

Appendix A
Instruments for Substance Use Assessment

ASSIST   Alcohol, Smoking, and Substance Involvement Screening Test (Source: World
Health Organization (WHO) ASSIST Working Group)

Question 1
(if completing follow-up please cross check the patient's answers with the answers given for Q1 at baseline. Any differences on this question should be queried)

In your life, which of the following substances have you <u>ever used</u>? *(NON-MEDICAL USE ONLY)*	No	Yes
a. Tobacco products (cigarettes, chewing tobacco, cigars, etc.)	0	3
b. Alcoholic beverages (beer, wine, spirits, etc.) .	0	3
c. Cannabis (marijuana, pot, grass, hash, etc.)	0	3
d. Cocaine (coke, crack, etc.)	0	3
e. Amphetamine type stimulants (speed, diet pills, ecstasy, etc.)	0	3
f. Inhalants (nitrous, glue, petrol, paint thinner, etc.)	0	3
g. Sedatives or Sleeping Pills (Valium, Serepax, Rohypnol, etc.)	0	3
h. Hallucinogens (LSD, acid, mushrooms, PCP, Special K, etc.)	0	3
i. Opioids (heroin, morphine, methadone, codeine, etc.)	0	3
j. Other - specify:	0	3

Probe if all answers are negative:
"Not even when you were in school?"

If "No" to all items, stop interview.
If "Yes" to any of these items, ask Question 2 for each substance ever used.

Scoring: A 'specific substance involvement score' is calculated for each substance endorsed, based on the sum of responses to Q2–Q7. For illicit drugs and tobacco, scores of 0–3 constitute low risk; 4–26 moderate risk; 27 + high risk/possible dependence.

ASSIST is validated in multiple languages, including Spanish.
Available at: http://www.who.int/substance_abuse/activities/assist_test/en/index.html

R. Saitz (ed.), *Addressing Unhealthy Alcohol Use in Primary Care*,
DOI 10.1007/978-1-4614-4779-5, © Springer Science+Business Media New York 2013

NM-ASSIST   NIDA-Modified Alcohol, Smoking, and Substance Involvement Screening Test
             (Source: National Institute on Drug Abuse)

Print and electronic versions available, including online 'NIDA Quick Screen'

NIDA Home > NIDAMED > Screening for Drug and Alcohol Abuse > NM Assist

Hide Instructions | Print this Page

NIDA QUICK SCREEN ➕

Clinician's Screening Tool for Drug Use in
General Medical Settings*

Note: This website collects no personally identifiable
information and does not store your responses to any of the
following questions.

Instructions: Ask your patient each question,
then mark answers affirmative when appropriate
(the default setting is a negative response). At
the end of the survey, the screening tool will
tally the responses to generate a substance
involvement score, determine risk and
recommended level of intervention, and provide
additional resources.

Quick Screen   Start   Quick Results ① ② ③ ④ ⑤ ⑥ ⑦ ⑧ Results

In the *past year*, how many times have you used the following?

Drug Type	Never	Once or Twice	Monthly	Weekly	Daily or Almost Daily
Alcohol For Men ▾ more than 5 drinks in a day	●	○	○	○	○
Tobacco products	●	○	○	○	○
Prescription Drugs for Non-Medical Reasons	●	○	○	○	○
Illegal drugs	●	○	○	○	○

⊙ Give Feedback   Next ▶

Scoring: Alcohol assessment follows NIAAA guidelines. Illicit drug use is scored identically to the
ASSIST. For tobacco, no further assessment following the initial screen; cessation advised for all
current tobacco users.

Available at: http://www.drugabuse.gov/nidamed/screening/
NIDA Quick Screen: http://ww1.drugabuse.gov/nmassist/

DAST-10© Drug Abuse Screening Test (Source:)

In the past 12 months...		Circle	
1.	Have you used drugs other than those required for medical reasons?	Yes	No
2.	Do you abuse more than one drug at a time?	Yes	No
3.	Are you unable to stop abusing drugs when you want to?	Yes	No
4.	Have you ever had blackouts or flashbacks as a result of drug use?	Yes	No
5.	Do you ever feel bad or guilty about your drug use?	Yes	No
6.	Does your spouse (or parents) ever complain about your involvement with drugs?	Yes	No
7.	Have you neglected your family because of your use of drugs?	Yes	No
8.	Have you engaged in illegal activities in order to obtain drugs?	Yes	No
9.	Have you ever experienced withdrawal symptoms (felt sick) when you stopped taking drugs?	Yes	No
10.	Have you had medical problems as a result of your drug use (e.g. memory loss, hepatitis, convulsions, bleeding)?	Yes	No
Scoring: Score 1 point for each question answered "Yes," except for question 3 for which a "No" receives 1 point.		Score:	

Scoring: Score 1 point for each 'yes' response, except on question 3 for which a 'no' response receives 1 point. Scores of 0–2 indicate low-level or no substance use problems; 3–5 indicates moderate problems; 6–8 indicates substantial and 9–10 severe problems.

DAST is also validated in Spanish[1]

Available at: http://archives.drugabuse.gov/diagnosis-treatment/DAST10.html

Copyright 1982 by Harvey A. Skinner, PhD, and the Centre for Addiction and Mental Health, Toronto, Canada. May be reproduced for non-commercial use with permission of Dr. Harvey Skinner (harvey.skinner@yorku.ca)

---

[1] Pérez Gálvez B, García Fernández L, de Vicente Manzanaro MP, Oliveras Valenzuela MA, Lahoz Lafuente M. Validación espaola del Drug Abuse Screening Test (DAST-20 y DAST-10). Health and Addictions/Salud y Drogas. 2010;10:34–50

DUDIT   Drug Use Disorders Identification Test (Source: Berman, 2005)

DUDIT Drug Use Disorders Identification Test

Here are a few questions about drugs. Please answer as correctly and honestly as possible by indicating which answer is right for you.

☐ Man ☐ Woman		Age [ ]

	Never	Once a month or less often	2-4 times a month	2-3 times a week	4 times a week or more often
1. How often do you use drugs other than alcohol? (See list of drugs on back side.)	☐	☐	☐	☐	☐
2. Do you use more than one type of drug on the same occasion?	☐	☐	☐	☐	☐

	0	1-2	3-4	5-6	7 or more
3. How many times do you take drugs on a typical day when you use drugs?	☐	☐	☐	☐	☐

	Never	Less often than once a month	Every month	Every week	Daily or almost every day
4. How often are you influenced heavily by drugs?	☐	☐	☐	☐	☐
5. Over the past year, have you felt that your longing for drugs was so strong that you could not resist it?	☐	☐	☐	☐	☐
6. Has it happened, over the past year, that you have not been able to stop taking drugs once you started?	☐	☐	☐	☐	☐
7. How often over the past year have you taken drugs and then neglected to do something you should have done?	☐	☐	☐	☐	☐
8. How often over the past year have you needed to take a drug the morning after heavy drug use the day before?	☐	☐	☐	☐	☐
9. How often over the past year have you had guilt feelings or a bad conscience because you used drugs?	☐	☐	☐	☐	☐

	No	Yes, but not over the past year	Yes, over the past year
10. Have you or anyone else been hurt (mentally or physically) because you used drugs?	☐	☐	☐
11. Has a relative or a friend, a doctor or a nurse, or anyone else, been worried about your drug use or said to you that you should stop using drugs?	☐	☐	☐

Scoring: Items 1–9 are scored on scale of 0-1-2-3-4 points and Items 10 and 11 are scored on scale of 0-2-4 points. The DUDIT score is the sum of all points. Cut-off score to distinguish drug-related problems is 6 points for men and 2 points for women. Scores of 25 + points likely reflect dependence on one or more drugs.

Available at: http://www.emcdda.europa.eu/attachements.cfm/att_10455_EN_DUDIT.pdf
Also see the manual at: http://www.penalreform.ro/fileadmin/pri/projects/documente/
DUDITManual.pdf

Note: The layout of the DUDIT forms the basis for the evaluation of its psychometric properties and should not be altered.

| CRAFFT | CRAFFT is a mnemonic for the 6 items in the assessment: Car, Relax, Alone, Forget, Friends, Trouble (Source: Knight, 1999) | 1. Have you ever ridden in a **CAR** driven by someone (including yourself) who was high or had been using alcohol or drugs?
2. Do you ever use alcohol or drugs to **RELAX**, feel better about yourself, or fit in?
3. Do you ever use alcohol or drugs while you are by yourself (**ALONE**)?
4. Do you ever **FORGET** things you did while using alcohol or drugs?
5. Do your family or **FRIENDS** ever tell you that you should cut down on your drinking or drug use?
6. Have you ever gotten into **TROUBLE** while you were using alcohol or drugs?

Scoring: 2 or more 'yes' answers indicates substance use, abuse, or dependence.
Available at: http://www.slp3d2.com/rwj_1027/webcast/docs/screentest.html |

The on-line instrument library of the Alcohol and Drug Abuse Institute, University of Washington, has information and links to copies of questionnaires for these and many other substance use screening and assessment instruments. This resource is located at http://lib.adai.washington.edu/instruments/

Appendix B
Useful Tools and Online Materials

Helping Patients Who Drink Too Much: A Clinician's Guide. Published at http://www.niaaa.nih.gov/Publications/EducationTrainingMaterials/Pages/guide.aspx

A practical guide for generalist clinicians that addresses screening, assessment, brief intervention and pharmacotherapy. The website includes a free printable and downloadable guide and resources (progress note example, educational videos). A pocket guide is available and reproduced here.

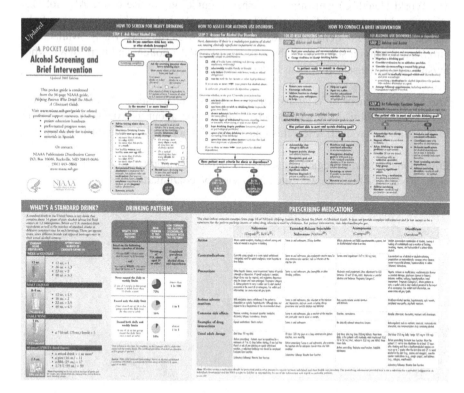

Rethinking Drinking is also published online by the National Institute on Alcohol Abuse and Alcoholism and is a site geared towards the general public. It includes useful tools for self-assessment and materials useful for self-change. http://rethinkingdrinking.niaaa.nih.gov/

Alcohol, Other Drugs and Health is a free bimonthly e-newsletter that publishes brief clinically relevant summaries from the medical literature with expert commentary. The site also provides slide sets for presentation (grand rounds type and journal club). www.aodhealth.org

www.mdalcoholtraining.org posts slides and videos of alcohol screening and brief intervention.

The National Institute on Drug Abuse has also published clinical tools for indentifying and managing drug use at http://www.drugabuse.gov/nmassist/

Two websites for patient self-screening are www.alcoholscreening.org and www.drugscreening.org

The World Health Organization published a guide on the use of the Alcohol Use Disorders Identification Test (AUDIT) and the Alcohol Smoking and other Substance Involvement Screening Test (ASSIST). Materials are freely available at http://www.who.int/substance_abuse/publications/alcohol/en/ and http://www.who.int/substance_abuse/activities/assist/en/index.html

The US Department of Veterans Affairs Quality Enhancement Research Initiative has a very useful website with detailed information about the AUDIT-C screening tool at http://www.queri.research.va.gov/tools/alcohol-misuse/alcohol-faqs.cfm

Educational materials regarding screening and brief intervention are also available at the BNI-ART Institute web site http://www.bu.edu/bniart/

Addiction Research Foundation Clinical Institute Withdrawal Assessment for Alcohol, Revised (CIWA-Ar)

Appendix: Addiction Research Foundation Clinical Institute Withdrawal Assessment for Alcohol (CIWA-Ar)

Patient_____   Date |_|_|_| Time____:____
                               y m d   (24 hour clock, midnight=00:00)

Pulse or heart rate, taken for one minute: _____   Blood pressure: _____/_____

NAUSEA AND VOMITING—As "Do you feel sick to your stomach? Have you vomited?" Observation.
0 no nausea and no vomiting
1 mild nausea with no vomiting
2
3
4 intermittent nausea with dry heaves
5
6
7 constant nausea, frequent dry heaves and vomiting

TREMOR—Arms extended and fingers spread apart. Observation.
0 no tremor
1 not visible, but can be felt fingertip to fingertip
2
3
4 moderate, with patient's arms extended
5
6
7 severe, even with arms not extended

PAROXYSMAL SWEATS—Observation.
0 no sweat visible
1 barely perceptible sweating, palms moist
2
3
4 beads of sweat obvious on forehead
5
6
7 drenching sweats

ANXIETY—Ask "Do you feel nervous?" Observation.
0 no anxiety, at ease
1 mildly anxious
2
3
4 moderately anxious, or guarded, so anxiety is inferred
5
6
7 equivalent to acute panic states as seen in severe delirium or acute schizophrenic reactions

AGITATION—Observation.
0 normal activity
1 somewhat more than normal activity
2
3
4 moderately fidgety and restless
5
6
7 paces back and forth during most of the interview, or constantly thrashes about

TACTILE DISTURBANCES—Ask "Have you any itching, pins and needles sensations, any burning, any numbness or do you feel bugs crawling on or under your skin?" Observation.
0 none
1 very mild itching, pins and needles, burning or numbness
2 mild itching, pins and needles, burning or numbness
3 moderate itching, pins and needles, burning or numbness
4 moderately severe hallucinations
5 severe hallucinations
6 extremely severe hallucinations
7 continuous hallucinations

AUDITORY DISTURBANCES—Ask "Are you more aware of sounds around you? Are they harsh? Do they frighten you? Are you hearing anything that is disturbing to you? Are you hearing things you know are not there?" Observation.
0 not present
1 very mild harshness or ability to frighten
2 mild harshness or ability to frighten
3 moderate harshness or ability to frighten
4 moderately severe hallucinations
5 severe hallucinations
6 extremely severe hallucinations
7 continuous hallucinations

VISUAL DISTURBANCES—Ask "Does the light appear to be too bright? Is its colour different? Does it hurt your eyes? Are you seeing anything that is disturbing to you? Are you seeing things you know are not there?" Observation.
0 not present
1 very mild sensitivity
2 mild sensitivity
3 moderate sensitivity
4 moderately severe hallucinations
5 severe hallucinations
6 extremely severe hallucinations
7 continuous hallucinations

HEADACHE, FULLNESS IN HEAD—Ask "Does your head feel different? Does it feel like there is a band around your head?" Do not rate for dizziness or lightheadedness. Otherwise, rate severity.
0 not present
1 very mild
2 mild
3 moderate
4 moderately severe
5 severe
6 very severe
7 extremely severe

ORIENTATION AND CLOUDING OF SENSORIUM—Ask "What day is this? Where are you? Who am I?"
0 oriented and can do serial additions
1 cannot do serial additions or is uncertain about date
2 disoriented for date by no more than 2 calendar days
3 disoriented for date by more than 2 calendar days
4 disoriented for place and/or person

Total CIWA-A Score_____
Rater's Initials_____
Maximum Possible Score 67

This scale is not copyrighted and may be used freely.

Index